D0856117

Pediatric Compliance

A Guide for the
Primary Care Physician

**CRITICAL ISSUES IN
DEVELOPMENTAL AND BEHAVIORAL PEDIATRICS**

SERIES EDITOR: MARVIN I. GOTTLIEB, M.D., Ph.D.

*Hackensack Medical Center
Hackensack, New Jersey
and University of Medicine and Dentistry of New Jersey—
New Jersey Medical School
Newark, New Jersey*

DEVELOPMENTAL-BEHAVIORAL DISORDERS: Selected Topics
Volumes 1–3
Edited by Marvin I. Gottlieb, M.D., Ph.D., and John E. Williams, M.D.

PEDIATRIC COMPLIANCE: A Guide for the Primary Care Physician
Edward R. Christophersen, Ph.D.

A Continuation Order Plan is available for this series. A continuation order will bring delivery of each new volume immediately upon publication. Volumes are billed only upon actual shipment. For further information please contact the publisher.

Pediatric Compliance

A Guide for the Primary Care Physician

Edward R. Christophersen, Ph.D.

Chief, Behavioral Pediatrics Section, and
Professor of Pediatrics
University of Missouri at Kansas City
School of Medicine, and
Children's Mercy Hospital
Kansas City, Missouri

Plenum Medical Book Company ● New York and London

Library of Congress Cataloging-in-Publication Data

Christophersen, Edward R.
    Pediatric compliance : a guide for the primary care physican /
Edward R. Christophersen.
        p.   cm. -- (Critical issues in developmental and behavioral
pediatrics)
    Includes bibliographical references and index.
    ISBN 0-306-44454-2
    1. Pediatrics--Psychological aspects. 2. Behavior disorders in
children. 3. Health behavior in children. 4. Patient compliance.
I. Title. II. Series.
    [DNLM: 1. Child Behavior Disorders. 2. Patient Compliance--in
infancy & childhood. 3. Primary Health Care.   WS 350.6 C556p 1994]
RJ47.5.C47   1994
618.92'89--dc20
DNLM/DLC
for Library of Congress   93-41063
                                                               CIP

ISBN 0-306-44454-2

© 1994 Edward R. Christophersen
233 Spring Street, New York, N.Y. 10013

Plenum Medical Book Company is an imprint of Plenum Publishing Corporation

All rights reserved

No part of this book may be reproduced, stored in a retrieval system, or transmitted in any form or by any means, electronic, mechanical, photocopying, microfilming, recording, or otherwise, without written permission from the Publisher.

Printed in the United States of America

Preface

As long as there have been children, parents have had questions about raising them. Primary care physicians and nurses are often approached for answers. A good portion of the time the answers given, however, have been based on prior experience rather than objective, scientific studies.

In 1974, when I joined the Department of Pediatrics at the University of Kansas Medical Center, my colleagues and I embarked on a systematic program of research on the common, everyday problems faced by parents and, in turn, by their primary care physicians. We studied well-child visits, otitis media, urinary tract infections, injury control, and anticipatory guidance. At that time we discovered, as did many of our fellow researchers around the country, that parents don't necessarily change their behavior just because we make an impassioned plea for them to do so. We learned that we could encourage parents, scare parents, and repeat ourselves at one visit after another, but the parents' behavior did not change. Their verbal behavior—what they said to us—often changed, but their behavior with and toward their children did not.

Like other researchers, we were first upset, then disappointed, and then challenged. We were upset because we knew these parents wanted to do a better job of parenting and, at the time, we didn't know how to help them do so. We were disappointed because our initial attempts at changing their behavior failed, and we knew that new procedures probably would have to be developed. And we were challenged because we knew it was going to take a lot of work before we were able to successfully teach parents to change their parenting skills or strategies.

Later, in our research on common pediatric illnesses, we discovered exactly the same phenomenon—we could change verbal behavior much more easily than we could change actual behavior. But in our illness-oriented work, we demonstrated we were more effective as teachers of parents if we communicated with them in plain English instead of using the jargon of the medical and psychological community, if we provided written summaries of our treatment recommendations to supplement what we said to them during office visits, and if we provided them with more structured strategies for implementing our treatment recommendations. Later, we discovered that we could systematize the data gathering that is such an important part of an office visit if we used written intake forms; they made it easier for us to take a comprehensive history without errors and without omissions. Much of what you read in this book reflects these findings.

About this time a colleague introduced me to a classic book written over a hundred years ago by Claude Barnard, who was later to become known as the "Father of the History of Experimental Medicine." In the book, Barnard described what he termed the "clinician's fallacy": in short, when a patient comes to a clinician's office with a problem and receives advice on coping with that problem, and the problem then lessens or is eliminated, it is a fallacy to conclude this improvement was the result of what the clinician said or did. Rather, the clinician must demonstrate experimental control over the condition before he can say he has an effective treatment for it.

Faced with the temptation to commit our own "clinician's fallacy," and knowing from experience that what Barnard so eloquently stated in his book was true, we decided to systematically evaluate our treatment recommendations prior to disseminating them to other clinicians.

Our program of research, then, has been conceptualized in order to demonstrate that the procedures we recommend are, in fact, responsible for whatever clinical improvement patients and their parents experience. Many of the treatment recommendations made in this book have been scientifically evaluated, with the results of the evaluations published in journals in pediatrics and in psychology.

I also have distributed the written handouts included in this book at literally hundreds of continuing education meetings where I have had the privilege of speaking. The feedback I've received from speaking at these meetings has been very gratifying, verifying that we have not only passed the scientific scrutiny of our peers but also allayed the skepticism of the clinicians who come to continuing education meetings seeking effective treatment strategies.

Over the years, I have noted it is relatively easy to get information and training on dealing with children who have serious problems and with children from dysfunctional families—pediatric training programs based in tertiary-care centers are always addressing these types of situations. It is much harder to get information and training about raising normal children. Much of the literature on normal childhood development appears in psychology or child development journals, publications not usually read by primary care physicians; hence, the need for the field called Behavioral Pediatrics, a field in which knowledge about normal child development is made available to clinicians who see normal families every day during well-child visits and acute care office visits. This is where I think the collaboration between pediatrics and psychology has been symbiotic.

This book is written for those clinicians who want to incorporate information on normal child development into their primary care practices—those clinicians who want answers to the questions parents raise every day. This book summarizes the clinical experience gathered treating thousands of children using previously evaluated treatment protocols. These procedures were developed in and intended for use in busy clinical care settings.

Over the past 20 years, I've received thousands of letters from clinicians (primarily from around the United States, but from many other places around the world as well). Based on their continuing requests for more information about the strategies and procedures developed in our office, let me presume that we continue to make an impact on the field of Behavioral Pediatrics.

I'd like to acknowledge the challenge presented to me by the child psychologists, nurses, pediatric residents, child psychiatry residents, and practicing pediatricians and family physicians who have either trained here in Kansas City or who have registered for any of the hundreds of workshops and continuing education meetings at which I have presented over the years. Their thirst for more information, their questions, and their skepticism have kept me on my toes.

And I'd like to acknowledge more than anyone else the children and the parents to whom I've had the pleasure of delivering clinical services. They are my nurturants, my reason for being. I love it every time parents come in for a return appointment and tell me how grateful they are, how I've made their lives and the lives of their children more pleasant. As long as parents are as pleased with the services they receive as I am in delivering those services, I will continue to practice.

EDWARD R. CHRISTOPHERSEN

Acknowledgments

The writing of this book would never have been initiated without the encouragement and insistence of the Series Editor, Dr. Marvin Gottlieb. He has been the one with the vision, the overview, the knowledge of existing gaps in the literature in Behavioral and Developmental Pediatrics, and the persistence to seek out individuals who were qualified to fill these gaps. Without his kind and gentle nurturing, this book never would have come to fruition.

Barbara Cochrane-Wood has edited almost every manuscript that I have written. She has learned how I write and what I want to say, and, although not a pediatric practitioner, she has helped to make my writing more intelligible, more understandable. She edited the first version of this book.

Jane F. Christophersen, Business and Technical Communications, in Walnut Creek, California, has provided excellent and timely editorial services that made this book a reality.

My family, Miki, Hunter, and Catherine, have tolerated months of my working on the word processor. They have gone to movies and dinners without me during the entire time that I have written this book, giving up what every family of an author gives up—their time, one on one, with the author. They have waited, ever patiently, for this project to be completed.

I typed every word in this book on a microcomputer. The chapters were sent by modem back and forth between JFC Communications and me with amazing speed and clarity. I'm certain that authors' entire lives have been changed forever by the microcomputers that have become their companions.

During my entire professional career, I have been in the enviable position of loving what I do for a living. The parents and children whom I see in my practice have made this possible, and to them I am forever grateful.

Contents

V. Office Management Strategies

VI. Postscript

Appendixes

Sample Handouts

Chapter 5

Chapter 6

Chapter 7

Chapter 8

Chapter 9

Chapter 10

Chapter 11

Chapter 12

Chapter 13

Chapter 14

Chapter 15

Chapter 17

Chapter 1

Introduction

"My mother's proud of me. My father's proud of me. I'm even proud of me." So wrote a young girl we once treated for enuresis. Thank-you notes like these are gratifying, and they demonstrate that Behavioral Pediatrics can be as fun and rewarding as any other clinical service provided to children and their families.

Primary-care practitioners who see pediatric patients in their practice are bound to encounter problems, like enuresis, that are an integral part of a child's development. While individual providers may elect not to offer pediatric behavioral services, incorporating procedures for encouraging compliance into a primary-care practice can be an exciting and rewarding endeavor. Problems that were previously referred, ignored, or undertreated can now be handled routinely, using practical, effective, and economically feasible techniques that have not been readily available to the medical community.

The protocol for teaching children to swallow pills, discussed in Chapter 3, "Behavioral Problems," for example, is so simple to implement and so effective that it is surprising that no one addressed the issue of pill swallowing prior to the time this protocol appeared in the research literature.

A year or so before the procedures for pill swallowing appeared in the published literature, I was fortunate enough to be asked to review the study for publication by an associate editor of the journal in which it ultimately appeared. I was immediately struck by the eloquent simplicity of the procedures.

Within a week of the time I reviewed the manuscript, I had an opportunity to try the procedures with a young child, referred by one of our pediatric neurologists. It worked then, and it has worked ever since. It works so well that my partners, Drs. Linda Ross and Patty Purvis, have put together a "pill-swallowing kit" that looks like a small package of soda pop bottles or milk bottles. In the bottles are cake sprinkles of increasing sizes, beginning with a size so small that virtually any child could swallow them and progressing upward, in eight steps, to candies that are larger than most pills a child would ever have to ingest.

Similarly, our protocols for getting children to bed at night, to wear their glasses, and to use the toilet properly are all quite simple—simple enough that they will work with a majority of children—provided that the initial assessment rules out more serious problems and allows us to conclude that children simply need to learn how to self-quiet, wear their glasses, or independently toilet.

This book describes a variety of procedures that I and my colleagues have used for a number of years. Because any given practitioner is unlikely to implement all of the suggestions, the book is written so that practitioners can refer only to those sections of interest to them.

Our policy of summarizing our protocols in brief, one- or two-page handouts can be deceptive. Some practitioners get the impression on seeing our protocols that the practice of Behavioral Pediatrics is easy. As one of our Pediatric Mini-Fellows said in 1985 after completing the Fellowship and having time to pause and reflect on the experience, "My reading and research led me to believe that under your tutelage I would learn highly effective short-term techniques for particular behaviorally based problems of early childhood. I did indeed acquire such knowledge. However, in addition, I absorbed a functional, humane philosophy of behavior management."

Behavioral Pediatrics is a very personal endeavor, probably as personal as anything the physician or the psychologist does. It is personal in that the parents' interactions with their children are under review. The way they talk to and play with their children is under scrutiny, as well as the places they take their children and how they interact with them when they get there.

The primary message in this book is that Behavioral Pediatrics is at once a simple, straightforward, and humane specialty that must deal with intimate details while putting a parent at ease. As Dr. Barbara Korsch has said many times, we must be able to listen to what parents have to say, both to what they tell us and to what they don't tell us.

BEHAVIORAL PROBLEMS

The Chapters in Part I address the main issues in Behavioral Pediatrics: compliance and noncompliance, assessment, learning and cognitive development in children, and common behavior problems.

Compliance, in terms of both the parents' compliance with the health-care provider's recommendations regarding treatment and the child's compliance with parental requests, is central to whether intervention in Behavioral Pediatrics is effective. As we in the field of Behavioral Pediatrics develop skills for encouraging higher levels of compliance from parents, we, in turn, have a greater impact on the children we serve. Without compliance, behavioral interventions cannot and will not be effective.

Chapter 2, "Learning, Discipline, and Compliance in Children," discusses the process of children's cognitive development and the optimal ways of promoting learning in children; both are central to Behavioral Pediatrics. Without a working knowledge of how to optimize children's learning, behavioral procedures are difficult to develop and implement, and the likelihood of the procedures producing therapeutic gains is remote.

The most important part of Chapter 3, "Behavioral Problems," discusses certain skills, referred to as "survival skills," that form the foundation for much of what parents want to teach their children. To me, these skills, self-quieting and independent play, are critical to what a child must learn at home and in school in order to be a productive member of society. My experience has been that it is far easier to encourage the development of these skills during the early years than to try to play catch up in later years.

Chapter 3 also contains a section on spanking that addresses why parents spank, reviews the research literature on spanking from the standpoint of its effectiveness, presents the religious roots of spanking, and gives the available alternatives to spanking.

Assessment, versus the amount of time that assessment takes, has long been a problem in well-child care. The brevity of well-child office visits mandates that assessment be accomplished in very little time. Yet treatment outcomes usually depend on accurate assessment. Chapter 4, "Recognition and Assessment of Compliance Problems," discusses readily available assessment devices that are relatively inexpensive to purchase and simple to administer and score—two qualities that are essential if the devices are to be used in a primary-care office or, for that matter, in the office of a pediatrician or psychologist who specializes in Behavioral Pediatrics.

Many written handouts are included throughout this book. These handouts were developed with the practitioner in mind, and the practitioner can copy and distribute the handouts to parents.

Chapter **2**

Learning, Discipline, and Compliance in Children

Although the majority of adult-oriented health education strategies rely almost exclusively on verbal and printed instructions, research has demonstrated that these predominantly verbal strategies are ineffective at producing lifestyle changes in adults and children (Haynes, Taylor, and Sackett, 1979). From birth to about 6 years of age, a child interacts with his* environment in concrete or preabstract ways. Therefore,

*I have alternated the use of gender throughout the text to maintain fair, nonsexist terminology.

abstract explanations or warnings about impending consequences of behavior cannot have much impact during these early years. Knowing that children under the age of 6 cannot benefit from verbal abstractions helps to explain many problems parents report having with children of this age group. The absence of abstract thinking in young children has clear ramifications for both child rearing and health education.

2.1. HOW CHILDREN LEARN

Children generally learn in the same basic manner that adults do—through repetition. Whether children are learning how to snow ski or to do mathematics, only by doing something over and over again can they learn how to do it. Watching a child learning to walk after pulling herself up to stand is a good example of this learning process. During a period of several weeks, the child makes hundreds—if not thousands—of attempts to walk and tries many approaches, pulling herself up and holding on to secure objects, letting go, and taking as many steps as possible before falling down.

The more often children have the opportunity to practice a given behavior, the more quickly they will learn how to do it. Thus, when parents say they "don't want to see a child do something again," they are actually choosing an option that will only prolong the length of time it takes to teach the child a new skill. It would be far better for the parent to monitor the child's behavior very closely and to provide appropriate consequences every time the child performs the behavior either appropriately or inappropriately. Much like children learn to ski by skiing and falling numerous times, they can learn many other skills.

The more dramatic the contrast between the outcomes of appropriate behaviors and inappropriate behaviors, the more quickly learning occurs. Often this contrast between appropriate and inappropriate behaviors can be emphasized by making the enjoyment derived from appropriate behaviors more dramatic. While there is always the temptation to make punishment more severe when a child is engaging in an inappropriate behavior, the more effective procedure is to emphasize the results of appropriate behavior. To continue with the skiing example, nobody goes skiing to avoid falling; people go skiing because they enjoy the activity and they are willing to accept occasional falls in order to continue with the enjoyment of skiing.

Another important variable affecting a child's learning is the amount of time that passes between learning opportunities. In the examples above of learning how to walk or how to ski, the child usually gets up immediately after a fall and tries again. This repetition makes for efficient learning. If children engage in a behavior only once every month or two, it will take substantially longer to teach them than if it occurs repeatedly.

When a coach is teaching a child a new sport, he typically has the child practice the same skill over and over again, with the knowledge that the child may need many opportunities before she masters the skill. In fact, coaches often have children practice only one or two parts of a skill and, even when working with one or two skills, the coach sets up conditions that maximize the child's learning.

For example, when a child is learning to do back flips in gymnastics, the coach may have the child practice by bending over a large cylinder on a mat. As the children bend backward over the cylinder, time after time, they develop a sense of balance and learn to use muscles that they may not have even known they had. Thus, when a task is broken down into smaller parts and those parts are practiced under circumstances that promote learning, children can learn complicated skills without much fear of failing or of getting injured. Parents must be able to maintain this kind of perspective on children's learning. A child may have to learn many smaller skills, through practice, before he has mastered a more complicated set of skills.

Children don't learn to clean a house or clean their room as readily as they learn the component parts of such a complex task. If parents practice each of the components of "cleaning" over and over again, they set up a situation where the child is learning how to clean her room without ever being cognizant that the learning is going on.

Many parents will express concern to their pediatrician that their child "doesn't care about treating his diabetes properly." They might even say to their physician, "I told Jeffrey exactly what he was supposed to do for his diabetes, but he just doesn't seem to care. He won't do what I tell him to do." Because Jeffrey doesn't yet have the ability to operationalize his parents' instructions, he is virtually certain to disappoint them by not following what they've asked him to do.

Unfortunately, many parents don't understand, or have never learned, that making the outcome for appropriate behaviors more pleasant not only teaches children much more quickly, it also avoids many of the side effects of punishment procedures. The primary side effects of punishment have been well documented in the research literature (e.g., Azrin and Holz, 1966), and include the child:

- Trying to avoid or get away from the parent.
- Acting more aggressive toward the parent.
- Becoming intimidated by the parent.
- Becoming more anxious when near the parent.

While many practitioners and parents favor the use of punishment in child rearing, most would never use punishment procedures in the workplace or in their recreational activities.

It's ironic that a father can go to a driving range and putting green many times to improve his golf game, without ever encountering any punishment more severe than seeing that the way he hit the ball did not result in the direction and distance he wanted; then he returns home from his practice and reprimands and punishes his child for doing something incorrectly, such as not picking up his room correctly. Although both the parent and the child may have to practice the same behaviors over and over again before they truly master them, the child must endure some form of punishment because he "knew" how to do something and still did it wrong. Conversely, the father will return to the practice range week after week, sometimes for years, in an effort to make a small improvement in his golf game.

Children, like adults, learn from repetition or practice, not from lectures or explanations. They may have to repeat a task dozens of times before they become proficient at it, regardless of the nature of the task. That's why many practitioners have family members practice injecting oranges as a way of becoming more proficient at injecting their child. If both the parents and the child become proficient at injecting an orange, there are two results. First, their skill at injecting increases. Second, their anxiety at having to give an injection decreases. This example is applicable to many learning situations with children.

2.2. MINIMIZING FRUSTRATION FROM CHILD REARING

If a parent tells her child that a certain behavior is unacceptable, and the child is unable, because of his level of cognitive development, to act on the parent's comment, two entirely separate and distinct processes occur in the parent and the child.

The parent repeats the rule, assuming the child "didn't hear the rule" the first time. After repeating a request numerous times, the parent begins to feel frustrated because her child "refuses" to do what he is told or because he "acts" defiant. Over time, the parent will make such statements as, "I don't know what it's going to take to get him to . . .," "If I've told her once, I've told her a hundred times," or "I'm not going to tell him again."

If parents assume the child is capable of following verbal rules, they usually begin to discipline the child for rule violations; the discipline, however, will probably be ineffective. After repeating this process over and over again, many parents conclude their children are intentionally not following the rules and become even more frustrated. While the parent is developing a sense of frustration, his child is going through a very different process. After hearing numerous explanations and seeing his parent getting more and more frustrated, the child perceives that her mother or father is "mad" at her. If her parents get so frustrated that they discipline her for "not doing what she was told," the child has even more reason to feel her parents don't like her. Parental threats then, aimed at forcing children to comply with commands, only serve to strengthen the child's belief that mommy or daddy is "mad at me." In time, the parental nagging can take its toll on a child's self-esteem.

2.3. THE ROLE OF THE PHYSICIAN

The physician can begin teaching parents about children's cognitive development at the 6-month well-child visit. Introducing such topics as discipline and cognitive development at these early ages is one way physicians have to reduce the anxiety and frustration parents experience in raising children. As a result, parents may be spared the anguish of attempting procedures that are almost destined to fail, such as yelling at an infant or slapping his hand for touching things. In Handout 2.1, the description of how children learn has been prepared for physicians or primary caregivers to give to parents.

A discussion of children's behavior that is initiated for the first time when the child is 6 or 7 months old may catch many parents before they have begun to use ineffective parenting strategies; it is hoped this will prevent or minimize parental frustration.

By introducing such topics as discipline at an early age, the physician can identify parents who have unrealistic expectations of what a child is capable of or who already are experiencing problems handling their own emotions. The parent who begins to work on compliance with a child less than 1 year of age is in the best position to prevent problems from escalating.

Too often, parents are unconcerned with the issue of behavioral compliance until it becomes mandatory, as in the case of a child who is essentially untrained until the time comes to toilet train him or, worse yet, until the child is diagnosed with a chronic illness. Then it becomes paramount that the child consistently do what he is told to do, even though he may have a long history of noncompliant behavior.

Whether the child has a history of noncompliance or the parents are interested in working on compliance early, before there is any actual need for compliant behavior, the approach to obtaining compliance is basically the same.

2.4. FOSTERING INDEPENDENCE

Parents are often so concerned about their child's day-to-day behavior that they do not take the time or the initiative to focus on specific skills their children will need as they grow older and become more independent. To explain this concept, we use an example that appeals to many parents: the driver's education programs offered by many high schools.

Most new drivers have a tendency to look at the road directly in front of their vehicle. This results in erratic driving that is anxiety provoking. Parents, analogously, concentrate on the behavior their child is exhibiting today, rather than on the skills their child will need 5 and 10 years from now. In driver's education, instructors train students to look farther down the road, to give the student a wider perspective as well as time to react to unexpected situations. If you can convince parents to focus on skills their children will need later, two areas are enormously important: self-quieting skills and independent play skills. These skills will be discussed in detail here.

Prior to any attempt to instruct parents on parenting strategies, the practitioner would be well advised to assess how well developed the child's skills are for self-quieting and independent play. These two skills, or sets of skills, play a large role in determining whether attempts at instructing the parents will be successful.

2.4.1. Infant Self-Quieting Skills

Brazelton's Neonatal Behavioral Assessment Scale (1973) contains a set of procedures designed to assess the self-quieting or self-consoling skills of newborns prior to any learned interaction with adult caregivers. The individual performing the testing begins with a quiet infant who is less than 1 month of age (see Handout 2.2). Typically, the exam is performed for the first time during the first week of life to reduce any previous learning that many have taken place on the part of the infant.

The assessment begins when an adult has purposely startled an infant to begin crying. For the first 2 minutes after the startled infant has begun crying, the tester leaves the infant completely alone. If the infant quiets down during this time, she has excellent self-quieting skills. About 20% of infants can self-quiet, completely alone, in 2 minutes.

If the infant doesn't self-quiet during the first 2 minutes alone, the tester positions himself so that his face is approximately 10 to 12 inches directly above the infant for 1 full minute. If there isn't any self-quieting, the tester begins talking to the infant in a normal voice tone and volume, keeping his head about 10 to 12 inches above the infant. Next, the tester places his hand firmly on the infant's chest, while continuing to have facial contact and talking in a normal voice.

The earlier in the test the infant quiets down, the better the infant's self-quieting skills. An infant with excellent self-quieting skills will presumably be a happier, more contented infant, an infant who is better able to cope with minor upsets without the assistance of an adult. Just as self-quieting skills are important in the infant, they are important in children of all ages. While Brazelton's early writings (1973) seemed to imply that babies either had self-quieting skills or did not have these skills, now it is becoming increasingly more obvious that babies can learn self-quieting skills just like they learn many other behaviors.

2.4.2. Toddler Self-Quieting Skills

Self-quieting skills are very important in older children—they equip the child to better deal with disappointment, disruption, and discomfort. Fortunately, self-quieting skills can be fostered, or even taught, in a relatively short period of time if learning conditions are optimal.

Indications are that a toddler has good self-quieting if she can:

• Accept "No" as an answer without fussing and whining.
• Deal with frustration when playing alone.
• Deal with frustration when playing with other children.
• Self-quiet after being scared or having received a minor injury.
• Self-quiet when in a fearful situation.

Interestingly, Anders, Halpern, and Hua (1992) reported that parents who, with the best of intentions, assist their young children with sleep onset may very well end up with a child who cannot independently deal with night awakening. That is, the child who is assisted in falling to sleep at bedtime will usually require the same assistance if he should awaken in the middle of the night.

In our own work, we have gone one step further and correlated children's ability to self-quiet during the day with their ability to deal with sleep onset independently. The advantage of working on self-quieting skills during the daytime, rather than working on helping a child return to sleep after a night awakening, is that the parents have not been awakened themselves. Additionally, there are potentially more opportunities during the day to work on self-quieting skills.

2.4.3. Practices That Encourage Self-Quieting Skills

Two instances during the child's day present opportunities for parents or caregivers to encourage children in the development of self-quieting skills: naturally occurring situations that promote self-quieting skills and the use of time-out to promote self-quieting skills.

2.4.3a. Naturally Occurring Situations That Promote Self-Quieting Skills

First, if a child is sitting on the floor playing with a toy, and he drops that toy so that it is just barely out of his reach, many parents retrieve the toy for the child. In this way, although the parents may lessen the child's distress at dropping the toy, what they are doing to help him is actually counterproductive to the child's developing sense of independence. That is, if the child is left to his own means, and, after a brief period of fussing, he reaches or stretches forward and retrieves the toy himself, he not only has retrieved his toy but also is beginning to learn he can reduce his own distress with skills that are already in his repertoire.

While this procedure requires the parent to stifle a natural tendency, the advantage for the child is significant. The child's sense of independence and self-esteem are far more important than any temporary distress he may have had to endure to develop that sense.

2.4.3b. Using Time-Out to Encourage Self-Quieting Skills

Another way to help a child to develop self-quieting skills is through the use of a very brief time-out (see Handout 2.3). If the child is engaging in a behavior such as whining that is aggravating to the parent and maladaptive to the child, the child should be placed in time-out until she has self-quieted for 2 to 3 seconds. As soon as the child self-quiets, the parent tells her the time-out is over and asks her what it was she wanted.

When the child begins whining, the parent should simply say, "Time-out, whining," and ignore the child until he stops whining. The parent should be prepared for an initial increase in whining (Drabman and Jarvie, 1977); sometimes the increase is dramatic. But if the parents can learn to tolerate an initial increase in whining and fussing, their child can learn self-quieting skills.

Repetition is vitally important to a child's learning. If the child is placed in time-out every time she whines, and if she is released from time-out every time she self-quiets, she will learn very quickly that whining does not result in getting anything she wants and, conversely, self-quieting can help obtain much of what she wants.

The contrast between being "timed-out" for whining and getting parental attention as soon as he self-quiets presents the child with two remarkably different and mutually exclusive choices. He can continue whining and spend a great deal of his day in time-out, or he can calm himself down and receive a lot of attention from his parents.

The child who learns self-quieting skills can usually generalize these skills to other times and places. Basically, once a child has learned self-quieting skills, she is no longer at the mercy of other people to comfort her; she no longer has to depend on someone else every time she encounters a situation that is not to her liking.

2.5. INDEPENDENT PLAY SKILLS

A separate, but equally important, set of skills comes under the general heading of independent play skills. Dr. Robert Wahler, of the University of Tennessee, Department of Psychology, has conducted research for over a decade that highlights the importance of children learning independent play skills. In one of his early research papers (Wahler and Fox, 1980), he reported that interventions with behavior-disordered children had lasting effects with children who had independent play skills, whereas the same interventions, when used with children who had poor independent play skills, would not produce lasting effects.

We now know that children can be taught independent play skills much like we would teach them anything else. Whenever the child is playing appropriately for his age, the parent should provide the child with a great deal of brief, nonverbal, physical contact ("time in," as we've referred to it here). Over the course of several months, the child will be able to entertain himself for increasingly longer periods of time. When a child is able to entertain himself for long periods of time—we look for 1 to 2 hours of independent play by 4 years of age—there is much less need for discipline.

2.5.1. Teaching Independent Play Skills to Infants

The demand characteristics of infants are such that parents must interact with them frequently to provide routine care. However, as the child develops and matures, she should become less dependent on her caregivers and increasingly more independent.

Because infants require so much assistance, their parents will usually need to be encouraged to provide the child with attention and physical contact *when they don't need it* (see Handout 2.4). This means, for example, if an infant is on a blanket on the floor, sucking on his hand and otherwise quite content, the caregiver should provide him with a good deal of brief, nonverbal, physical contact. In this way, the infant learns to enjoy independent activities while receiving a lot of physical contact from important adults. Instead of waiting until the infant has finished an activity and begins to fuss or cry, the caregiver should be encouraged to provide physical comfort prior to the onset of fussing and crying.

2.5.2. Teaching Independent Play Skills to Toddlers

Many toddlers already have independent play skills—it's just that their parents don't do anything to encourage these skills. Rather, many parents will intentionally ignore their child when she is playing quietly. Or, alternatively, they will go to "check up" on their toddler because he is quiet and they suspect he "might be up to something."

The essence of encouraging independent play skills is to provide attention while the child is playing—before she interrupts or terminates her play and goes looking for an adult (see Handout 2.5). Over time, the judicious attention paid to a child engaged in independent play can encourage him to play for increasingly longer periods of time. From playing for increasingly longer periods of time, the child learns to enjoy independent play activities. Whether he is organizing his baseball cards, reading a book, or working on his bike, he is learning a healthy degree of independence that can benefit him for the rest of his life.

A child engaged in independent play is much less likely to get into trouble, and parents will find the need for discipline is much less in children who have good independent play skills. When there is much less need for discipline, and a child is deriving a good deal more enjoyment from her independent play activities, self-esteem improves. The improvement in self-esteem, in turn, makes it easier for the child to try new things, and so on. In this way, the child naturally builds up both her confidence and her independence.

When a child has self-quieting skills and independent play skills, the issue of behavioral compliance becomes much easier. For one thing, when parents rely on discipline to keep a child out of trouble, instead of relying on competing activities the child truly enjoys, the parents must maintain a high level of vigilance. In the long run, it is far easier to encourage the development of self-quieting and independent play skills than it is to monitor a child's every activity.

2.6. TEACHING CHILDREN TO BEHAVE APPROPRIATELY

The vast majority of leaders in the field of parent training, while differing in their particular approach to solving behavior problems, all seem to agree with two major points. First, concentrating on a child's acquisition of appropriate behaviors is more important than disciplining or punishing him for inappropriate behavior. Second, punishment, even when it is effective, only teaches a child what *not* to do—it does not teach a child what to do. Thus, much of the parent training effort should be devoted to teaching children appropriate ways of behaving. Children learn a great deal from what they see their parents do: This is called modeling.

If parents are constantly getting angry with their child, he is likely to learn a great deal about how to behave ineffectively when he is angry. If parents are calm, exhibit a matter-of-fact manner, and approach tasks in a consistent and orderly fashion, their children will be more likely to approach problems in a calm and matter-of-fact manner. Modeling, whether of appropriate behaviors or inappropriate behaviors, seems to be an effective teaching method.

2.7. USING TIME-OUT

Perhaps the most often mentioned and best researched approach to discipline is the use of "time-out." Over the years, the term "time-out" has come to mean many things to many people. When the concept of time-out was introduced into child development literature in the 1960s, the term referred to the deliberate removal of a pleasant or rewarding state of affairs. More specifically, the original technical term was "time-out from positive reinforcement."

In early research on time-out, researchers created an artificially pleasant environment from which they could remove the child who was behaving inappropriately. For example, the researchers may have arranged for a child to receive many rewards over a short period of time (this has come to be referred to as "time-in" [Handout 2.6]). The time-out, then, simply consisted of removing the child from the opportunity to receive all of the rewards. Unfortunately, the popular use of the term "time-out" has come to mean that a child should sit quietly in a chair or should go to her room. The act of sit-ting is somehow supposed to have taken on almost magical properties for discouraging certain types of behavior. Often, little attention is given toward making the time-in more rewarding for the child.

Along this same line, sometimes parents unwittingly encourage their child to misbehave. For example, if a parent is talking on the telephone while the child is watching TV quietly, reading a book, or playing with his sibling, most parents will simply ignore the child. Many parents adhere to the adage, "Let sleeping dogs lie," when managing their children's behavior. Yet, when the child engages in any behavior the parent finds objectionable, the parent moves quickly to correct the behavior. The message the child receives is quite clear—if you want to get mommy or daddy off the phone, you should misbehave.

These examples point out one major problem: Parents may have been instructed about the use of time-out without being instructed about the importance of time-in. Whenever the child is not misbehaving, the parent should be lavishing the child with brief, nonverbal, physical contact—teaching the child the easiest way to get attention from a parent is by behaving appropriately (Solnick, Rincover, and Peterson, 1977).

Physical contact, rather than verbal praise, can often be used without interrupting such parental activities as talking on the telephone (Christophersen, 1990). For exam-ple, parents can maintain frequent physical contact with their children while continu-ing their telephone conversations—especially if they have a long telephone cord or a cordless phone.

2.8. DISCIPLINING THE INFANT AND YOUNG TODDLER

The younger a child is when she first experiences discipline, the easier it seems to be to get parents to use it. If parents begin unemotional discipline around or before the first birthday, children usually catch on very quickly and the parents are rewarded for their efforts by seeing an improvement in their child's behavior. Conversely, when parents put off establishing any rules about discipline until a child is 5 or 6 years old, the parents typically find it difficult to follow through with the discipline.

The use of a brief period of time-out in a playpen immediately after the inappropri-ate behavior, coupled with a great deal of time-in for appropriate behavior (brief, nonverbal, physical contact from parent to child), usually results in improvements in the child's behavior within 1 to 3 days.

Fortunately, parents do not have to be concerned whether the child will dislike his playpen from using these procedures. In fact, just the opposite is true. Because the child is removed from the playpen only when quiet, he begins to associate the playpen with quiet play and learns to quiet more quickly with each passing day.

When we have taught parents to use brief time-outs with children below 1 year of age, both the parents and the child usually learn the appropriate skills very quickly. We have demonstrated that young children not only learn to enjoy time-in quickly but also learn to avoid behaviors that resulted in their being sent to time-out (Mathews, Friman, Barone, Ross, and Christophersen, 1987). Also, parents tend to rate the use of time-out as much more satisfactory than such traditional forms of physical punishment as spanking. Handout 2.7 describes the major points for parents to remember when using time-out with a young child.

The major consideration in using time-out with a young child is to make sure the time-in is as rewarding and enjoyable as possible and that the time-out is not over until the child has self-quieted.

If the child can experience repeated time-in and time-out, he can quickly learn to choose time-in over time-out. Although other authors may use a myriad of terms to refer to what I am calling time-in, there is almost universal agreement that parents must provide their children with a nurturing, loving relationship. Even professionals who abhor the use of any type of punishment, including time-out, can hardly recommend that parents refrain from pleasant interactions with their children.

If is important to remember that time-in does not require exclusivity in order to be effective. Rather, just the opposite may be true. Instead of the parent devoting an entire morning to sitting on the floor and playing with the child, or just observing the child's play, it is imperative that parents learn to engage in their own activities while also providing time-in for their children.

Thus, a mother who is fixing dinner or balancing the checkbook needs to continuously monitor her child, frequently providing brief, nonverbal, physical contact. This is usually much easier to accomplish if the mother arranges the environment so that the child is playing in her immediate vicinity. Throughout Mom's activity, she should briefly interrupt what she is doing to provide brief, nonverbal, physical contact with her child. While this whole process may take days or weeks to establish, the benefit derived from it, for both parent and child, is substantial.

2.8.1. Side Effects of Time-Out

Many children will object to the use of time-out when it is first introduced. The first 2 or 3 days after a parent introduces time-out for discipline, there is a high probability the child will have a tantrum during the time-out. Therefore, parents must know the importance of encouraging the development of self-quieting skills in their children. They need to know not only that time-in and time-out discourage children from engaging in certain inappropriate behaviors, but, together, these procedures also greatly facilitate the development of self-quieting skills.

2.9. MINI-TIME-OUTS

Some young children get so adept at fussing and demanding attention that adult caregivers find it almost impossible to get physically close to the child before the fussing starts. A parent working in the kitchen can notice if the child is playing quietly on the floor and, as soon as he begins walking over to the child to provide brief physical contact, the child starts crying. In these types of situations, I recommend the use of "mini-time-outs."

The parent should remain in the immediate vicinity of the infant—within 1 to 2 feet—to provide physical contact with the infant the instant he stops crying. Sometimes the situation is so bad the only break the infant takes from crying is occasional breaths between cries. Every time the infant is not crying, the parent should be instructed to touch the infant and maintain frequent touching—for example, stroking the baby's hair—until the baby begins crying again. For extremely difficult babies, these pleasant touches may last only 1 to 3 seconds before the crying resumes and the parents must ignore the child again.

The combination of brief physical touches for being quiet and removal of all contact when the crying starts again usually reduces the infant's crying within a day or two. Mini-time-outs should be practiced three or four times each day for about 20 minutes each time. Whenever possible, the practitioner should demonstrate this procedure for the parent during an office visit.

The procedures outlined in Handouts 2.8 and 2.9, preventing and managing excessive crying, respectively, teach the child she can get all the attention she desires without crying all of the time. Usually, not only does the crying diminish within 24 hours, but the parents report an improvement in the baby's general disposition at the same time. This is a sign that the parents are following the procedures properly and that the child is responsive to them. As the child learns to enjoy playing, while getting generous physical contact from a parent, parents learn they can get important activities completed while enjoying their child. The process is mutually beneficial.

2.10. DISCIPLINING THE TODDLER

The major difference between disciplining a toddler and disciplining an older child is that a playpen can be used with a toddler but not with an older child. The obvious advantage of the playpen—the child cannot get out, which greatly facilitates learning a self-quieting behavior—is absent once the child is old enough to climb out of the playpen. Time-out with older children, then, requires a good deal more restraint on the parents' part because they must ignore the child's inappropriate behavior rather than engage in lengthy power struggles over time-out. (Handout 2.10 presents guidelines for use of time-out.)

If a child already has some self-quieting skills, then parents can use a chair for time-outs. However, if the child refuses to sit in a chair, it's not a good idea to attempt to force him to do so. The resulting power struggle isn't won by either the parent or the child, and it's usually very unpleasant for both. Rather, we recommend that the parents begin time-outs by simply ignoring the child until he self-quiets. (See Handout 2.11 for ways to increase the effectiveness of time-out.)

The parents must be reminded that the absence of time-in is what makes a time-out effective—not the place or what he's doing. Therefore, as long as the parents can completely ignore the child, regardless of what he is doing, the child will eventually self-quiet. As soon as he can self-quiet for 2 to 3 seconds, the parents should be instructed to gradually increase the length of time the child is quiet by several seconds every day or two. In this way, the child is learning to self-quiet for increasingly longer periods of time. After the child can self-quiet consistently, then the parents can be instructed to begin using a chair or a stair step for the time-outs. As stated in Handout 2.10, while the child is in time-out the parents should not talk to him, look at him, or talk about him. They should not attempt to hold him in time-out or use any other coercive

procedure in conjunction with time-out. Rather, it is far more important that the child learn self-quieting skills. By definition, if the parent must help the child to quiet, it can't be considered self-quieting.

The parents may need to work on their coping skills, as discussed in Chapter 14, so that they can continue to ignore the child while he's in time-out. There is no such thing as a time-out within a time-out. Any interaction that the parents direct toward a child in time-out will only encourage the child to act up in time-out. Self-quieting requires that the child be left alone during a time-out.

2.11. REDIRECTING A CHILD

Many parents become very uncomfortable when their child is clearly becoming frustrated with a particular activity or a particular toy. In a well-intentioned effort to reduce both their child's frustration and their own frustration, they will redirect the child's activity while the child is fussing. Unfortunately, all this does is make the child more dependent on the parent in these kinds of situations. Teaching children how to redirect their own activities, when they are frustrated or bored, is valuable (see Handout 2.12). Doing so teaches the child a skill that he can use all of his life. However, doing the redirecting for him only makes him more dependent. For this reason, I suggest that parents *always* wait until their child has self-quieted before they redirect him. In this way, the child is more receptive, because he was calm when the redirecting took place. Over time, the child will learn how to redirect his own activities when he begins to feel frustration or boredom.

The real essence of redirecting is that it should be child initiated, not parent initiated. If the parent can wait until the child has self-quieted before redirecting, the child will learn how to implement this strategy before his parent comes to the rescue. In time, redirecting his own activities will become natural and the parent will no longer need to be concerned about the child's ability to do so.

2.12. TEACHING PEER INTERACTION SKILLS

Children need to be taught how to interact appropriately with their siblings and their peers. If parents take a proactive, educational approach to teaching their children these skills, they know their children have these skills, and they have the satisfaction of watching as the skills continue to develop. Rather than leave such an important skill area up to chance, it's better to schedule times specifically for teaching peer interaction skills. Handout 2.13 summarizes the steps for teaching peer interaction skills. Although it can take months to teach a child peer interaction skills, these are skills that a child can use for years to come.

2.13. CONCLUDING REMARKS

The health-care provider should begin discussing with parents the importance of time-in during the prenatal period and continue emphasizing it until she is certain the

parents know what it is and use time-in on a daily basis. This may be one of the most effective ways of minimizing later behavior problems.

Any time the provider is discussing with a parent how to teach an infant or child a new behavior, the importance of practice as a learning technique should be emphasized again and again. Practice is not only to be expected, it should be welcomed, for it is only through such practice that a child learns any new behavior.

REFERENCES

Anders TF, Halpern LF, Hua J: Sleeping through the night: A developmental perspective. *Pediatrics* 90(4):554–560, 1992.

Azrin NH, Holz WC: Punishment, in Honig WK (ed.), *Operant Behavior: Areas of Research and Application.* New York: Appleton-Century-Crofts, 1966.

Brazelton TB: *Neonatal Behavioral Assessment Scale.* Philadelphia: Spastics International Medical Publications, 1973.

Christophersen ER: *Beyond Discipline: Parenting That Lasts a Lifetime.* Kansas City, MO: Westport Publishers, 1990.

Drabman RS, Jarvie BA: Counseling parents of children with behavior problems: The use of extinction and time-out techniques. *Pediatrics* 59:78–85, 1977.

Haynes RB, Sackett DL, Taylor DW (eds.): *Compliance in Health Care.* Baltimore: Johns Hopkins University Press, 1979.

Mathews JR, Friman PC, Barone VJ, Ross LV, Christophersen ER: Decreasing dangerous infant behaviors through parent instruction. *J Appl Behav Anal* 20(2):165–169, 1987.

Solnick JV, Rincover A, Peterson CP: Some determinants of the reinforcing and punishing effects of time-out. *J Appl Behav Anal* 10:415–424, 1977.

Wahler RG, Fox JJ: Solitary toy play and time-out: A family treatment package for children with aggressive and oppositional behavior. *J Appl Behav Anal* 13(1):23–39, 1980.

Sample Handouts

HANDOUT 2.1

Cognitive Development in the Toddler and Preschooler as It Relates to Discipline

Children who are 7 years of age or younger are at the preabstract level of cognitive development, meaning they are unable to deal with abstractions like reasoning.

If a parent tells her 3-year-old daughter, Jennifer, not to go into the street because there are cars and she might get hit and be hurt, Jennifer may be perfectly capable of repeating the instruction back to her mom and dad, but that is where her ability ends. It is extremely unlikely she will actually be able to do what her parent instructed her to do.

Because reasoning with young children doesn't work, it usually results in a parent repeating the instruction over and over again, using threats and nagging such as, "If I have to tell you one more time," or "If I've told you once, I've told you a hundred times." Her parent ends up telling her the same thing over and over again, since Jennifer is unable to comply with the instructions because of her level of cognitive development.

When Mom continually has to repeat the instruction, she may begin to feel frustrated or angry. Jennifer, unable to comply, begins to feel that Mom doesn't like her because she threatens and yells at her. Over time, repeated attempts to reason with a child can result in lowering the child's self-esteem. As this process goes on, day after day, the parent gets more and more frustrated and the child develops a very poor self-image.

Children learn through repetition. They must have the opportunity to practice the same thing over and over again.

If Jennifer needs to be taught not to go into the street, she must be shown this lesson repeatedly. Every time Jennifer goes near the street, she needs to be disciplined in an unemotional way. Every time she starts to go toward the street, but stops short of doing so, she needs to be praised. After Jennifer has experienced 20 or 30 trips toward the street, with some resulting in discipline and some in praise, she will learn from the contrast to stay out of the street.

Parents cannot tell small children only once not to do something and realistically expect the child never to do it again.

Parents need to understand that teaching involves many repetitions before something is learned. Children must do something both the right way and the wrong way many times before they learn to do it right consistently. Rather than becoming frustrated because learning takes place over a long period of time, parents should understand that they are in the process of teaching their child an important skill. The more times the child can experience the contrast between what happens when something is done the right way and when it is done the wrong way, the quicker and more thoroughly the child will learn what the right way is.

Edward R. Christophersen, *Beyond Discipline: Parenting That Lasts a Lifetime*. Kansas City, MO: Westport Publishers. ©Edward R. Christophersen, 1990.

HANDOUT 2.2

Testing Your Infant's Self-Quieting Skills

This test measures the number of activities you must perform that interrupt your baby's fussing and allow your baby to move to a quieter state.

To test your baby's self-quieting skills, pick a time during the first month of life when your baby is happy, content, and sleeping.

Wake your baby up either with a loud clap of your hands, above the crib or bassinet, or by moving him around enough to start him crying. As soon as he has been fussing or crying for 15 seconds, progress through the following steps.

Step 1. *The baby alone.* Leave your baby completely alone for a full 2 minutes to see if she is capable of quieting alone. Although the 2 minutes may seem like an eternity, wait the full time. The baby is considered to have self-quieting skills if she is quiet for at least 5 seconds. If she is still crying at the end of 2 minutes, progress to the next step.

Step 2. *Parent's face alone.* Lean over your baby so that your face is about 10 inches from your baby's face. If your baby is still crying at the end of 30 seconds, progress to the next step.

Step 3. *Parent's voice and face alone.* While leaning over your baby, talk to him in a normal voice (both voice level and intonation). If your baby is still crying at the end of 30 seconds, progress to the next step.

Step 4. *Hand on belly steadily.* While continuing to look at your baby, talk softly and place your hand steadily on her belly. If your baby is still crying at the end of 30 seconds, progress to the next step.

Step 5. *Hand on belly and restraining one or both arms.* While continuing to look at your baby, talk softly and hold one or both of his hands firmly against his chest. If he is still crying at the end of 30 seconds, progress to the next step.

Step 6. *Picking up and holding.* Pick up your baby and hold her snugly against your chest while continuing to look at and talk to her. If your baby is still crying at the end of 30 seconds, progress to the next step.

Step 7. *Holding and rocking.* While talking softly to your baby, begin rocking him back and forth. If he is still crying at the end of 30 seconds, progress to the next step.

Step 8. *Dressing, holding in arms, and rocking.* Pick up your baby and place her on a receiving blanket. Wrap the blanket snugly around your baby and rock her gently while talking to her softly. If your baby is still crying at the end of 30 seconds, progress to the next step.

Step 9. *Pacifier or finger to suck in addition to dressing, holding, and rocking.* With your baby still wrapped in the receiving blanket, offer him your finger or a pacifier while continuing to rock him gently and talking to him softly.

Step 10. *Not consolable.* If none of the nine steps above works, you have a baby who is very difficult to console. Before jumping to any drastic conclusions, be sure to repeat the test at least two additional times, on different days. If you still apparently have a baby who is very difficult to console, make sure to tell your pediatrician at the first well-baby visit.

Edward R. Christophersen, *Beyond Discipline: Parenting That Lasts a Lifetime*. Kansas City, MO: Westport Publishers. ©Edward R. Christophersen, 1990.

HANDOUT 2.3

Teaching Self-Quieting Skills to Toddlers

In addition to using brief time-outs to encourage your child to develop self-quieting skills, you should discipline yourself to take advantage of every naturally occurring opportunity to teach your child self-quieting skills.

If your child comes to you with his feelings hurt or after falling off his tricycle, try to refrain from saying anything. Instead, hold him against you, without saying a word, while you rub his back and pat him. Your child will learn you are a great source of comfort when he needs you. He will also learn that you don't quiet him down—he will learn to quiet himself down.

Using time-outs for discipline is another way of teaching toddlers self-quieting skills. Every time you tell your toddler she is in time-out and she quiets down, she is learning self-quieting skills. While there may only be one or two opportunities each day to let your child naturally quiet herself down, using time-outs can create many additional opportunities to practice these skills.

If you keep reminding your toddler he must be quiet when he is in time-out, he will never have the opportunity to self-quiet. Toddlers must learn to quiet down without any help from you whatsoever. That means if they are having a horrendous tantrum, you must let them quiet down. Comforting a child who is having a tantrum only encourages him to continue having them.

Remember, the more opportunities there are, and the closer the opportunities are to each other, the quicker your toddler will learn self-quieting.

Edward R. Christophersen, *Beyond Discipline: Parenting That Lasts a Lifetime*. Kansas City, MO: Westport Publishers. ©Edward R. Christophersen, 1990.

HANDOUT 2.4

Teaching Independent Play Skills to Infants

To encourage independent play activities:

Step 1. Look for times when your infant is playing quietly by herself. Provide her with a lot of brief, nonverbal, physical contact when she doesn't need it or demand it.

Step 2. Try to find an activity you can engage in while you also are providing your infant with brief physical contact—reading the paper or a magazine, working on paperwork you brought home from the office, or making a telephone call.

Step 3. Learn to discipline yourself to provide the physical contact while you are engaged in a productive activity.

Step 4. Gradually begin using slightly longer periods of time between touching your infant. The increases should be very small so that your infant never notices the increases are occurring.

Step 5. Over time, perhaps 2 to 4 weeks, gradually decrease the frequency of your physical contact. Don't be surprised if it takes you months to substantially increase your infant's independent play skills.

Remember:

- Gradually wait for longer and longer amounts of time between physical touches.
- Your infant will get enjoyment out of playing alone and getting affection from you—all from the same activity!

Edward R. Christophersen, *Beyond Discipline: Parenting That Lasts a Lifetime*. Kansas City, MO: Westport Publishers. ©Edward R. Christophersen, 1990.

HANDOUT 2.5

Teaching Independent Play Skills to Toddlers

Teaching independent play is a very slow process but well worth the time and effort. But it is not accomplished overnight; it is a gradual process.

Your child's age determines the type of activities you will use to increase his attention span. Select a behavior or several behaviors that your child likes when you first begin.

For toddlers, playing quietly by themselves is a good behavior to use.

For older, school-age children, homework or reading can be used.

FOLLOW THESE EASY STEPS

Step 1. Determine how long your child is now playing or engaging in any specific behavior like coloring, playing quietly, or reading. This may be a very short time, like 1 to 5 minutes.

Step 2. Pick a time to work on increasing your toddler's attention span each day. Your child will need the structure of a specific time each and every day to make the process easier.

Step 3. Begin by instructing your child to engage in the behavior you have chosen, for example, playing quietly, for an amount of time you feel certain she can manage—for as long as 5 minutes, for example. Set a portable kitchen timer for that amount of time.

Step 4. Give your child very brief love pats—but don't distract him—as often as possible during this time.

Step 5. Gradually increase the time, though the exact amount depends on your toddler. When beginning, try 3 or 4 days at each time. You may need to stay at one length of time for more than 3 to 4 days, depending on your child's progress. Don't lengthen the time until your child is doing well at the shorter period.

Step 6. If your child is enjoying these quiet types of activities at any other time during the day, be sure to give her lots of physical contact.

Step 7. If your child has tantrums before or during the time you are working on this behavior, place him in time-out. After the time-out is over, instruct him again to engage in the activity. Praise getting started and trying. Make this situation as pleasant as possible, but do not give in to the tantrum by allowing you child to get out of working for the specified time.

Step 8. Equally important is modeling the kind of behavior you expect your child to exhibit. If you would like your child to read more, it's very important that she see you enjoying reading. Don't make the mistake of "waiting until the kids are in bed" to do your reading.

Step 9. Provide praise and recognition for your child's appropriate behavior for as long as he lives at home.

Edward R. Christophersen, *Beyond Discipline: Parenting That Lasts a Lifetime*. Kansas City, MO: Westport Publishers. ©Edward R. Christophersen, 1990.

HANDOUT 2.6

Time-In

By their very dependent nature, newborns and young infants receive a lot of physical contact from their parents. As infants grow to become toddlers and preschoolers, their demand characteristics change, and parents usually touch their children much less often. By the time children are 4 years old, they are usually toilet trained, and they can dress and undress and feed and bathe themselves. If parents don't conscientiously put forth an effort to maintain a great deal of contact with their older child, he will be touched much less than at earlier ages.

Parents can do several things to offset these natural changes.

1. *Physical proximity.* During boring or distracting activities, place your child close to you where it is easy to reach her. At dinner, in the car, in a restaurant, when you have company, or when you are in a shopping mall, keep your child near you so that physical contact requires little, if any, additional effort on your part.

2. *Physical contact.* Frequent and brief (1 or 2 seconds) nonverbal physical contact will do more to teach your child that you love him than anything else you can do. Try to touch your child at least 50 times each day for 1 or 2 seconds—touch him any time he is not doing something wrong or something you disapprove of.

3. *Verbal reprimands.* Children don't have the verbal skills that adults do. Adults often send messages that are misunderstood by children, who may interpret verbal reprimands, nagging, pleading, and yelling as signs that their parents do not like them. Always keep in mind the old expression, "If you don't have anything nice to say, don't say anything at all."

4. *Nonverbal contact.* Try to make most of your physical contact with children nonverbal. With young children, physical contact usually has a calming effect, whereas verbal praise, questioning, or general comments may only interrupt what your child was doing.

5. *Independent play.* Children need to have time to themselves—time when they can play, put things in their mouths, or stare into space. Generally speaking, children don't do nearly as well when their parents carry them around much of the time and constantly try to entertain them.

Keep in mind that, although your baby may fuss when frustrated, she will never learn to deal with frustration if you are always there to help. Give children enough freedom to explore the environment on their own, and they will learn skills they can use the rest of their lives.

Remember:

- Children need lots of brief, nonverbal physical contact.
- If you don't have anything nice to say, don't say anything at all.

Edward R. Christophersen, *Beyond Discipline: Parenting That Lasts a Lifetime*. Kansas City, MO: Westport Publishers. ©Edward R. Christophersen, 1990.

HANDOUT 2.7

Discipline for Toddlers: Time-Out

Time-out involves placing your child in his playpen for a short period of time following each occurrence of a negative behavior. This procedure has been effective in reducing such problem behaviors as tantrums, hitting, and other aggressive acts; failure to follow directions; and jumping on furniture. Parents have found this works much better than spanking, yelling, and threatening children. It is most appropriate for children aged 9 months through 2 years.

A. PREPARATIONS

Step 1. Select a place for time-out. This could be your child's playpen. It needs to be a dull place, but not a dark, scary, or dangerous place. The aim is to remove the child to a place where not much is happening, not to make the child afraid.

Step 2. Discuss with your spouse or other primary caregiver which behaviors will result in time-out. Then discuss these behaviors with your child in an unemotional, matter-of-fact manner.

B. PROCEDURES

Step 1. Following the negative behavior, say to the child, "No, don't." Say this calmly; no screaming, talking angrily, or nagging is allowed. Carry the child to the playpen without talking to her. Carry her facing away from you.

Step 2. When the child is in the playpen, wait until he has stopped crying for about 10 to 15 seconds. Do not look at him, talk to him, or talk about him until he has stopped crying. After he is finally quiet, go over to the playpen, pick him up without saying a word, and set him on the floor near some of his toys. Do not reprimand him or mention what he did wrong.

Step 3. After each time-out episode, children start with a "clean slate." No discussions, nagging, threatening, or reminding are necessary. At the first opportunity, look for and praise positive behaviors: "Catch 'em being good!"

C. SUMMARY OF THE RULES FOR PARENTS

- Decide which behaviors you will use time-out for ahead of time, and discuss this with your child.

- Don't leave your child in time-out and forget about her.

- Don't nag, scold, or talk to your child when he is in time-out. All family members should follow this rule.

- Remain calm, particularly when your child is being testy.

Edward R. Christophersen, *Little People: Guidelines for Commonsense Child Rearing*. Kansas City, MO: Westport Publishers. ©Edward R. Christophersen, 1988.

HANDOUT 2.8

Preventing Excessive Crying

Virtually all babies cry a lot. However, there are specific things parents can do to help reduce the amount of crying their babies do and, in turn, make the first few months a more pleasant experience for both the parents and the infant.

Here are some suggestions according to the age of your infant.

NEWBORN

Establish Consistent Routines

If you can discipline yourself to develop consistent routines for such caregiving as diapering, bathing, and shampooing your baby, you will probably find that you relax more and your baby fusses less.

Love Pats

When your baby is quietly watching what you are doing or entertaining himself by sucking on his hand or fingers, give him many brief, physical love pats without saying a word. Try to give him 50 to 100 love pats every day. Over time, your child will learn skills for keeping busy, because when he is busy he gets the enjoyment out of playing and also getting physical contact from important adults.

Brief, Boring Night Feedings

When feeding your baby at night, leave the lights off and don't talk. You can very gently caress or hold her; just refrain from providing any more stimulation than is necessitated by feeding.

Quiet Time

Try to have time every day when all noisy appliances, such as TVs and radios, are off, and you aren't talking on the phone or talking to your baby—just plain quiet time.

2 MONTHS OF AGE

Pick Up Calm Babies

When your baby awakens from a nap or from his nighttime sleep, he will begin babbling and cooing immediately instead of crying. Make sure you are up in time to pick up your baby *before* the crying actually starts. Under about 8 weeks of age, the baby's transition from sleeping to crying is simply too short for you to expect to get to him in time.

After 8 to 10 weeks of age, babies wake up and make cute noises before beginning to cry. If you consistently get to them before they cry, they learn you will take care of them when they babble and coo, and they will have no need to cry every time they awaken.

Put Your Baby to Bed Awake but Drowsy

In the newborn period, babies typically fall asleep while nursing. After the baby is 8 to 10 weeks of age, you will probably notice that he finishes nursing without falling asleep. If you put your baby to bed awake but drowsy, and be sure there are several things in the crib your baby can look at and reach out to, she will learn "transition skills" to help her make the transition from waking to sleeping.

These transition skills can be helpful to your baby for years to come. Babies with good self-quieting skills usually learn these transitions earlier and more quickly than do babies with poor self-quieting skills.

Quiet Time

Try to have time every day when all noisy appliances, such as television sets and radios, are off, and you aren't talking on the phone or talking to your baby—just plain quiet time.

Edward R. Christophersen, *Beyond Discipline: Parenting That Lasts a Lifetime*. Kansas City, MO: Westport Publishers. ©Edward R. Christophersen, 1990.

Managing Excessive Crying

Some babies seem to cry all or most of the time. Most of their parents' efforts—cuddling them, carrying them, talking softly to them, or holding them—do not reduce their crying. With these babies, attempts to let them "cry it out" don't seem to help either. They just can't seem to be consoled. Because the procedures we recommend usually reduce crying within 3 days, there is little risk to the parent who wants to try them.

There are two sharply contrasting activities parents can do to reduce an infant's crying. These procedures are best begun shortly after your baby has awakened and has been fed, burped, diapered, and generally attended to for a little while.

Step 1. Place your baby on a blanket on the floor, near enough to you so that you can engage in an everyday activity that takes a while to complete. This activity could be paying bills, reading, or doing paperwork. Stay very near your baby, but do not interact with her in any way as long as she is crying. Just maintain your activity and wait for the second there is a break in her crying.

Step 2. The instant the crying lets up, briefly rub your baby's head or back with your hand without saying a word. The second she starts crying again, immediately go back to your activity.

Step 3. Keep up these two contrasting actions for at least 30 minutes at a time, performing the exercise at least three times a day. If you can rub the baby's head or back for longer than 1 or 2 seconds without him crying, do so. But remember, the instant he starts crying, stop your touching.

Step 4. When you first begin these procedures, pick up your baby at the end of a session immediately following a quiet spell. It is best to have only one parent use these procedures at first until your baby becomes accustomed to them.

Step 5. Over a period of time, you should notice that the breaks between your baby's crying episodes get longer and longer, and the crying itself also lasts for shorter periods. As this happens, spend more and more time touching your baby. Always remember to stop touching her the second she starts crying again.

Step 6. As you see a decrease in the amount of crying, increase the number of times you touch your baby. You can then begin to carry your baby around and talk to him, but be prepared to place the baby gently on the floor and to stop your physical interaction with him the second he starts crying again.

Do not give up on these procedures until you have tried them consistently at least three times a day for 3 consecutive days. Follow these procedures as carefully as you possibly can. The parent with the most patience should be the one who initially tries these procedures. Do not encourage visiting from your relatives or friends during these 3 days, so that you have fewer distractions.

Edward R. Christophersen, *Little People: Guidelines for Commonsense Child Rearing*. Kansas City, MO: Westport Publishers. ©Edward R. Christophersen, 1988.

Using Time-Out for Behavior Problems

A. PREPARATIONS

Step 1. Purchase a small portable kitchen timer.

Step 2. Select a place for time-out: a chair in the hallway, kitchen, or corner of a room. Time-out needs to be in a dull place—not in your child's bedroom—where your child cannot watch TV or play with toys. It should not be a dark, scary, or dangerous place; the aim is to remove your child to a place where not much is happening, not to make him feel afraid.

Step 3. Discuss with your spouse or other caregiver which behaviors result in time-out. Consistency is very important.

B. PRACTICING (IF YOUR CHILD IS 3 OR OLDER)

Step 1. Before using time-out for discipline, practice using it with your child at a pleasant time.

Step 2. Tell your child the time starts only after she is quiet. Ask your child what would happen if she talks or makes noises when in time-out. Your child should say the timer will be reset or something similar. If she does not say this, remind her of the rule.

Step 3. After explaining the rules and checking your child's understanding of them, go through the steps under "C" below. Tell your child you are "pretending" this time.

Step 4. Mention to your child you will be using the time-out technique instead of spanking, yelling, or threatening.

C. PROCEDURES

Step 1. Following an inappropriate behavior, describe what your child did in as few words as possible. For example, say, "Time-out for hitting." Say it calmly and only once. Do not lose your temper or begin nagging. If your child has problems getting to the designated time-out chair quickly, guide him with as little effort as needed. This can range from leading him by the hand part way, to carrying him all the way to the chair. If you have to carry him, hold him facing away from you. Do not talk during time-out.

Step 2. Practice initially with 2-second time-outs until you are certain the child understands she must be quiet before getting up. Gradually increase the length of time the child must sit. After you are using time-outs that are at least a minute long, begin to use the timer to signal the end of time-out.

Step 3. The rule of thumb is a *maximum* of 1 minute of quiet time-out for each year of age. A 2-year-old would have 2 minutes; a 3-year-old, 3 minutes; and a 5-year-old, 5 minutes. For children 5 years old and older, 5 minutes remains the maximum amount of time.

If your child makes noises, screams, or cries, reset the timer. Do this each time the child makes any annoying noises. If your child gets off the chair before the time is up, replace him on the chair and reset the timer. Do this each time the child gets off the chair.

Two to 3 seconds of time-out is used to teach your child self-quieting skills. After your child can self-quiet for 2 to 3 seconds, increase the time to 3 to 5 seconds. In this fashion, it may take you 4 to 6 months before she is staying in time-out for a minute or 1.5 minutes. It may take a full year until she is staying in time-out for the full minute per year of life. *Do not confuse the maximum amount of time that a child is to be quiet in time-out with the fact that you should start out with time-outs that end with 2 to 3 seconds of quiet.*

Step 4. After your child has been quiet and seated for the required amount of time, the timer will ring. Walk over to him, place your hand on his back, and simply say "OK." Apply gentle pressure with your hand on his back for a second to let him know it's all right to get up. Do not comment on the time-out.

Step 5. After a time-out period, your child should start with a "clean slate." Do not discuss, remind, or nag about what the child did wrong. Within 5 minutes after time-out, look for and praise good behavior. It's wise to take your child to a different part of the house and start her in a new activity.

Edward R. Christophersen, *Beyond Discipline: Parenting That Lasts a Lifetime*. Kansas City, MO: Westport Publishers. ©Edward R. Christophersen, 1990.

Ways to Increase the Effectiveness of Time-Out

Parents may, unwittingly, decrease the effectiveness of time-out. The following suggestions will help you maximize the effectiveness of time-out.

Step 1. Be sure you are not warning your child one or more times before sending him to the time-out chair. Warnings only teach your child he can misbehave at least once (or more) before you'll use time-out. Warnings make children's behavior worse, not better.

Step 2. All adults who are responsible for disciplining your child at home should be using the time-out chair. You should agree when and for what behaviors to send your child to time-out. You will want new sitters, visiting friends, and relatives to read and discuss the time-out guidelines.

Step 3. To maximize the effectiveness of time-out, you must make the rest of the day ("time-in") pleasant for your child. Remember to let your child know when she is well-behaved, rather than taking good behavior for granted. Most children prefer to have you put them in time-out than ignore them completely.

Step 4. Your child may say, "Going to the chair doesn't bother me," or "I like time-out." Don't fall for this trick. Many children try to convince their parents that time-out is fun and therefore is not working. You should notice over time that the problem behaviors for which you use time-out occur less often.

Step 5. When you first begin using time-out, your child may act like time-out is a game. She may put herself in time-out or ask to go there. If this happens, give your child what she wants—that is, put her in time-out and require her to sit quietly for the required amount of time. She will soon learn time-out is not a game. Your child may also laugh or giggle when being placed in time-out or while in time-out. Although this may aggravate you, it is important for you to ignore her completely when she is in time-out.

Step 6. You may feel the need to punish your child for doing something inappropriate in the chair (for example, cursing or spitting). However, it is very important to ignore your child when he behaves badly in time-out. This will teach him that attention-getting strategies will not work. If your child curses when out of the chair and it bothers you, be sure to put him in time-out.

Step 7. TV, radio, or a nice view out of the window can make time-out more tolerable, but it may prolong the length of time your child must stay in the chair by encouraging her to talk or misbehave in other ways. Try to minimize such distractions.

Step 8. You must use time-out for major as well as minor behavior problems. Parents have a tendency to feel that time-out is not enough of a punishment for big things, like loud backtalk or hitting. Consistency is most important for time-out to work for both big and small problems.

Step 9. Be certain your child is aware of the rules that, if broken, result in time-out. Frequently, parents will establish a new rule like, "Don't touch the stereo," without telling their children. When children unwittingly break a new rule they weren't told about, they don't understand why they are being put in time-out.

Step 10. Review the time-out guidelines to make certain you are following the recommendations.

When your child is in time-out:

• Don't look at him or her.
• Don't talk to him or her.
• Don't talk about him or her.
• Don't act angry.
• Do remain calm.
• Do follow the written guidelines.
• Do find something to do (read a magazine, phone someone).

When your child is crying and talking in time-out:

• He should be able to see you.
• She should be able to tell you're not mad.
• He should be able to see what he is missing.

Edward R. Christophersen, *Beyond Discipline: Parenting That Lasts a Lifetime*. Kansas City, MO: Westport Publishers. ©Edward R. Christophersen, 1990.

HANDOUT 2.12

Redirecting Your Child's Activities

After your child has learned how to self-quiet, he needs to learn how to redirect. Waiting until after the child knows how to self-quiet is critical because, if he cannot self-quiet, he will never be able to redirect. Thus, if you work on teaching children redirecting skills before they have self-quieting skills, chances are you are only doing it to protect yourself from the unpleasant feelings that you get when they can't self-quiet or redirect.

Step 1. When you see your child playing with one toy or engaging in one activity for a period of time, and you sense that she may be just about finished with that activity or that she may be getting frustrated with it, then it's a perfect time to work on teaching her how to redirect her energies.

Step 2. Begin by gradually joining the activity, either by playing with the child or by talking to him while he is playing.

Step 3. Try substituting another toy or activity that you know, from prior experience, the child might easily become interested in. In this way, she will begin to learn how to redirect from one activity to another.

It is critical that you put off teaching your child how to redirect until he has well-established self-quieting skills.

Edward R. Christophersen, *Beyond Discipline: Parenting That Lasts a Lifetime*. Kansas City, MO: Westport Publishers. ©Edward R. Christophersen, 1990.

HANDOUT 2.13

Peer Interaction Skills

There are many children who don't have anyone to play with because they tend to drive other children away. They need a lot of supervised practice in playing nicely with other children. This can be done using the following steps.

Step 1. You must have time-in and time-out well established before you begin trying to teach interaction skills. To begin without a good time-in/time-out base is almost foolhardy.

Step 2. Call another child's parents and invite their child over to your house to play with your child, giving the parent the assurance that you will be monitoring the play activity.

Step 3. The children will be playing inside. Decide ahead of time how long the play will last, and convey this to the other child's parents. Don't schedule or plan any other competing activities for yourself—most of your time will be taken up with the children's playing.

Step 4. Monitor the play very closely. Use as much brief, gentle contact (time-in) as you can with your son or daughter whenever he or she is playing nicely.

Step 5. Be prepared to use time-out as quickly as possible for any objectionable behavior, such as obnoxious talk, refusing to share, or withdrawing from the activity.

Step 6. During your child's time-outs, be prepared to continue the play with the other child so that he isn't sitting doing nothing while your child is in time-out.

Step 7. Don't give your child any benefit of the doubt—if in doubt, put him in time-out.

Step 8. If your child is thoroughly used to time-in and time-out, the first play session should go much better than past play sessions. Begin by having several play sessions each week.

Step 9. The more experience your child gets playing nicely with other children, the easier this will get for you to handle. After your child is consistently doing well with one child at a time, then you can begin inviting more than one child over. However, don't press your luck. Invite one child at a time until your child is really good at playing cooperatively.

Step 10. Expect to have to continue monitoring your child very closely during play for a long time to come.

Edward R. Christophersen, *Little People: Guidelines for Commonsense Child Rearing*. Kansas City, MO: Westport Publishers. ©Edward R. Christophersen, 1988.

Chapter 3

Behavioral Problems

Although the term "behavioral pediatrics" has been around since about 1930, not much attention was paid to it until the mid-1970s. Since that time, numerous books and articles have chronicled advances made in the assessment and improvement of compliance with both behavioral and biomedical regimens. After almost 20 years of delivering clinical services to children of all ages from infancy to adolescence, it has become obvious to me that most compliance problems encountered with medical regimens have as their root either the complexity of the medical regimen or general problems with compliance.

The research literature on compliance has identified several characteristics of medical regimens that are predictive of problems with compliance: multicomponent regimens, regimens requiring lifestyle changes, long-term regimens, and regimens for very young patients and the elderly. Yet, there are many occasions when children seem to defy the epidemiological data and comply with their treatment regimens.

One parsimonious explanation for these findings is that patients who have compliance problems with medical regimens probably exhibited problems with compliance prior to being placed on a medical regimen. And, conversely, those patients who have no problems complying with a medical regimen probably did not have compliance problems before being placed on the regimen.

There are several strategies for obtaining and maintaining behavioral compliance in children. These strategies can be used in the absence of a medical regimen and to improve compliance with a medical regimen. Generally, it is easier for a practitioner to begin compliance-improvement training prior to diagnosis and management of a medical disorder than it is to begin once the child is ill. The strategies for general behavioral compliance are just as appropriate for parents who simply prefer better levels of compliance from their children as they are with children placed on medical regimens.

3.1. NONCOMPLIANCE AS THE ROOT OF MOST BEHAVIOR PROBLEMS

The issue of child compliance is the root cause of most of the behavioral problems parents bring to the attention of their pediatrician. Whether the problems involve bedtime, dressing, or eating habits, the parents will have a difficult, frustrating, or seemingly impossible task on their hands unless they have the skills to routinely get the child to comply with reasonable verbal requests.

Primary care providers interested in incorporating behavioral pediatrics into their practice should begin by developing skills for teaching parents how to obtain general compliance. Once the provider is able to routinely teach parents how to obtain compliance when there are no complicating extraneous factors, the remaining interventions appropriate for the primary care setting are relatively straightforward.

3.1.1. The Role of the Primary Care Provider

Providing general compliance training typically involves the primary care provider explaining and demonstrating the procedures, having parents practice the

procedures in the office so that corrective feedback can be given, giving parents written handouts that summarize the practitioner's recommendations, and doing appropriate follow-up.

The written handouts included in Chapter 2 on cognitive development were written specifically for distribution by the primary care physician, nurse practitioner, or physician's assistant, after the practitioner has had enough discussion with the parents to ascertain that they understand the principles involved and after the provider has obtained enough history to rule out family problems that might interfere with the parents' ability to implement the treatment recommendations. Simply handing out the protocols, without taking an adequate history and without discussing any recommendations with the parents, is unlikely to remedy many problems.

Rather than rely on the parents' verbal report, the practitioner should observe the parent-child interaction during the examination or in the interview room to ascertain whether the parents can effectively manage such common pediatric behaviors as opening exam room drawers, climbing on furniture, and playing with the otoscope on the wall.

If the parents cannot deal effectively with these behaviors, then, in this author's experience, there is little chance they can effectively intervene with more difficult problems. Depending on the time remaining in the appointment and the parents' ability to learn the procedures, we teach the procedures at that time or schedule a return appointment for training. After the parents have effectively implemented the compliance program, we schedule a return appointment to deal with specific problems, such as those described in the remainder of this chapter.

3.1.2. Treating Children with Physiological Problems

A recent study by Anders, Halpern, and Hua (1992) suggests that many problems with sleep onset can be related to the mother-child interaction style. Children who present with behavior problems that have a strong physiological component, such as eating, sleeping, and toileting, should therefore be given general compliance training before an attempt is made to remediate the presenting problem.

By delaying training for the specific problem area, parents can be trained to work with the child's general behavior without much concern for exacerbating the difficulties encountered with the presenting problem. If the parents were to work unsuccessfully on a sleeping or toileting problem first, they may unintentionally exacerbate the sleep problem. If, however, they begin by working on the child's general compliance, encountering minor difficulties as they do, they probably will not make the sleep problems worse.

3.2. PRIORITIZING CLINICAL INTERVENTIONS

The pediatrician must be aware of three critical areas before attempting to intervene with common behavior problems.

First, many specific problems, like problems with sleeping, toileting, and eating,

should not be directly addressed until the parents have effectively obtained general compliance from their children. These three problem areas are discussed in Chapter 7 on problems with sleep onset and eating and Chapter 8 on toileting problems.

Second, problems that have a strong time component, such as dressing in the morning prior to leaving for preschool or mother's day out, should not be addressed without prior compliance training.

Third, the practitioner must be able to implement the treatment procedures herself prior to any attempts to teach them to parents. Just as no physician would ever attempt to teach a parent to give an insulin injection without first having the skills himself, compliance training should not be attempted prior to the provider personally learning the skills.

3.3. OPPOSITIONAL BEHAVIOR

Beyond crying in infants and young children, the most commonly encountered problem is oppositional or noncompliant behavior.

Oppositional Defiant Disorder (ODD), the common occurrence of a child refusing to do what he is asked to do or to stop doing, is estimated to range from 3% to 8.7% (Christophersen and Finney, 1993). Sometimes ODD takes the form of the child actually verbally stating that he refuses to do something, sometimes it takes the form of a temper tantrum, and sometimes the child behaves as though she never heard the instruction or request in the first place. Each of these behaviors comes under the general heading of noncompliance or oppositional behavior.

Children who are classified as oppositional often have such problems as temper outbursts, argumentiveness, noncompliance, and negativism. Children with oppositional problems vary in terms of the severity of their presenting symptoms.

3.3.1. Diagnostic Criteria for Oppositional Disorder

The criteria used by the *Diagnostic and Statistical Manual* of the American Psychiatric Association (Version III-R, 1987) define Oppositional Defiant Disorder as:

> A disturbance of at least six months during which the child often demonstrates at least five of the following behaviors:
> (1) Loses temper.
> (2) Argues with adults.
> (3) Actively defies or refuses adult requests or rules, e.g., refuses to do chores at home.
> (4) Deliberately does things that annoy other people, e.g., grabbing other children's hats.
> (5) Blames others for his own mistakes.
> (6) Touchy or easily annoyed by others.
> (7) Angry and resentful.
> (8) Spiteful and vindictive.
> (9) Swears or uses obscene language.
>   A criterion should be considered as being met only if the behavior occurs considerably more frequently than in most children of the same mental age.

3.3.2. Intervention with Oppositional Behavior

Early intervention is critical with children who present with oppositional behavior. Many of our interventions with children 18 to 24 months of age have been successful within 2 to 3 weeks of the first office visit, whereas working with a 10- to 12-year-old child takes substantially more time. Based on our experience, the following points must be covered with parents prior to giving them the recommended written handouts.

3.3.2a. Children Who Lack Self-Quieting Skills

Attempts to deal with oppositional behavior when a child doesn't have adequate self-quieting skills can be very frustrating for both the practitioner and the caregiver. Fortunately, the procedure for using time-out to encourage self-quieting skills can also be used to deal with oppositional behavior. Thus, although the initial intervention may be difficult for the caregiver, who is teaching the child self-quieting skills while trying to encourage more appropriate behavior, the payoff for the caregiver is significantly greater.

3.3.2b. Children Who Lack Independent Play Skills

Children who lack independent play skills typically are disciplined more, with less effect, than children with good independent play skills. Implementation of time-in for the child, which involves much greater interaction between the parents and the child, also can work to make the use of time-outs more effective. Thus, the child is taught independent play skills as he is discouraged from engaging in inappropriate behaviors.

3.3.2c. Limiting Attempts at Reasoning

Encourage parents to limit their use of warnings, threats, and attempts at reasoning. We emphasize to the parents the expression, "*If you don't have anything nice to say, don't say anything at all.*" Many parents have told me they frequently use this expression with their children, which is ironic, since, in doing so, they are breaking the basic tenet of the expression.

3.3.2d. The Need for Enriched Time-In

Encourage parents to start enriched time-in (frequent brief physical contact without talking). Time-in should be provided whenever the child is *not* engaging in a behavior the parents consider unacceptable or offensive—they don't have to wait for "good behavior." Encourage the parents to provide time-in whenever their child is not doing something wrong.

Time-in is not to be confused with praise, which is used only when a child has done something "good." We discourage the use of praise for two major reasons. First, parents who have not been good at praising their children, once taught to praise, usually do not continue to do so. Second, praise very often results in the parent disrupting exactly the behavior he was trying to praise.

The best time to use verbal praise is during natural breaks in an activity. For example, if a child is coloring, the parent should provide lots of brief, nonverbal, physical contact. When the child has finished coloring, or stops coloring to show it to one of her parents, verbal praise is appropriate.

Simple physical contact, without any praise, is much less likely to distract your child, as discussed in detail in Handout 2.6.

3.3.2e. Giving Directions Properly

Emphasize to parents the need to be careful about how and when they give directions to their children. The manner in which a direction is given can, in part, determine whether a child complies (see Handout 3.1). Most children respond better if they are given one instruction at a time in a calm, matter-of-fact manner. Although many parents will tell you that their child responds better if they raise their voice or "give him that look," children learn to follow directions by repeatedly being given directions to follow. We routinely use Handout 3.1 with parents.

3.4. SPANKING

Whether or not parents ask, the vast majority want to know what role spanking should play in child rearing. Although the average parent believes spanking plays at least a minor role in child rearing, the American Academy of Pediatrics (1991) has repeatedly taken a position against spanking, both in task force reports and in published articles and commentaries.

I do not believe it is adequate simply to tell parents they should never spank their children. To do so may result in a brief period of time when parents don't spank their children, only to be followed by a return to spanking with a renewed conviction that it is important and that spanking works. Each time the health-care provider convinces a parent to stop spanking, and the parent tries to stop spanking only to return to spanking again, the health-care provider is faced with a more difficult task of stopping it the next time.

What, then, is the practitioner to do if he or she really believes, as the Academy does, that spanking does not work and should not be a part of child rearing?

3.4.1. Introducing the Topic of Discipline

In my 1980 invited commentary on corporal punishment in *Pediatrics*, I recom-mended that providers introduce the topic of discipline early, discourage parents from spanking their children, *and provide them with a viable alternative to spanking*. I still believe this is the key to educating parents so that they don't start using spanking in the first place.

The topic of discipline should be discussed and parents should be given written handouts on discipline at the 6-month well-child visit—before parents have begun to make their decisions about what form of discipline they are going to use. I don't think most parents use spanking because they are intellectually committed to it. I think they use it because they have no alternative that they understand and think might work; they use it because they have tried spanking and, as best they could tell, it worked. If parents had an effective alternative to spanking, most parents, I believe, would have tried it and, finding it effective, would have continued to use it.

The key point then, is to introduce the topic of discipline prior to the time it is necessary and to give parents an effective alternative to spanking. One alternative is the use of time-out and the concomitant development of a rich time-in.

In my 1986 chapter in *Pediatric Clinics of North America*, I discussed how to introduce the topic of discipline prior to the time parents felt they needed it. If the practitioner not only tells parents about the use of time-in and time-out but also demonstrates, during an office visit, that the combination does work, parents are much more likely either to refrain from spanking altogether or at least to use it very infrequently.

3.4.2. The Truth about Spanking

Literally thousands of parents will tell you spanking does work. For the most part, they are correct. Because parents have no alternative to spanking, and never know in advance when their child is going to engage in a behavior the parents think must be stopped, they resort to spanking almost by default. Parents will start spanking their children and will find it is effective. Later, when the practitioner tries to discourage the use of spanking, the parent is not motivated to take the effort to switch from spanking to the use of time-in and time-out.

The research literature on punishment (most of which has been done with animal models) demonstrates that behavior can be discouraged by the use of physical punishment (Azrin and Holz, 1966). Research on punishment has shown that it is most effective if it is immediate, if it is strong, and if it is administered every time the behavior occurs.

3.4.3. Side Effects of Physical Punishment

The side effects of using physical punishment include the child trying to avoid the person administering the punishment, or escaping the situation in which the punishment is administered. The child also may become more aggressive when subjected to physical punishment. Virtually every summary account of punishment research has appended the warning statement that the use of punishment is contraindicated when dealing with applied problems of human behavior (Risley, 1968). Recent research suggests long-term detrimental effects do result from physical punishment; children who are subjected to spanking as a routine form of discipline are more physically aggressive when they are older.

3.4.4. Religious Support for Spanking

Through the years, numerous religious leaders have advocated spanking, predicating their argument on the use of spanking as reported in the Bible. Readers interested in an opposing viewpoint should consult the recent book *Spare the Child*, by Greven

(1992). Greven presents a thought-provoking review of the arguments based on the Bible as a basis for physical punishment of children and shows, through biblical citations, that the Bible does not support physical punishment of children.

3.4.5. Alternatives to Spanking

With normal children who exhibit typical behavior problems, the alternatives to physical punishment have been so effective that there is virtually no justification for resorting to such physical punishment as spanking. By using currently available disciplinary techniques, it is possible to raise a child without any form of physical punishment.

Perhaps the primary reason parents resort to physical punishment is that they themselves lack adequate coping skills to deal effectively with their child's inappropriate behaviors and, as mentioned above, they don't have any alternatives they understand well enough to use. In situations where the practitioner suspects parents lack adequate coping skills, she can introduce the strategies discussed in Chapter 14 on coping skills or refer the parents to a practitioner who is experienced in dealing with parents who lack adequate coping skills.

3.5. JOB GROUNDING

There are times when the behavior that a child has engaged in is more serious than the daily behaviors that should result in using time-out. If a child is 6 years of age or over, if time-out is already well established as a disciplinary procedure, and if the child can routinely self-quiet during time-outs, then, with infractions of more important rules, job grounding may be more appropriate than using time-out (see Handout 3.2). An example of such behavior would be a child going to a shopping center, on his bike, without informing his parents about it and without getting permission to do so. Another example would be a 7-year-old who refuses to get ready for bed and appears to be using time-out as a way of getting out of going to bed.

Job grounding, unlike the more traditional time-based grounding, does not punish parents as much as it does the child. Instead of grounding a child for a day, a week, or a month, we recommend that children be grounded until they have completed one job either selected by their parents or drawn at random from a list of jobs that can be done in order to "work off" the grounding. We recommend that parents allow the child to select one job from a list of jobs the parents usually do, such as vacuuming the family room or taking out the garbage, jobs that the child could be expected to do.

3.6. OVERCORRECTION

Occasionally, children need many opportunities to practice a behavior until they "get it right." Again, like job grounding, overcorrection should not be used until after a child has learned self-quieting skills and after he has learned to accept time-outs matter-of-factly.

One of the best known uses of overcorrection is described in the book *Toilet Training in Less Than a Day*, by Drs. Nate Azrin and Richard Foxx (1974). When a child has a toileting accident, they recommend having the child "practice" the behavior that he should have engaged in instead of having the accident. The basis for overcorrection is giving the child many opportunities to practice a behavior that she had not been using in the past. With the toileting example, which is described in detail in Chapter 8 on toileting problems, the child who has a toileting accident, after being toilet trained, is told that he must "practice." The child practices the correct behavior, walking to the bathroom and using the toilet. Azrin and Foxx (1974) recommend having the child practice 10 times after each accident. Usually, a child doesn't have to practice on very many occasions before he decides that he would rather walk to the toilet once prior to an accident than 10 times after an accident.

Examples of incidents where overcorrection would be appropriate include children slamming their bedroom door or stomping up the stairway when they are unhappy with a decision made by one of their parents. In the case of the child slamming her bedroom door, the parent would ask the child to "come back here," and, when the child returned, the parent would say something like, "I think you need to practice shutting your bedroom door a little more quietly. Please shut it for me quietly now." As soon as the child shuts the door quietly, the parent would say, "Yes. That's right. Now, please shut the door again." This procedure would be repeated until the child had practiced shutting the door 10 times. At the conclusion of the practicing, the parent could state, "I hope that you know how to shut your door now. I guess we'll see."

3.6.1. Cautions with Grounding and Overcorrection

With both grounding and overcorrection, the child must first be able to self-quiet. If parents are merely looking for more unpleasant or more aversive forms of punishment, we usually say that they are going in the wrong direction. Children will misbehave. The manner in which the parents handle the misbehavior usually determines how much further misbehavior the child exhibits.

The advantage with both job grounding and overcorrection is that the child gets practice performing skills that he probably needed practice in anyway. The advantage for the parents is that, rather than inflict pain or humiliation on the child, they encourage the child to engage in a much more educational procedure.

Also, the message that we, as professionals, convey to parents when we recommend procedures such as time-out, job grounding, and overcorrection is that there are options that are available to parents that do not require the parents to be upset or angry. We convey that parents are teachers and, when their child continues to exhibit inappropriate behaviors, it just means that the child needs more practice—not that he is a "bad child" or that we are "unhappy with him."

3.7. FOLLOW-UP

Whether a family is scheduled for a return office visit 1 to 2 weeks later or followed by telephone, parents need an opportunity to discuss their progress with their practitioner. Just as parents are scheduled for follow-up appointments to recheck otitis or urinary tract infections, they should receive the same conscientious follow-up when dealing with their child's behavior.

3.8. DEVELOPING WRITTEN PROTOCOLS FOR SPECIFIC BEHAVIOR PROBLEMS

If you observe the parents spanking the child for unacceptable behavior in the office (or observe the child spanking her doll in the office), you can assume that the child is spanked at home. Similarly, when you observe the parents matter-of-factly placing the child in time-out for inappropriate behavior (or observe the child placing her doll in time-out), you can assume that the parents use time-out at home. Once you have observed the parents following through with the procedures you have discussed with them, and once you have seen that the child has clearly been exposed to the procedures, the use of written treatment protocols for specific problems is appropriate. Such intervention protocols must include several important characteristics. They must

1. Be easy to explain.
2. Be standardized so that they can be printed in the form of an instruction sheet for parents.
3. List some of the possible side effects of the procedures, with an indication of their severity and duration (Drabman and Jarvie, 1977).

Several of the written protocols we use in our clinic—for such common problem areas as crying at bedtime, getting out of bed, dressing, mealtime behavior, behavior in public places, noncompliance, and guidelines for child automobile-seat use—can be found in Christophersen (1988) and are included here for your convenience.

3.8.1. Separation Anxiety

Of all the problems parents bring to the attention of their practitioner, probably none is more closely related to self-quieting skills than separation anxiety.

Most separation anxiety presents with both the child and the parent having difficulty separating. Thus, in a typical scene where a parent drops a child off at a day-care center, you can usually see both the child and the parent having a difficult time dealing with the separation. It's a good idea to give anxious parents strategies for reducing their own anxiety, such as the recommendations made in Chapter 14 on coping skills, prior to or while they are encouraging the development of self-quieting skills in their child.

For the parent who has difficulty dropping off her child at day care, for example, we recommend that the parent practice going to the day-care center without the child until she can do so without any anxiety. It has been interesting to me to see how surprised parents are that they get anxious at the day-care center even when their child isn't with them. The rationale behind this strategy is to give the parents an opportunity to reduce their anxiety and time to develop the skills necessary to "pretend it doesn't bother them to drop their child off."

Handout 3.3 details the author's recommendations for handling separation problems in young children.

For the child with poor self-quieting skills, which is quite common with separation anxiety, parents should be prepared to drop the child off at many different places and times for a week or two while both the parent and the child learn the coping skills for separating.

3.8.2. Dressing Problems

Some children never do seem to learn how to get themselves dressed in a timely fashion. Handouts 3.4 and 3.5 address the two problems commonly associated with dressing: behavior problems while dressing and how to teach dressing skills.

3.8.3. Public Places

One problem area usually not addressed in discussions of infants' and toddlers' behavior has to with their behavior in public places. Handout 3.6 makes recommendations for managing children's behavior in public places.

The essence of our recommendations for behavior in public places concerns parents beginning compliance training in the home and extending it to public places in a systematic fashion. Many parents allow children too much leeway at home, then expect them to behave in public.

We recommend that parents practice taking their children out in public until the children have learned to behave more appropriately. The first couple of trips out in public, after establishing firmer limits at home, could be to places like a public park, where some whining and fussing on the child's part would be barely noticeable. When the child can handle the limits set in the park, the parents can take him to smaller open areas. In this fashion, the parents gradually take the child into situations that are more typical of their day-to-day activities.

3.8.4. Glasses Wearing

The child who is accustomed to doing what her parents request of her will usually adapt to wearing glasses very easily. Conversely, the child who is accustomed to doing what he wants to do may have a lot of trouble adapting to having to wear glasses. Because these parents must deal with both general compliance and glasses wearing at the same time, we usually recommend the parents begin by working on general compliance, using a combination of time-in and time-out. Once the behavioral procedures are effective with more general kinds of behavior, the procedures may be extended to include glasses. Handout 3.7 on glasses wearing includes references to the handouts on cognitive development (Handout 2.1), time-in (Handout 2.6), and time-out (Handout 2.10).

This is just one instance where we recommend that parents be given multiple handouts. In the case of glasses wearing and similar problem areas, the most appropriate thing to do might be to work with the parents, at the first appointment, on behavioral compliance training; then, at the second appointment, when you can see that the parents have implemented your recommendations from the first appointment, introduce the specific procedures for improving compliance with wearing glasses.

3.9. MULTICOMPONENT TREATMENT REGIMENS

Some problems involve compliance at several different levels. As such, multicomponent treatment regimens are more likely to be complicated by compliance problems. Many of the additional problems stem from the simple fact that multicomponent treatment regimens require lifestyle changes that are unnecessary with less complicated regimens. Multicomponent treatment regimens are discussed in Chapter 6 on compliance in health education.

3.9.1. Staged Introduction of Regimens

Anytime a multicomponent treatment program is necessary, the practitioner must bear in mind that it is more difficult for the parents to follow the treatment recommendations than it would be with a simpler regimen. For this reason, as has often been suggested in the research literature, treatment should be introduced in stages or phases.

The parents of a child with diabetes, for example, can be started out with procedures for testing blood-sugar levels and insulin injections. When the parents return to the office, usually within 1 or 2 weeks, the provider can discuss the progress made with the first two procedures. If satisfied that the blood-sugar testing and insulin injections are progressing satisfactorily, the practitioner can introduce such additional treatment components as diet or exercise.

In this way, the parents and the child aren't faced with an almost incomprehensible amount of responsibility all at once. If parents encounter compliance problems with the first step or two of the multicomponent regimen, the provider can help the parents to deal with these prior to introducing the rest of the treatment regimen.

Finally, giving parents written materials to read about the medical disorder gives them time to read and digest the material and puts them in a much more informed position to ask questions on their return visit.

3.10. CONCLUDING REMARKS

Much is now known about compliance training and oppositional behavior in children. It is now possible to introduce standardized treatment regimens with predictable therapeutic outcomes for common compliance problems. The initial assessment of compliance problems is discussed in Chapter 4 on assessment. After the initial assessment is completed, compliance training should be introduced for common behavior problems. After a therapeutic effect is evidenced with common behavior problems, the procedures can be expanded to cover some of the more difficult problem areas. Chapter 7 extends compliance training to cover simpler problems such as sleeping and mealtimes. Chapter 8 extends the compliance recommendations to toileting problems, and Chapter 9 on Attention Deficit Hyperactivity Disorder extends these recommendations to the hyperactive child.

REFERENCES

American Psychiatric Association: *Diagnostic and Statistical Manual of Mental Disorders*, 3rd ed. Washington, DC: American Psychiatric Association, revised, 1987.

Anders TF, Halpern LF, Hua J: Sleeping through the night: A developmental perspective. *Pediatrics* 90(4):554–560, 1992.

Azrin NH, Foxx RM: *Toilet Training in Less Than a Day*. New York: Simon and Schuster, 1974.

Azrin NH, Holz WC: Punishment, in Honig WK (ed.), *Operant Behavior: Areas of Research and Application*. New York: Appleton-Century-Crofts, 1966.

Christophersen ER: Anticipatory guidance on discipline. *Pediatr Clin N Am* 33(4):789–798, 1986.

Christophersen ER: The pediatrician and parental discipline. *Pediatrics* 66(4):641–642, 1980.

Christophersen ER: *Little People: Guidelines for Commonsense Child Rearing*. Kansas City, MO: Westport Publishers, 1988.

Christophersen ER, Finney JW: Oppositional defiant disorder, in Ammerman RT, Last CG, Hersen M (eds.), *Handbook of Prescriptive Treatments for Children and Adolescents*. New York: Pergamon Press, 1993, pp. 102–114.

Committee on School Health, American Academy of Pediatrics: Corporal punishment in schools. *Pediatrics* 88:173, 1991.

Drabman RS, Jarvie BA: Counseling parents of children with behavior problems: The use of extinction and time-out techniques. *Pediatrics* 59:78–85, 1977.

Greven P: *Spare the Child: The Religious Roots of Punishment and the Psychological Impact of Physical Abuse*. New York: Random House, 1992.

Risley TR: The effects and side effects of punishing the autistic behavior of a deviant child. *J Appl Behav Anal* 1:21–34, 1968.

Sample Handouts

Teaching Your Child to Follow Instructions

Parents frequently have problems getting their children to follow instructions. Your child's compliance can improve if you follow the suggestions given below.

GIVING INSTRUCTIONS OR COMMANDS

Step 1. Get your child's attention when giving a direction: Say the child's name and request that he look at you (for example, "Bob, look at me").

Step 2. Thank the child when she has complied by looking at you.

Step 3. Give the child a simple, clear command, like, "Please shut the door."

THINGS TO REMEMBER

1. Be realistic. Give your child instructions that you know he is *physically* and *developmentally* capable of following.

2. Be direct. Say things like, "Joey, please put your shoes in the closet" and "Open the door." Avoid questions that imply choice when there really is no choice, like, "Won't you go to your room?" or "Don't you want to go downstairs?"

3. Give one instruction at a time, and allow your child 5 seconds to begin to obey. Do not repeat the same instruction a second time.

4. Avoid giving a second command while the child is working on the first command.

5. *Avoid giving your child a command unless you are prepared to use time-out for not minding.*

WHEN YOUR CHILD OBEYS

Step 1. When your child begins to comply, praise and encourage her so that she will continue the desired behavior.

Step 2. Thank the child immediately for following the direction by saying something like, "Thank you for putting your bear in the toy box, Joey."

Step 3. Kids love hugs and pats, so be sure to touch your child as well as praise his behavior.

WHAT TO DO IF YOUR CHILD DOES NOT BEGIN TO OBEY WITHIN 5 SECONDS

Step 1. Put her in time-out immediately (see Handout 2.10).

Step 2. Be careful not to unintentionally give your child attention for not obeying or for behaving unacceptably.

Step 3. After time-out, require your child to complete the requested task. This will give her a chance to receive attention when she obeys and will teach her that you are serious when you give a command.

©Edward R. Christophersen, 1992.

HANDOUT 3.2

Grounding as a Method of Discipline

Grounding is a method of discipline that may be used to teach your child the consequences of breaking rules (inappropriate behavior). Grounding also provides your child with an opportunity to learn how to do various jobs around your home and receive your instructive feedback.

The following instructions describe how to use grounding.

Step 1. Sit down with your child at a pleasant time and develop a list of at least 10 jobs that need to be done regularly around the house. The individual jobs should be about equal in difficulty and the amount of completion time required. Be sure your child is physically capable of doing each job. Examples of jobs are washing the kitchen floor, cleaning the bathroom, sweeping out the garage, raking the front yard, and vacuuming the living and dining rooms.

Step 2. Each job should be written on a separate index card with a detailed description of what is required to complete the job correctly. For example:

Wash kitchen floor

The floor should be swept clean first. Remove all movable pieces of furniture. Fill a bucket with warm, soapy water, and wash the floor with a clean rag, squeezed dry. Dry the floor with a clean, dry rag. Replace the furniture that was moved.

Step 3. Explain to your child that when she has broken a rule, for example, not returning home from school on time or fighting with her brother, she must randomly select a job card from the deck of written job cards. Until the assigned job described on the card is completed correctly, your child will be grounded from all privileges.

Step 4. Being grounded means (child's rules):
- Attending school.
- Performing required chores.
- Following house rules.
- Staying in your own room unless eating meals, working on chores, or attending school.
- No television.
- No telephone calls.
- No record player, radio, and so on.
- No video games or other games or toys.
- No bike riding.
- No friends over or going to friends' houses.
- No snacks.
- No outside social activities like movies or going out to dinner.

You will need to have a baby-sitter available on short notice in case your child is grounded and unable to accompany you on a planned family outing.

Step 5. Grounding does *not* mean (parents' rules):
- Nagging.
- Reminding about jobs to be done.
- Discussing the grounding.
- Explaining the rules.

Step 6. When the jobs are completed, you should check to be sure they have been done correctly. Praise your child for completing the chores correctly and, thus, ending the grounding. If a job is not completed correctly, review the job description and provide feedback on parts done correctly and incorrectly. Without nagging, instruct your child to redo the incorrect tasks in order to end the grounding.

Step 7. Your child determines how long he is to be grounded. The grounding lasts only as long as it takes to complete the assigned jobs. It could last from 5 minutes to several hours. The child determines the duration of the grounding by the speed with which he tackles the chores. If used correctly, without any nagging from you, it's rare for job grounding to last beyond the end of the day.

Step 8. If the grounding seems to be lasting an excessively long period of time, more than an hour or two, check to be sure your child's life is dull during the grounding. Be sure you are not providing a lot of attention in the form of nagging.

Step 9. Grounding is effective when your child follows the rules more often and is aware of the consequences of breaking the rules.

Edward R. Christophersen, *Little People: Guidelines for Commonsense Child Rearing*. Kansas City, MO: Westport Publishers. ©Edward R. Christophersen, 1988.

HANDOUT 3.3

Separation Anxiety

The first couple of times you leave your child with a sitter or drop him off at a day-care center will probably be a very emotional experience for you. If you can treat these separations matter-of-factly, your child will learn to separate rather easily, making the whole process much less draining on both of you.

ADDITIONAL SUGGESTIONS

1. Do not discuss the separation before it occurs. Doing so will not help, but it may make separating more difficult.

2. Plan ahead so that you can separate quickly. Have all of your child's things together in one bag or her toys out in one place so that you won't prolong the act of separating.

3. When it comes time to do so, separate as quickly and as matter-of-factly as possible.

4. If separating is hard for you, set up artificial opportunities to practice separating. For example, arrange to drop your child off at a friend's or relative's house several additional times each week until you become more proficient at it.

5. When you pick your child up, don't be overly emotional. It's OK to act glad to see him, but don't start crying and hugging him excessively—doing so only shows him how hard the separation was for you.

6. Generally, the way children handle separation is a direct reflection of how their parents handle it. Do well and your child will do much better.

Edward R. Christophersen, *Beyond Discipline: Parenting That Lasts a Lifetime*. Kansas City, MO: Westport Publishers. ©Edward R. Christophersen, 1990.

HANDOUT 3.4

Dressing Problems: Poking and Stalling

1. Make sure your child is capable of completing the task you are asking him to do. Once he has shown you he has the skills necessary to dress himself, it is reasonable to expect him to do so within a specific amount of time (20 minutes) every morning. Preschool-age children may occasionally need some assistance.

2. Establish a morning routine; for example, get up, go to the bathroom, get dressed, make the bed, and eat breakfast. The routine will help your child know what you expect on a daily basis.

3. Allow your child enough time (20 to 30 minutes before breakfast—you can set a timer to keep track of the time) to complete her dressing.

4. Initially, praise him very frequently for dressing. "Catch em being good" (dressing appropriately) as often as possible.

5. Ignore stalling—don't nag.

6. Use the time-out chair for each tantrum.

7. Do not allow the TV to be turned on until after the child is completely dressed.

8. Remember to praise *any* appropriate dressing behavior *often*. Check on your child every 2 to 5 minutes.

9. Have breakfast ready after the 20-minute dressing time.

10. If your child is completely dressed when the timer rings, *praise her* and have her eat breakfast. Reward her with 10 to 15 minutes of your time doing whatever she would like to do (play a game, read a story, and so on) after she gets home from school, or immediately if your child is a preschooler.

11. If your child did not complete dressing:
    a. Have him stay in his room to complete dressing. If he is not done 5 to 10 minutes before it is time to leave for school, dress him, but don't talk to him except to give instructions.
    b. Regardless of whether your child finishes dressing 2 minutes or 30 minutes after the timer has gone off, she has *not* finished in time to eat breakfast. (Although it's terribly hard to send your child to school without breakfast, she won't starve. You will only have to do this once or twice before your child is getting dressed within the allowed amount of time.)
    c. You may want to call the school to briefly explain the situation so that the school won't be calling you to ask why you didn't provide breakfast for your child.

12. Don't give in, and remember to praise all appropriate dressing behaviors.

Edward R. Christophersen, *Little People: Guidelines for Commonsense Child Rearing*. Kansas City, MO: Westport Publishers. ©Edward R. Christophersen.

Teaching Dressing Skills

Before your child is capable of dressing himself, you can begin teaching him the skills he will need. Dressing your child or helping him get dressed can and should be a very pleasant interaction.

Step 1. Praise your child when she tries to put something on—even if it's wrong—and begin teaching her how it should be.

Step 2. Explain briefly what you're doing by saying something like, "Here's the tag. It belongs in the back." Later you'll be able to ask him which is the back, and he'll show you. Make it fun, but remember to praise any attempts to do things by himself and later for successfully accomplishing the task, regardless of how much you helped. Your help should be gradually decreased as your child acquires dressing skills.

Step 3. Set a kitchen timer so that your child can learn that the dressing job must be completed within a certain time period, for example in 20 minutes; then gradually have your child use a clock rather than a timer.

Step 4. Establish a set routine and follow it as consistently as possible. This will make it easier if your child knows what you expect. For example:

Get up at 7:30 A.M.
Go to the bathroom.
Get dressed.
Eat breakfast.
Brush your teeth.
Play or go to school.

Step 5. All children get distracted from dressing by siblings, toys, animals, and such. Establish reasonable rules concerning dressing, discuss them with your health-care provider, and then stick to them. Be consistent—time-out can be used for inappropriate behaviors. For example:

Dressing must be done in the bedroom.
The TV cannot be turned on.
Dressing must be completed before breakfast.

Step 6. Remember to praise staying with the job (getting dressed) frequently at first, gradually reducing the frequency of your praising as your child gets better at dressing. For example, at first you should praise each movement involved in putting on a pair of pants. As your child learns each movement, just praise her for correctly putting on her pants.

Step 7. Don't expect your child to learn shoe-tying as readily as he learns the other dressing skills. Children frequently have more difficulty with shoe-tying, so just have your child put the shoes on, with you tying them until your child offers to help and has acquired the necessary manual dexterity.

Edward R. Christophersen, *Little People: Guidelines for Commonsense Child Rearing*. Kansas City, MO: Westport Publishers. ©Edward R. Christophersen, 1988.

HANDOUT 3.6

Behavior Problems in Public Places

Taking children to restaurants and to grocery, discount, and department stores can be both fun and educational for them. To make trips to these public places more enjoyable, begin by taking numerous training trips. These are best described as short trips made for the sole purpose of teaching appropriate store behaviors.

TRAINING TRIPS

1. Trips should not exceed 15 minutes and can be as short as only 5 minutes.

2. Choose a time when the store or restaurant is not very busy.

3. Trips should be for teaching, not for shopping or eating.

4. Rules should be stated prior to leaving the house or apartment, as matter-of-factly as possible, and restated immediately prior to entering the "training area." Suggested rules include:

   a. Stay with Mom or Dad. Do not walk alone.
   b. Do not pick up or touch things without permission from Mom or Dad.
   c. Nothing will be purchased on the trip.

5. Provide your child with a lot of brief, nonverbal, physical contact (at least once every minute or half-minute) for appropriate behaviors. Occasionally offer verbal praise, such as "Mike, you sure are being good," "You're staying right next to Mommy," "Thank you for not picking up any candy," or "It's easier to shop when you don't pick up things."

6. Maintain frequent physical contact with your child. Touch him gently on the back, rough up his hair, or briefly give him a hug, pulling him next to you.

GENERAL GUIDELINES

1. Involve your child in the activity as much as possible. Have her get groceries for you or place them in the cart. Give her educational instructions, like, "Get the green can, please," or "Bring me the bag of pretzels, please." Don't forget to say "please" and "thank-you" when appropriate.

2. Include your child in pleasant conversation regarding what you're doing, like, "We're going to make sloppy joes with this hamburger meat. You really like sloppy joes, don't you?"

3. This is also a good time to teach your child about his world: "Bananas grow on trees. What else can you think of that grows on trees? All fruits have a skin or cover on them to protect them from rain and from bugs."

4. By frequent physical contact, praise, teaching, and pleasant conversation, your child will remain much more interested in the trip. By actually helping you, he will learn that stores are a fun place to visit.

5. If your child breaks one of your rules, immediately make her sit in time-out. This can be any place that is generally out of the normal flow of foot traffic. In a grocery store, you can point to one of the tile-floor squares and firmly tell your child to sit on that square because she walked away from you. In a restaurant, you can simply turn your child's chair around, or, if the restaurant is not very crowded, place her on another chair about 3 to 4 feet away from you. As soon as your child is quiet for one-half to one minute, tell her it is OK to get up or to turn her chair back to the table.

6. Remember, praise and attention, coupled with firm discipline, are the tools you have to teach your child. Discipline alone will not work. Using the two together will make your trips to stores and restaurants much more enjoyable for both of you. Generally, the better your child does at home, the better he'll do in public. When you are having trouble in public, step up your efforts at home.

Edward R. Christophersen, *Little People: Guidelines for Commonsense Child Rearing*. Kansas City, MO: Westport Publishers. ©Edward R. Christophersen, 1988.

Instructions for Improving Glasses Wearing

Several basic steps are essential to getting young children to wear their glasses. Each of these steps is described in detail below, with written handouts of specific information provided where we think it will help.

1. *Refrain from nagging.* By the time most parents see us, they have already found out that nagging, reasoning, explaining, and the like do not improve glasses wearing. Therefore, we request that you refrain from such reminders. Handout 2.1 (on cognitive development) describes this feature in more detail.

2. *Provide lots of love pats.* Children, like adults, thrive on affection. While we cannot say children will not wear their glasses *because* they are not loved enough, we can say providing lots of love pats (50 to 100 per day per parent) can provide much of the foundation for getting a child to wear his glasses. Handout 2.6 describes this feature (time-in) in more detail.

3. *Discipline must be calm and matter-of-fact.* The only form of discipline we use for glasses wearing is called time-out. You should practice using time-out with many other behaviors *before* you ever try to use it for glasses wearing. *Our rule of thumb is that you should do at least nine love pats for each time-out.* Only after you are successful at using it for other behaviors (*for at least 1 to 2 weeks*) do we recommend that you attempt to use it for glasses wearing. Handout 2.10 describes time-out. If you have been using time-out, please make careful note of any differences between the way you have been doing it and the way we recommend you do it.

4. *Your questions.* We cannot be expected to guess when you are having difficulty implementing our treatment recommendations. The first week or two, when you and your child are just learning how to do time-in and time-out correctly, is the most important. Please contact our answering service if you encounter any difficulties or if you have questions. The doctor on-call knows these procedures and can help you.

5. *Your follow-up appointment.* Please plan on keeping the return appointment you scheduled for a week or two from now. While it may be tempting to go ahead on your own, we would like to help you to resolve the glasses-wearing problem permanently, and we cannot do so without your cooperation. We can hardly be expected to do so in only one office visit. If we agree that a third appointment appears necessary, please plan on keeping it.

6. On completion of the glasses-wearing treatment, we will send a letter to your referring doctor to inform her or him of our efforts on your child's behalf as well as the results. The Written Consent Form is a formality that allows us to communicate with your physician.

©Edward R. Christophersen, 1994.

Chapter 4

Recognition and Assessment of Compliance Problems

The very nature of interactions between parents and their children allows multiple opportunities for parents to request or expect compliance from their children. There also are innumerable opportunities for parents to avoid or sidestep the need for compliance by making few, if any, demands on the children. Minor behavioral problems that have gone unchecked by parents may gain increased importance when they prevent compliance with a critically important medical regimen. For example, while a normal child's noncompliance might be considered a minor inconvenience, the same child's noncompliance becomes exceedingly important if the child is diagnosed with insulin-dependent diabetes.

Two distinctly different levels of compliance must therefore be addressed:

- Behavioral compliance with routine or reasonable parental instructions
- Compliance with medical regimens for the treatment of acute or chronic disease

4.1. SCREENING FOR BEHAVIORAL PROBLEMS

While screening for medical problems is a well-established practice, formal screening for pediatric behavioral problems, particularly by health-care providers, is a relatively new procedure. Pediatric health-care providers, through the provision of well-child care, are in an excellent position to detect both medical and behavioral problems.

Physicians are well acquainted with taking medical case histories. In diagnosing otitis media, for example, a physician may ask the parent if the child has been pulling at his ear, if he has been running a fever, and if his sleeping patterns have been disrupted. After asking a standard set of questions, the physician usually performs a complete physical examination, including the use of an otoscope to visualize the tympanic membrane and, perhaps, tympanotomy, prior to arriving at a clinical diagnosis of otitis media. The physician's training includes substantial experience with otitis, including the medications available for treatment.

The same screening procedure can be used by physicians to detect behavioral problems. During a well-child visit for a 3-year-old, for example, a health-care provider can ask the parent or caregiver:

- What time the child gets ready for bed
- Where and how the child goes to bed
- How long it takes the child to quiet down
- What time the child falls asleep
- Whether the child awakens during the night
- What time the child rises in the morning

The answers to these questions offer the health-care provider a basis on which to decide whether the 3-year-old is experiencing any difficulties in developing appropriate habits for sleep onset. Similar questions can be asked about a variety of other behaviors. As with the otitis media example, it is rare for a physician to ask a parent if his child has otitis—it would be just as inappropriate, in most instances, to ask a parent if her child has behavior problems. The parent is not always aware that a problem or a potential problem exists, so it is often up to the physician to decide at what point to be concerned and to intervene.

The author, on numerous occasions, for example, has interviewed parents who spend 2 hours a night "helping" a child settle at bedtime (e.g., reading story after story, accompanying the child on a number of trips to the kitchen or bathroom, or "falling asleep" with the child). Many of these behaviors develop over a period of time and are so ingrained that parents do not clearly perceive the magnitude of such problems. Both in my own writing (Christophersen, 1990) and in a recent article by Anders, Halpern, and Hua (1992), parents are encouraged to refrain from assisting infants with sleep onset.

Under the auspices of "early detection," that is, deciphering clues that parents are troubled by their child's behavior, we suggest that a standard set of questions be asked. In principle, these questions parallel the routines that form a large part of the work-up for such organic problems as otitis media. Asking specific questions regarding discrete behaviors, rather than merely asking the parents whether a behavior problem exists, overcomes the reluctance some parents may have in admitting that their child has a behavior problem. The possibility also exists, as the work on sleep onset shows, that parents may be engaging in behaviors with their children that, no matter how well intentioned, may result in behaviors that the parents were specifically trying to prevent or avoid.

In practice, the physician must remain flexible about screening. Some children obviously need a comprehensive evaluation; for them, an initial screening would be insufficient. For children who are obviously developing normally, an initial screening also would be unnecessary, except perhaps to document for the medical record the child's attainment of developmental milestones. An initial screening is appropriate when a new family transfers into a practice, to compensate partially for the lack of prior contact, and when the physician is unsure about or unfamiliar with the child.

4.2. FIRST-STAGE SCREENING TESTS

In a review of popular screening tests, Frankenburg (1983) indicated that the typical test takes from 10 to 30 minutes to administer. Even if the average well-child visit included no physical examination, no immunizations, no history taking, and no interview, the physician still would not have time to administer many of the accepted standardized tests that screen developmental or behavioral problems. Frankenburg suggested a plausible solution: a two-stage screening process.

The first stage, done in the physician's office, involves quick, simple testing that preferably would overestimate the number of children in need of further screening (to reduce false negatives, test scores that suggest no problems exist when, in fact, one does exist). These children would be considered for second-stage screening that could be done either in the physician's office or by referral to another health-care professional (one who does not have the serious time constraints of the physician).

4.2.1. Eyberg Child Behavior Inventory

Over the years, the author has used a brief, caretaker-completed test with well over a thousand patients—the Eyberg Child Behavior Inventory (ECBI) (Robinson, Eyberg, and Ross, 1980). The inventory (Handout 4.1) has been standardized on children between the ages of 2 and 12 and, more recently, with adolescents.

The inventory, which consists of 36 questions on one side of a piece of paper, typically can be completed in 5 minutes by the parent while she waits with her child, either in the waiting room or in an exam room. Or, as is the case in many offices, the inventory can be mailed to a family at the time their appointment is made, completed ahead of time, and brought to the appointment by the parent. The ECBI includes questions about the child's behavior during such standard caregiving times as bedtime and mealtime, and is useful as an initial screening test for detecting children with behavior problems (Robinson et al., 1980).

Providers could use the ECBI as the first stage of the two-stage screening process. This type of screening tool also can help identify parents who may benefit from parent education. The primary advantages of the ECBI are that it can be completed fairly quickly by the parents, the questions are phrased in a way that parents find easy to understand, and it is easy to score (the mean intensity and mean problem scores can be calculated simply by adding up the number of items checked by the parent (Handout 4.2). The practitioner can visually scan the completed ECBI to ascertain, in a matter of seconds, whether further evaluation for psychosocial problems is indicated.

In practice, the ECBI can be used to screen children with conditions such as encopresis, where the practitioner believes that, from the interview and prior history with the patient, no medical problems are present that may interfere with management of the encopresis. Handout 4.3 is an actual ECBI from a child successfully treated (no soiling for 3 successive months after 1 month of treatment) for encopresis.

Further information on the ECBI can be obtained from Dr. Sheila Eyberg, Department of Clinical Psychology, University of Florida, Box J-165 Health Sciences Center, Gainesville, FL 32610.

4.3. SECOND-STAGE SCREENING TESTS

Second-stage screening tests are those instruments that take considerably longer to administer but have yielded significantly greater clinical data for the practitioner. Several examples of such instruments will be reviewed here.

4.3.1. Conner's Parent Symptom Questionnaire

One second-stage screening test relatively easy for parents to complete (48 questions) and providers to score is Conner's Parent Symptom Questionnaire (Handout 4.4), also referred to as the PSQ (Goyette, Conners, and Ulrich, 1978). Scoring the PSQ yields individual scores for conduct problems, learning problems, psychosomatic problems, impulsivity-hyperactivity, anxiety, and a hyperactivity index. The PSQ has a teacher form that provides an assessment of how the child is behaving in the school classroom.

To score the PSQ, add up the total numerical equivalent for each of the loaded factors, then compare the resulting scores with the standardized samples. Each item checked in the first column received a score of "0"; each item in the second column received a "1"; each item in the third column received a "2"; and each item in the fourth column received a "3." If the resulting scores exceed one standard deviation above the mean for the child's age and sex, the results are considered to be significant. Handout 4.5 gives the means and standard deviations for the Conner's PSQ for boys and girls at each age level.

The PSQ is relatively easy to administer and score, uses forms for parents and for teachers, and is standardized for children from 2 to 17 years of age.

The PSQ is widely used to assess children for possible Attention Deficit Hyperactivity Disorder. Office staff can be trained to score the PSQ in a brief time, probably less than 10 minutes. Copies of the tests and additional information on the PSQ are available in Russell Barkley's book, *Hyperactive Children: A Handbook for Diagnosis and Treatment*. MultiSystems Health, Inc., 908 Niagara Falls Boulevard, North Tonawanda, NY, 14120, markets both a "quick scoring" form and a computer scoring program for the PSQ. These forms reduce the scoring time to about two minutes.

4.3.2. Behavioral Pediatrics Intake Form

In our office, we send the ECBI or PSQ to all families scheduling a first appointment, along with a Behavioral Pediatrics Intake Form (Handout 4.6). The intake form covers most of the questions we would normally ask during the initial interview with a family referred for either behavior problems or medical compliance problems.

The intake form provides a comprehensive set of questions that becomes a permanent part of the medical-legal record, with answers provided directly by the parents. Because the material is provided by the parents, there is little chance that the provider recorded the answer inaccurately.

When both the intake form and a parent-rated scale are available at the beginning of an initial examination, the health-care provider has the advantage of having to spend less time acquiring this information, leaving more time to spend on other historical issues, or, as is the case in our office, leaving more time for explaining to parents the suggested intervention. While the information requested varies from office to office, the practice of having a complete intake form in each child's medical record is well established.

4.3.3. Achenbach Child Behavior Checklist

For those children who have remarkable scores on the ECBI, a second-stage evaluation, using a measurement device such as the Achenbach Child Behavior Checklist (CBCL) (Handout 4.7), is indicated (Achenbach and Edelbrock, 1983). The CBCL consists of 113 parent-completed items for children and youth from 2 to 16 years of age (there are separate forms for the 2- and 3-year-olds). We routinely ask that a CBCL be completed and brought to the appointment when children are referred for a wide variety of problems, including oppositional behavior, Attention Deficit Hyperactivity Disorder, and adjustment reactions.

The CBCL can be scored by hand, template, or computer, to arrive at scores on a variety of subscales, including attention problems, social problems, thought problems, anxiety, delinquent behavior, aggressive behavior, and somatic complaints, depending on the age and the sex of the child. Handout 4.8 shows a profile of a 14-year-old girl suspected of having Attention Deficit Disorder without Hyperactivity.

Additional CBCL forms are available for completion by teachers and for self-reporting by youths. Also available is a direct-observation form, which is completed while a child is being observed in a classroom for a standard length of time. The CBCL is a much more sophisticated instrument than the ECBI and, although it takes longer to administer and score, yields much more information. Results from this measure can be used to decide whether the child should receive a comprehensive psychological evaluation and/or treatment. Many studies have been conducted using the CBCL. Further information is available in Barkley's (1981) book, or directly from T. M. Achenbach, University Associates in Psychiatry, One South Prospect Street, Burlington, VT 05401.

4.4. SELECTING A SCREENING TEST

The ECBI, PSQ, and CBCL are examples of the myriad of tests currently available to practitioners who need simple instruments to screen children for behavioral problems. Selecting any one of them can be based on personal preference. Any screening tool that helps health-care providers identify the child who presents with significant behavior problems can be a valuable aid in delivering well-child care.

Whatever test is chosen for first- or second-stage screening, it must be cost-effective to administer and must assist the provider in deciding whether a further work-up is indicated. The reader who is interested in obtaining comprehensive information on available tests is referred to the book *Tests*, by Sweetland and Keyser (1986). This valuable resource book lists most of the testing materials that are currently available, including information on standardization, administration, scoring, and the research base for each test.

4.5. ADDRESSING BEHAVIORAL COMPLIANCE ISSUES

In our experience, children who present with significant behavior management problems following any serious medical event or diagnosis (e.g., burns, cancer treatment, diabetes) typically presented with management problems prior to the medical event or diagnosis.

In a study conducted in our office (Friman, Mathews, Finney, Christophersen, and Leibowitz, 1988), we compared 50 children referred to us for behavior problems and 50 children referred to us for encopresis with 50 children, matched for age and sex, from the original standardization sample of normal children for the ECBI. There was no difference between the children from the normal sample and the children with encopresis. There were significant differences between the normal children and the behavior-disordered children, and between the encopretics and the behavior-disordered children.

These results are consistent with the growing body of literature that suggests children with encopresis typically do not present with significant behavior problems (Gabel, Chandra, Shindledecker, 1988).

Regardless of whether a history of noncompliance is suspected from the clinical interview or from use of a screening device like the ECBI or the Conner's PSQ, practitioners would be well advised, when indicated, to consider addressing general compliance issues prior to attempting to implement a complex medical regimen. Obviously there are situations where a medical regimen must be implemented, but the health-care provider, knowing there is a history of noncompliance, can attempt to monitor the child's treatment protocol more carefully. The health-care provider who routinely monitors compliance in the well child has the obvious advantage that compliance improvement strategies can be discussed with the parents without the added pressure of a medical problem.

The author recommends that pediatric health-care providers introduce the issue of compliance at the 6-month well-child visit, which helps make parents aware of problems that can stem, either directly or indirectly, from parents feeling uncomfortable with discipline and not knowing when or how to address issues related to it (Christophersen, 1986).

4.6. ASSESSING COMPLIANCE WITH MEDICAL REGIMENS

The literature has shown that as pediatric health care becomes increasingly more sophisticated, more and more children will experience medical settings, personnel, and treatments. Most children will be hospitalized before they are 21 years old, and they will encounter potentially aversive experiences during their hospital stay (Rapoff and Christophersen, 1982; Wright, Schaefer, and Solomons, 1979).

Children who have chronic illnesses will require ongoing treatment at home, the physician's office, and/or the hospital for extended periods of time (Haggerty, Roghman, and Pless, 1975). Such prolonged treatment increases the likelihood of children's noncompliance. This noncompliance may involve either the child who is required to cooperate with medical procedures and regimens or the parent who is required to implement or oversee those medical regimens.

If behavioral compliance issues have been addressed prior to the need for implementing a medical regimen, the health-care provider and the parent will have a prior history of discussing discipline, and the parents are more likely to have had some experience dealing with their child's compliance.

When a child is initially diagnosed with either an acute illness or a chronic disease, one decision the practitioner must make is whether compliance may be an issue in treating that child. Unfortunately, the literature on medical compliance has already documented that physician estimates or predictions of who will be compliant are usually no better than chance guesses (Rapoff and Christophersen, 1982). For this reason, it is important, with pediatric patients who are seen over an extended period of time for well-child care and episodic acute care visits, to document not only what medical regimens a child has been placed on but also what kind of compliance the parents have had. Perhaps the best predictor of compliance problems, short of some of the sophisticated measurement strategies employed in research on medical compliance, is the child's general behavioral compliance. The child who is visibly out of control in the practitioner's office is not a good candidate for placement on a multicomponent medical regimen. If there is any doubt in the mind of the practitioner, one of the screening instruments discussed above could provide valuable information about existing behavior problems.

4.7. CONCLUDING REMARKS

While entire volumes have been written on behavioral and academic assessment of children, the average clinician has a relatively small number of assessment tools that he or she uses on a regular basis. To be useful, these tools must be easy to administer, easy to score, and standardized, and, probably most important, they must provide information to the clinician that can be summarized for the parent.

The assessment tools reviewed in this chapter fit each of these criteria. They have been in use in many offices over an extended period of time. They do what needs to be done—they provide first- and second-stage screening for behavioral problems in children. For a more detailed discussion of the types of assessment available through the public schools, see Chapter 11 of this book.

REFERENCES

Achenbach TM, Edelbrock CS: Behavioral problems and competencies reported to parents of normal and disturbed children aged four through sixteen. *Monogr Soc Res Child Develop* 46(1, Serial No. 188), 1983.

Anders TF, Halpern LF, Hua J: Sleeping through the night: A developmental perspective. *Pediatrics* 90(4):554–560, 1992.

Barkley RA: *Hyperactive Children: A Handbook for Diagnosis and Treatment*. New York: Guilford Press, 1981.

Christophersen ER: *Beyond Discipline: Parenting That Lasts a Lifetime*. Kansas City, MO: Westport Publishing Group, 1990.

Christophersen ER: Anticipatory guidance on discipline. *Pediatr Clin N Am* 33(4):789–798, 1986.

Finney JW, Friman PC, Rapoff MA, Christophersen ER: Improving compliance with antibiotic regimens for otitis media: Randomized clinical trial in a pediatric clinic. *Am J Dis Child* 139:89–95, 1985.

Frankenburg WK: Infant and pre-school developmental screening, in Levine MD, Carey WB, Crocker AC, Gross RT (eds.), *Developmental-Behavioral Pediatrics*. Philadelphia: WB Saunders, 1983, pp. 927–937.

Friman PC, Mathews JR, Finney JW, Christophersen ER, Leibowitz JM: Do encopretic children have clinically significant behavior problems? *Pediatrics* 82(3):407–409, 1988.

Gabel S, Chandra R, Shindledecker R: Behavioral ratings and outcome of medical treatment for encopresis. *J Develop Behav Pediatr* 9:129–133, 1988.

Goyette CH, Conners CK, Ulrich RF: Normative data on Revised Conners Parent and Teacher Rating Scales. *J Abnorm Child Psychol* 6:221–236, 1978.

Haggerty RJ, Roghman KJ, Pless IB: *Child Health and the Community*. New York: Wiley & Sons, 1975.

Rapoff MA, Christophersen ER: Improving compliance in pediatric practice. *Pediatr Clin N Am* 29:339–357, 1982.

Robinson EA, Eyberg SM, Ross AW: The standardization of an inventory of child conduct problem behaviors. *J Clin Child Psychol* 9(1):22–29, 1980.

Sweetland RC, Keyser DJ: *Tests*, 3rd ed. Kansas City, MO: Test Corporation of America, 1986.

Wright L, Schaefer AB, Solomons G: *Encyclopedia of Pediatric Psychology*. Baltimore: University Park Press, 1979.

Sample Handouts

HANDOUT 4.1

Eyberg Child Behavior Inventory

Date _____

Child's Name _____ Child's Age _____ Birthdate _____

Directions: Below is a series of phrases that describe children's behavior. Please (1) circle the number describing how often the behavior occurs with your child and (2) circle "yes" or "no" to indicate whether the behavior is currently a problem for you.

	How Often Does This Occur with Your Child?							Is This a Problem for You?	
	Never	Seldom	Sometimes	Often		Always			
1. Dawdles in getting dressed	1	2	3	4	5	6	7	Yes	No
2. Dawdles or lingers at mealtime	1	2	3	4	5	6	7	Yes	No
3. Has poor table manners	1	2	3	4	5	6	7	Yes	No
4. Refuses to eat food presented	1	2	3	4	5	6	7	Yes	No
5. Refuses to do chores when asked	1	2	3	4	5	6	7	Yes	No
6. Slow in getting ready for bed	1	2	3	4	5	6	7	Yes	No
7. Refuses to go to bed on time	1	2	3	4	5	6	7	Yes	No
8. Does not obey house rules on his own	1	2	3	4	5	6	7	Yes	No
9. Refuses to obey until threatened with punishment	1	2	3	4	5	6	7	Yes	No
10. Acts defiant when told to do something	1	2	3	4	5	6	7	Yes	No
11. Argues with parents about rules	1	2	3	4	5	6	7	Yes	No
12. Gets angry when he does not get his own way	1	2	3	4	5	6	7	Yes	No
13. Has temper tantrums	1	2	3	4	5	6	7	Yes	No
14. Sasses adults	1	2	3	4	5	6	7	Yes	No
15. Whines	1	2	3	4	5	6	7	Yes	No
16. Cries easily	1	2	3	4	5	6	7	Yes	No
17. Yells or screams	1	2	3	4	5	6	7	Yes	No
18. Hits parents	1	2	3	4	5	6	7	Yes	No
19. Destroys toys and other objects	1	2	3	4	5	6	7	Yes	No
20. Is careless with toys and other objects	1	2	3	4	5	6	7	Yes	No
21. Steals	1	2	3	4	5	6	7	Yes	No
22. Lies	1	2	3	4	5	6	7	Yes	No
23. Teases and provokes other children	1	2	3	4	5	6	7	Yes	No
24. Verbally fights with friends his own age	1	2	3	4	5	6	7	Yes	No

	How Often Does This Occur with Your Child?							Is This a Problem for You?	
	Never	Seldom	Sometimes		Often	Always			
25. Verbally fights with sisters and brothers	1	2	3	4	5	6	7	Yes	No
26. Physically fights with friends his own age	1	2	3	4	5	6	7	Yes	No
27. Physically fights with sisters and brothers	1	2	3	4	5	6	7	Yes	No
28. Constantly seeks attention	1	2	3	4	5	6	7	Yes	No
29. Interrupts	1	2	3	4	5	6	7	Yes	No
30. Is easily distracted	1	2	3	4	5	6	7	Yes	No
31. Has short attention span	1	2	3	4	5	6	7	Yes	No
32. Fails to finish tasks or projects	1	2	3	4	5	6	7	Yes	No
33. Has difficulty entertaining himself alone	1	2	3	4	5	6	7	Yes	No
34. Has difficulty concentrating on one thing	1	2	3	4	5	6	7	Yes	No
35. Is overactive or restless	1	2	3	4	5	6	7	Yes	No
36. Wets the bed	1	2	3	4	5	6	7	Yes	No

Note: Standardization data for the behavioral inventory is included in the original article. (From Robinson EA, Eyberg SM, Ross AD. The standardization of an inventory of child conduct problem behaviors. *J Clin Child Psychol* 9(1):22–29, 1980. Copyright 1980, Lawrence Erlbaum Associates, Inc.)

HANDOUT 4.2

ECBI Scores by Age

		Problem Score		Intensity Score	
Age	n	M	SD	M	SD
2	44	7.9	7.7	116.2	33.7
3	69	6.9	7.9	104.5	34.0
4	56	5.5	5.8	104.6	32.8
5	55	7.8	8.0	104.8	31.7
6	45	9.6	8.6	113.9	32.6
7	49	9.8	10.8	111.8	45.7
8	38	4.6	5.0	96.1	28.4
9	40	5.1	6.4	89.3	24.8
10	42	6.7	7.8	105.3	36.9
11	34	4.5	5.6	91.0	30.4
12	40	7.0	8.0	96.8	36.1
13	31	5.8	7.7	90.3	35.3
14	25	6.7	8.1	87.9	37.3
15	30	7.4	7.4	94.4	34.4
16	16	4.9	6.9	77.6	32.6

Sources: Eyberg S, Robinson E: Conduct problem behavior: Standardization of a behavior rating scale with adolescents. *J Clin Child Psychol* 12:347–354, 1983. Robinson EA, Eyberg S, Ross AW: The standardization of an inventory of child conduct problem behaviors. *J Clin Child Psychol* 9:22–28, 1980.

HANDOUT 4.3

Eyberg Child Behavior Inventory

Date _____

Child's Name _____ Child's Age _____ Birthdate _____

Directions: Below is a series of phrases that describe children's behavior. Please (1) circle the number describing how often the behavior occurs with your child and (2) circle "yes" or "no" to indicate whether the behavior is currently a problem for you.

	How Often Does This Occur with Your Child?							Is This a Problem for You?
	Never	Seldom	Sometimes	Often	Always			
1. Dawdles in getting dressed	1	2	③	4	5	6	7	Yes (No)
2. Dawdles or lingers at mealtime	1	2	③	4	5	6	7	Yes (No)
3. Has poor table manners	1	②	3	4	5	6	7	Yes (No)
4. Refuses to eat food presented	1	2	③	4	5	6	7	Yes (No)
5. Refuses to do chores when asked	①	2	3	4	5	6	7	Yes (No)
6. Slow in getting ready for bed	1	②	3	4	5	6	7	(Yes) No
7. Refuses to go to bed on time	①	2	3	4	5	6	7	Yes (No)
8. Does not obey house rules on his own	1	②	3	4	5	6	7	Yes (No)
9. Refuses to obey until threatened with punishment	1	②	3	4	5	6	7	Yes No
10. Acts defiant when told to do something	①	2	3	4	5	6	7	Yes (No)
11. Argues with parents about rules	1	2	③	4	5	6	7	Yes (No)
12. Gets angry when he does not get his own way	①	2	3	4	5	6	7	Yes (No)
13. Has temper tantrums	1	2	3	4	5	6	7	Yes (No)
14. Sasses adults	1	2	3	④	5	6	7	(Yes) No
15. Whines	1	2	③	4	5	6	7	Yes (No)
16. Cries easily	1	②	3	4	5	6	7	Yes (No)
17. Yells or screams	1	②	3	4	5	6	7	Yes (No)
18. Hits parents	①	2	3	4	5	6	7	Yes (No)
19. Destroys toys and other objects	①	2	3	4	5	6	7	Yes (No)
20. Is careless with toys and other objects	1	②	3	4	5	6	7	Yes (No)
21. Steals	①	2	3	4	5	6	7	Yes (No)
22. Lies	①	2	3	4	5	6	7	Yes (No)
23. Teases and provokes other children	1	②	3	4	5	6	7	Yes (No)
24. Verbally fights with friends his own age	1	②	3	4	5	6	7	Yes (No)

	How Often Does This Occur with Your Child?							Is This a Problem for You?
	Never	Seldom	Sometimes	Often		Always		
25. Verbally fights with sisters and brothers	1	2	③	4	5	6	7	Yes (No)
26. Physically fights with friends his own age	1	②	3	4	5	6	7	Yes (No)
27. Physically fights with sisters and brothers	1	②	3	4	5	6	7	Yes (No)
28. Constantly seeks attention	1	2	③	4	5	6	7	Yes (No)
29. Interrupts	1	2	③	4	5	6	7	Yes (No)
30. Is easily distracted	1	②	3	4	5	6	7	Yes (No)
31. Has short attention span	①	2	3	4	5	6	7	Yes (No)
32. Fails to finish tasks or projects	1	2	3	4	5	6	7	Yes (No)
33. Has difficulty entertaining himself alone	①	2	3	4	5	6	7	Yes (No)
34. Has difficulty concentrating on one thing	①	2	3	4	5	6	7	Yes (No)
35. Is overactive or restless	①	2	3	4	5	6	7	Yes (No)
36. Wets the bed	①	2	3	4	5	6	7	Yes (No)

Note: Standardization data for the behavioral inventory is included in the original article. (From Robinson EA, Eyberg SM, Ross AD. The standardization of an inventory of child conduct problem behaviors. *J Clin Child Psychol* 9(1):22–29, 1980. Copyright 1980, Lawrence Erlbaum Associates, Inc.)

Conner's Parent Symptom Questionnaire

Child's name _____ Date _____

Please answer all questions. Beside each item, indicate the degree of the problem by a checkmark (✔).

	Not at all	Just a little	Pretty much	Very much
1. Picks at things (nails, fingers, hair, clothing).				
2. Sassy to grown-ups.				
3. Problems with making or keeping friends.				
4. Excitable, impulsive.				
5. Wants to run things.				
6. Sucks or chews (thumb, clothing, blankets).				
7. Cries easily or often.				
8. Carries a chip on his shoulder.				
9. Daydreams.				
10. Difficulty in learning.				
11. Restless in the "squirmy" sense.				
12. Fearful (of new situations, new people or places, going to school).				
13. Restless, always "up and on the go."				
14. Destructive.				
15. Tells lies or stories that aren't true.				
16. Shy.				
17. Gets into more trouble than others same age.				
18. Speaks differently from others same age.				
19. Denies mistakes or blames others.				
20. Quarrelsome.				
21. Pouts and sulks.				
22. Steals.				
23. Disobedient or obeys but resentful.				
24. Worries more than others (about being alone, illness, or death).				
25. Fails to finish things.				
26. Feelings easily hurt.				
27. Bullies others.				
28. Unable to stop a repetitive activity.				
29. Cruel.				
30. Childish or immature (wants help he shouldn't need, clings).				

	Not at all	Just a little	Pretty much	Very much
31. Distractibility or attention span a problem.				
32. Headaches.				
33. Mood changes quickly and drastically.				
34. Doesn't like or doesn't follow rules or restrictions.				
35. Fights constantly.				
36. Doesn't get along well with brothers or sisters.				
37. Easily frustrated in efforts.				
38. Disturbs other children.				
39. Basically an unhappy child.				
40. Problems with eating (poor appetite, up between bites).				
41. Stomachaches.				
42. Problems with sleep (can't fall asleep; up too early).				
43. Other aches and pains.				
44. Vomiting or nausea.				
45. Feels cheated in family circle.				
46. Boasts and brags.				
47. Lets self be pushed around.				
48. Bowel problems (loose, irregular, constipation).				

HANDOUT 4.5

Category (Factor) Norms for the Conner's Parent Symptom Questionnaire

Age (years)	n[a]	I. Conduct Problems		II. Learning Problems		III. Psychosomatic Problems		IV. Impulsivity Hyperactivity		V. Anxiety		VI. Hyperactivity Index	
		x	SD	x	SD	x	SD	x	SD	x	SD	x	SD
Males by age													
3–5	45	.53	.39	.50	.33	.07	.15	1.01	.65	.67	.61	.72	.40
6–8	76	.50	.40	.64	.45	.13	.23	.93	.60	.51	.51	.69	.46
9–11	73	.53	.38	.54	.52	.18	.26	.92	.60	.42	.47	.66	.44
12–14	59	.49	.41	.66	.57	.22	.44	.82	.54	.58	.59	.62	.45
15–17	38	.47	.44	.62	.55	.13	.26	.70	.51	.59	.58	.51	.41
Females by age													
3–5	29	.49	.35	.62	.57	.10	.17	1.15	.77	.51	.59	.78	.56
6–8	57	.41	.28	.45	.38	.19	.27	.95	.59	.57	.66	.59	.35
9–11	55	.40	.36	.43	.38	.17	.28	.80	.59	.49	.57	.52	.34
12–14	63	.39	.40	.44	.45	.23	.28	.72	.55	.54	.53	.49	.34
15–17	34	.37	.33	.35	.38	.19	.25	.60	.55	.51	.53	.42	.34

Note. The norms are taken from "Normative Data on Revised Conner's Parent and Teacher Rating Scales" by C. H. Goyette, C. K. Conners, and R. F. Ulrich, *J Abnorm Child Psychol* 6:221–236, 1978. Copyright 1978 by Plenum Publishing Corp. Reprinted by permission. The scores are derived by assigning 0, 1, 2, and 3 points to the answers "not at all," "just a little," "pretty much," and "very much," respectively, for each item. The scores for those items assigned to each factor are then summed and divided by the number of questions assigned to or loading on that factor. The items assigned to each factor from the Conner's Parent Questionnaire are as follows: *conduct problems*—questions 2, 8, 14, 19, 20, 21, 22, 23, 27, 33, 34, and 39; *learning problems*—questions 10, 25, 31, and 37; *psychosomatic problems*—questions 32, 41, 43, 44, and 48; *impulsivity–hyperactivity*—questions 4, 5, 11, and 13; *anxiety*—questions 12, 16, 24, and 47; *hyperactivity index*—questions 4, 7, 11, 13, 14, 25, 31, 33, 37, and 38.

n[a] = number of subjects per age group.

HANDOUT 4.6

Behavioral Pediatrics Intake Form

Interviewer: _____ Date: _____ Family Name: _____

Patient's Hospital Number _____

I. GENERAL BACKGROUND

Child's Name _____ Nickname _____

Age _____ Birthdate _____ Sex _____

Address _____ Home Phone _____

City/State _____ Zip Code _____

Father's Name _____ Age _____ Work Phone _____

Mother's Name _____ Age _____ Work Phone _____

Relationship to Child (Circle 1)

Marital Status: Unmarried _____

Father: Natural   Adoptive   Foster   Step   Married _____ Divorced _____

Mother: Natural   Adoptive   Foster   Step   Married _____ Divorced _____

Other Children:

Name   *Age*   *Sex*

_____

_____

_____

_____

_____

_____

Who referred you? _____ Name of child's physician _____

Reason for referral: _____

_____

_____

_____

II. PARENT ASSESSMENT

Education—Highest Grade Completed

Father _____ Mother _____

Employment—Job Position

Father _____ Hours a week: _____

Mother _____ Hours a week: _____

Describe overtime work or second job, if any:

_____

_____

Do you think the family is under a financial strain? Yes _____ No _____

Are you receiving any type of financial assistance? Yes _____ No _____

Home Schedule of Parents

Father _____

Mother _____

Emotional Status

Describe a typical day experienced by your child: _____

_____

_____

_____

Has either parent ever received counseling or psychotherapy? Yes _____ No _____

If yes, describe problem, therapist, and dates:

_____

_____

How would you describe your marriage during the past 6 months? (Circle 1):

   Very Good   Good   Fair   Bad   Very Bad

How would you describe your marriage during the past month?

   Very Good   Good   Fair   Bad   Very Bad

Do you and your spouse agree on the two previous questions? Yes _____ No _____

If not, how does your spouse rate these questions?

_____

_____

III. ASSESSMENT OF OTHER CHILDREN
(Skip if you have only one child)

Emotional Status

Have any of your other children ever received counseling or psychotherapy?
Yes _____ No _____

If yes, describe problem, therapist, and dates:

_____

_____

_____

Do any of your other children have an emotional or behavioral problem that concerns you?

Yes _____ No _____

If yes, describe:

_____

_____

_____

Physical Health

Do any of your other children have a physical health problem that interferes with normal functioning? Yes _____ No _____

If yes, describe:

_____

_____

_____

IV. CHILD PHYSICAL ASSESSMENT

Growth and Development

Birth weight _____

Normal pregnancy: Yes _____ No _____

Normal labor delivery: Yes _____ No _____

Normal perinatal period (first month of life): Yes _____ No _____

General impression of infant development (Circle 1): Poor   Fair   Good

Note the month your child achieved the following activities:

   Sat alone _____ Crawled _____ Walked _____ Fed self _____ Spoke words _____

General appearance now:

Weight _____ Height _____

Physical Assessment of Vision, Hearing, and Speech:

Vision:	Normal _____	Abnormal _____	Corrected _____
Hearing:	Normal _____	Abnormal _____	Corrected _____
Speech:	Normal _____	Abnormal _____	Corrected _____

Does the child have a physical health problem that interferes with normal functioning?

Yes _____ No _____

If yes, describe:

_____

_____

Is your child on any medication at present? Yes _____ No _____

For what is it prescribed? _____ How long has the child been on it? _____

What kind and who prescribed it? _____

Does this affect his/her behavior? _____ How? _____

V. CHILD EMOTIONAL ASSESSMENT

Has the child ever received counseling or psychotherapy? Yes _____ No _____

If yes, describe problem, therapist, and dates:

_____

_____

Does the child have a behavioral or emotional problem that concerns you?

Yes _____ No _____

If yes, elaborate:

_____

_____

Is the relationship between this child and the father good? Yes _____ No _____

If no, elaborate:

_____

_____

Is the relationship between this child and the mother good? Yes _____ No _____

If no, elaborate:

_____

_____

Is the relationship between this child and any brothers/sisters good? Yes _____ No _____

If no, elaborate:

_____

_____

Which of the following *have been* or are now problems with your child?

	Yes	No	Sometimes		Yes	No	Sometimes
Won't mind	_____	_____	_____	Headbanging	_____	_____	_____
Too active	_____	_____	_____	Soiling	_____	_____	_____
Bad temper	_____	_____	_____	Bedwetting	_____	_____	_____
High-strung or nervous	_____	_____	_____	Clings to parents	_____	_____	_____
Breathholding	_____	_____	_____	Cries a lot	_____	_____	_____
Easily upset	_____	_____	_____	Toilet training	_____	_____	_____
Clumsy	_____	_____	_____	Too shy	_____	_____	_____
Nightmares	_____	_____	_____	Brothers/sisters	_____	_____	_____
Destructive	_____	_____	_____	Hyperactive	_____	_____	_____
Other							

Bedtime

What time do you usually begin getting your child ready for bed? _____

What time is s/he usually in bed? _____

What time is s/he usually asleep? _____

How many times does s/he usually wake up? _____

Do you go to her/him when s/he awakens? _____

Where does s/he fall asleep? _____

Who puts her/him to bed? _____

Meals

What are your child's favorite foods? _____

_____

What are some foods that s/he doesn't like? _____

_____

How long does a meal typically last? _____

How many times does s/he typically disrupt the meal? _____

What kinds of snacks does s/he prefer? _____

How often does s/he get snacks? _____

Temper Tantrums

Has your child ever had a tantrum? _____ How often? _____

What do her/his tantrums usually involve? Kicking _____ Crying/screaming _____

Throwing self on floor _____ Other _____

What usually starts a tantrum? _____

Dressing

Who picks out your child's clothes? _____

Are there any articles of clothing that s/he cannot put on alone? _____

What? _____

How long does dressing usually take? _____

VI. SCHOOL ASSESSMENT

What type, if any, of school does the child attend? (Circle 1):

   Preschool   Kindergarten   Grade School   Junior High

Describe school progress (Circle 1): Poor Fair Good Very Good

School Name _____ Principal's Name _____

School Address _____ Teacher's Name _____

Phone _____ Hours in Attendance _____

According to the teacher, your child:

	Yes	No	Sometimes
Has difficulty following instructions	___	___	___
Talks out of turn	___	___	___
Is a slow learner	___	___	___
Has a short attention span	___	___	___
Has trouble finishing work	___	___	___
Does not get along with other children	___	___	___

Have you had special or extra conferences with the teacher or school authorities for your

child's behavior or learning problems? Yes _____ No _____

What do they suggest is needed to help the child? _____

_____

Do you agree with the teacher, or what are your ideas about what is needed? _____

_____

VII. ASSESSMENT OF BEHAVIOR MANAGEMENT

Who ordinarily disciplines your child? _____

How is your child disciplined?

Spank _____ Yell _____ Reasoning _____ Take away privileges _____

Send to room _____ Other _____

How often do you need to use discipline? _____

Have your methods of discipline been effective? _____

Do you and the child's mother/father agree on discipline? _____

Parents: What does your daughter/son like to do with you?

Mom: _____

_____

_____

Dad: _____

_____

_____

Child: What do you like to do with mom/dad?

Mom: _____

_____

_____

Dad: _____

_____

_____

HANDOUT 4.7

Achenbach Child Behavior Checklist (CBCL)

Below is a list of items that describe children and youth. For each item that describes your child **now or within the past 6 months**, please circle the **2** if the item is **very true** or **often true** of your child. Circle the **1** if the item is **somewhat** or **sometimes true** of your child. If the item is **not true** of your child, circle the **0**. Please answer all items as well as you can, even if some do not seem to apply to your child.

0 = Not True (as far as you know)   **1 = Somewhat or Sometimes True**   **2 = Very True or Often True**

0 1 2	1. Acts too young for his/her age	0 1 2	31. Fears he/she might think or do something bad
0 1 2	2. Allergy (describe): _____		
		0 1 2	32. Feels he/she has to be perfect
		0 1 2	33. Feels or complains that no one loves him/her
0 1 2	3. Argues a lot		
0 1 2	4. Asthma	0 1 2	34. Feels others are out to get him/her
		0 1 2	35. Feels worthless or inferior
0 1 2	5. Behaves like opposite sex		
0 1 2	6. Bowel movements outside toilet	0 1 2	36. Gets hurt a lot, accident-prone
		0 1 2	37. Gets in many fights
0 1 2	7. Bragging, boasting		
0 1 2	8. Can't concentrate, can't pay attention for long	0 1 2	38. Gets teased a lot
		0 1 2	39. Hangs around with others who get in trouble
0 1 2	9. Can't get his/her mind off certain thoughts; obsessions (describe): _____		
		0 1 2	40. Hears sounds or voices that aren't there (describe): _____
0 1 2	10. Can't sit still, restless, or hyperactive		
0 1 2	11. Clings to adults or too dependent	0 1 2	41. Impulsive or acts without thinking
0 1 2	12. Complains of loneliness	0 1 2	42. Would rather be alone than with others
		0 1 2	43. Lying or cheating
0 1 2	13. Confused or seems to be in a fog		
0 1 2	14. Cries a lot	0 1 2	44. Bites fingernails
		0 1 2	45. Nervous, highstrung, or tense
0 1 2	15. Cruel to animals		
0 1 2	16. Cruelty, bullying, or meanness to others	0 1 2	46. Nervous movements or twitching (describe): _____
0 1 2	17. Day-dreams or gets lost in his/her thoughts		
0 1 2	18. Deliberately harms self or attempts suicide	0 1 2	47. Nightmares
0 1 2	19. Demands a lot of attention	0 1 2	48. Not liked by other kids
0 1 2	20. Destroys his/her own things	0 1 2	49. Constipated, doesn't move bowels
0 1 2	21. Destroys things belonging to his/her family or others	0 1 2	50. Too fearful or anxious
		0 1 2	51. Feels dizzy
0 1 2	22. Disobedient at home		
		0 1 2	52. Feels too guilty
0 1 2	23. Disobedient at school	0 1 2	53. Overeating
0 1 2	24. Doesn't eat well		
		0 1 2	54. Overtired
0 1 2	25. Doesn't get along with other kids	0 1 2	55. Overweight
0 1 2	26. Doesn't seem to feel guilty after misbehaving		
			56. Physical problems without known medical cause:
0 1 2	27. Easily jealous	0 1 2	a. Aches or pains (*not* headaches)
0 1 2	28. Eats or drinks things that are not food — *don't* include sweets (describe): _____	0 1 2	b. Headaches
		0 1 2	c. Nausea, feels sick
		0 1 2	d. Problems with eyes (describe): _____
0 1 2	29. Fears certain animals, situations, or places, other than school (describe): _____	0 1 2	e. Rashes or other skin problems
		0 1 2	f. Stomachaches or cramps
		0 1 2	g. Vomiting, throwing up
		0 1 2	h. Other (describe): _____
0 1 2	30. Fears going to school		

Please see other side

PAGE 3

105

0 1 2	57.	Physically attacks people
0 1 2	58.	Picks nose, skin, or other parts of body (describe): _____

_____

0 1 2	59.	Plays with own sex parts in public
0 1 2	60.	Plays with own sex parts too much
0 1 2	61.	Poor school work
0 1 2	62.	Poorly coordinated or clumsy
0 1 2	63.	Prefers being with older kids
0 1 2	64.	Prefers being with younger kids
0 1 2	65.	Refuses to talk
0 1 2	66.	Repeats certain acts over and over; compulsions (describe): _____

_____

0 1 2	67.	Runs away from home
0 1 2	68.	Screams a lot
0 1 2	69.	Secretive, keeps things to self
0 1 2	70.	Sees things that aren't there (describe):

_____

_____

0 1 2	71.	Self-conscious or easily embarrassed
0 1 2	72.	Sets fires
0 1 2	73.	Sexual problems (describe): _____

_____

_____

0 1 2	74.	Showing off or clowning
0 1 2	75.	Shy or timid
0 1 2	76.	Sleeps less than most kids
0 1 2	77.	Sleeps more than most kids during day and/or night (describe): _____

_____

0 1 2	78.	Smears or plays with bowel movements
0 1 2	79.	Speech problem (describe): _____

_____

0 1 2	80.	Stares blankly
0 1 2	81.	Steals at home
0 1 2	82.	Steals outside the home
0 1 2	83.	Stores up things he/she doesn't need (describe): _____

_____

0 1 2	84.	Strange behavior (describe): _____

_____

0 1 2	85.	Strange ideas (describe): _____

_____

0 1 2	86.	Stubborn, sullen, or irritable
0 1 2	87.	Sudden changes in mood or feelings
0 1 2	88.	Sulks a lot
0 1 2	89.	Suspicious
0 1 2	90.	Swearing or obscene language
0 1 2	91.	Talks about killing self
0 1 2	92.	Talks or walks in sleep (describe): _____

_____

0 1 2	93.	Talks too much
0 1 2	94.	Teases a lot
0 1 2	95.	Temper tantrums or hot temper
0 1 2	96.	Thinks about sex too much
0 1 2	97.	Threatens people
0 1 2	98.	Thumb-sucking
0 1 2	99.	Too concerned with neatness or cleanliness
0 1 2	100.	Trouble sleeping (describe): _____

_____

0 1 2	101.	Truancy, skips school
0 1 2	102.	Underactive, slow moving, or lacks energy
0 1 2	103.	Unhappy, sad, or depressed
0 1 2	104.	Unusually loud
0 1 2	105.	Uses alcohol or drugs for nonmedical purposes (describe): _____
0 1 2	106.	Vandalism
0 1 2	107.	Wets self during the day
0 1 2	108.	Wets the bed
0 1 2	109.	Whining
0 1 2	110.	Wishes to be of opposite sex
0 1 2	111.	Withdrawn, doesn't get involved with others
0 1 2	112.	Worries
	113.	Please write in any problems your child has that were not listed above:
0 1 2		

_____

0 1 2	

_____

0 1 2	

_____

PLEASE BE SURE YOU HAVE ANSWERED ALL ITEMS.   PAGE 4   UNDERLINE ANY YOU ARE CONCERNED ABOUT.

Copyright 1991 T. M. Achenbach, University of Vermont, 1 S. Prospect Street, Burlington, VT. Reprinted by permission.

Child Behavior Checklist Profile

```
_____Internalizing_____        TRF Profile - Girls 12-18 _____Externalizing_____  T Score
-|         17        35      25      15      39      |             48    |- ID# 123456
-|   17              33      24              38      |       17    47    |- IN:GIRL12.TES
-|         16                        14              |       16    46    |-95 Girl AGE: 12
-|   16    15        31      22      13      36      |             44    |-  DATE FILLED:
-|         14        30      21              35      |       15    42    |-  02/10/91
-|                   29              12              |             41    |-90 BY: Teacher
-|   15    13        28      20      11      34      |       14    40    |-  CARDS 02,03
-|         12        26      19              33      |       13    38    |-  AGENCY
-|   14                      18      10      32      |             37    |-85
-|         11        24      17       9      31      |       12    36    |-
-|   13    10        23      16              30      |       11    34    |-  # ITEMS    25
-|                   22               8              |             33    |-80 TOTSCORE  33
-|   12     9        21      14       7      28      |       10    31    |-  TOT T      61+
-|          8        19      13               27     |              29   |-  INTERNAL    4
-|          7                          6             |        9     28   |-75 INT T      53
%ILE-|  11              17      12       5      26     |        8     27   |-  EXTERNAL    5
-|          6        16      11              25      |              25   |-  EXT T      57
98 -|-- 10- - - - - 5 - - - -15 - - | - - -10- - - -  4 - - -24 - -|- - -7- - - - 24 - - - |-70 ++ Clinical
-|    8     3        12 _ _ | _ _ _ 7 _ _ _  3 _ _###_|_ _ _ _5_ _ _ _ 18_ _ _|-  + Borderline
-|    7             11               2       17     |             16    |-
93 -|          2        |       6               16     |        4     14   |-65  OTHER PROBS
-|    6              9        4               14     |             10    |-  0 5. ActOppSex
-|    5              7        3               12     |        3     7    |-  1 28.EatNonFood
84 -|    4              6                        11     |              6    |-60 0 30.FearSchool
-|  ###     ###       5       2       1       9      |      ###     4    |-  0 44.BiteNail
-|                    4                        7     |      ###          |-  0 46.Twitch
69 -|    2              3                        6      |        1          |-55 0 55.Overweight
-|                   |      ###              4     |              2    |-  0 56h.OtherPhys
-|    1              2                         2     |              1    |-  0 58.PickSkin
50 -|    0      0      ###|      0      ###     0-1    |        0     0    |-50 1 59.SleepClass
```

I WITHDRAWN	II SOMATIC COMPLAINTS	III ANXIOUS/ DEPRESSED	IV SOCIAL PROBLEMS	V THOUGHT PROBLEMS	VI ATTENTION PROBLEMS	VII DELINQUENT BEHAVIOR	VIII AGGRESSIVE BEHAVIOR	
								1 73.Irresponsb
								0 79.SpeechProb
0 42.Rather BeAlone	0 51. Dizzy	0 12.Lonely	1 1. Acts Young	0 9. Mind Off	1 1. Acts Young	0 26.NoGuilt	0 3. Argues	0 83.StoresUp
	1 54. Tired	0 14.Cries				1 39.Bad Compan	0 6. Defiant*	0 91.TalkSuicid
0 65.Won't Talk	0 56a.Aches	0 31.FearDoBad	0 11.Clings	0 18.Harms Self*	0 2. Hums*		0 7. Brags	0 96.SexPreocc
	0 56b.Head- aches	0 32.Perfect	0 12.Lonely*	2 4. Finish*	0 43.LieCheat	0 16.Mean	0 99.TooNeat
0 69.Secret- ive	0 56c.Nausea	0 33.Unloved	0 14.Cries*	0 29.Fears*	2 8.Concentr	0 63.Prefers Older	0 19.DemAttn	0 107.DislkSchl
0 75.Shy	0 56d.Eye	0 34.OutToGet	0 25.NotGet Along	0 40.Hears Things	0 10.SitStil		0 20.DestOwn	0 109.Whining
1 80.Stares	0 56e.Skin	0 35.Worthless	0 33.Unlove*	0 66.Repeats	1 13.Confuse	0 82.Steals	0 21 DestOthr	1 110.Unclean
0 88.Sulks	0 56f.Stomach	0 45.Nervous	0 34.OutTo Get*	Acts	0 15.Fidget*	0 90.Swears	0 23.DisbSchl	0 113.OtherProb
1 102.Under- active	0 56g.Vomit	0 47.Conforms*	0 35.Worth-	0 70.Sees Things	2 17.DaDream	1 98.Tardy*	1 24.Disturbs*	
0 103.Sad	1 TOTAL	0 50.Fearful	less*	0 84.Strange	2 22.Direct*	0 101.Truant	0 27.Jealous	
1 111.With- drawn	58 T SCORE	0 52.Guilty	0 36.GetHurt*	Behav	2 41.Impulsv	0 105.Alcohol Drugs	0 37.Fights	
	47 CLIN T	0 71.SelfConsc	0 38.Teased	0 85.Strange	2 45.Nervous		0 53.TalksOut*	
3 TOTAL		0 81.HurtCrit*	0 48.NotLiked	Ideas	2 49.Learng*	2 TOTAL	0 57.Attacks	
58 T SCORE		0 89.Suspic	0 62.Clumsy	2 61 Poor	43 CLIN T	1 67.Disrupts*	
43 CLIN T		0 103.Sad	0 64.Prefers	50 T SCORE	School		0 68.Screams	
		0 106.AxPleas*	Young		0 62.Clumsy		0 74.ShowOff	
		0 108.Mistake*	43 CLIN T		0 72.Messy*		0 76.Explosive*	
*Items not on Cross- Informant Construct		0 112.Worries			1 78.Inatten*		0 77.Demanding*	
		0 TOTAL	1 TOTAL		1 80.Stares		0 86.Stubborn	
		50 T SCORE	54 T SCORE		2 92.UnderAch*		0 87.MoodChng	
		34 CLIN T	37 CLIN T		1 100.Tasks*		1 93.TalkMuch	
					21 TOTAL		0 94.Teases	
Profile Type: WTHDR SOMAT SOCIAL DEL-AGG Att					68 T SCORE		0 95.Temper	
ICC: .002 -.555 -.812 -.323 .584**					55 CLIN T		0 97.Threaten	
** Significant ICC with profile type							0 104.Loud	
Copyright 1993 T. Achenbach							3 TOTAL	
							56 T SCORE	
							39 CLIN T	

Chapter **5**

Predicting Noncompliance with Medical Procedures

Most practicing clinicians have seen a variety of serious consequences resulting from noncompliance with medical procedures: These consequences include (1) diseases that result from noncompliance with immunization schedules and (2) life-threatening convulsions that result from abrupt discontinuation of anticonvulsant medication.

5.1. FACTORS INDICATIVE OF NONCOMPLIANCE

Numerous studies have attempted to identify demographic factors, predisposing factors such as health beliefs, and antecedent factors (for example, previous experience, parents' presence) that may be correlated with noncompliance with medical procedures. The obvious goal in identifying such factors is to know when to tailor treatment regimens to an individual child identified as at risk for noncompliance.

5.1.1. Demographic Factors

The primary-care provider cannot change demographic factors. Thus, while age (the very young and the very old) or socioeconomic status (families who lack resources) may be correlated with noncompliance, there may be little a practitioner can do after having ascertained that an individual patient may be at higher-than-normal risk for noncompliance. Cognizance that a patient is at high risk for noncompliance because of demographic factors often is not enough to foster changes that will reduce the risk.

As with medical procedures, a child's developmental level should be taken into consideration when making regimen recommendations. This may include adapting the complexity of instructions, the detail of explanations of the child's illness, or the degree of responsibility given to the child.

Explanations with young children should be short and concrete, providing simple information about what the procedure will entail.

Prior rehearsal or modeling with another child or a doll provides a much better explanation of what to expect and how to behave than do words alone. Having a child practice a procedure on a doll, much like adults practice such procedures as CPR on a dummy, can help the child learn the procedures and reduce whatever anxiety may have been expected because of lack of familiarity with the procedures.

Young children's behavior often generalizes from one procedure to another, and from procedures to people and settings in the hospital environment. The child therefore needs to be given clear delineations between invasive and noninvasive procedures, and to associate the staff with positive consequences as well as the inevitable unpleasant ones (Traughber and Cataldo, 1983).

While older children (near adolescence) are better able to understand explanations of their illness and upcoming procedures, caution should be taken not to overwhelm children with details beyond their language ability.

5.1.2. Illness Characteristics

Any illness that remains asymptomatic for some time is less likely to result in compliance. This often is seen with insulin-dependent diabetic children during what has long been referred to as the "honeymoon" phase. Right after diabetes has been diagnosed, when the disease is very easy to control, there are few real immediate consequences if the child is noncompliant with her medical regimen. If failing to comply with the prescribed medical regimen produces no change in the child's condition, and certainly no detrimental effects, the child is less likely to remain compliant (Rapoff and Christophersen, 1982). Conversely, an illness that responds dramatically to a child's attempts to be compliant is more likely to result in compliance. For example, medication that quickly eliminates or reduces a headache will reinforce a child's compliance. With hypertension, where there are no obvious, immediate differential effects of taking or not taking medication, a child is less likely to be compliant.

5.1.3. Regimen Characteristics

Generally, the more complex the regimen and the longer it must be followed, in terms of months or years, the higher the likelihood of noncompliance (Rapoff and Christophersen, 1982). Other factors contributing to noncompliance include:

1. Noxious-tasting medication
2. Adverse side effects
3. High cost of medicine
4. Medication that must be taken frequently
5. Multiple regimen components, such as arthritis regimens that combine medication, splinting, and exercise
6. Restrictions or interference with lifestyles

5.1.4. Barriers to Compliance

Research literature has identified several major barriers to compliance, including:

1. Transportation problems to the practitioner's office or to the treatment center
2. Long waiting times, both waiting for the day of the appointment and waiting to see the practitioner after arriving at the scheduled appointment time
3. Parents' knowledge; both lower formal education and poor parental knowledge of the disease, medication, or regimen
4. The child's behavior

Parents are more likely to be noncompliant with a medical regimen if their child resists the regimen, or if the child has a history of noncompliant behavior (Rapoff and Christophersen, 1982). The vast majority of our consultations for medical noncompliance are for children who were exhibiting behavioral noncompliance prior to their illness or injury, which helps to explain the noncompliance but also makes remediation of the medical noncompliance more difficult. This is the main reason why we emphasize the importance of identifying behavioral noncompliance as early as possible—preferably prior to the time that a child is injured or becomes chronically ill. Behavioral noncompliance is much easier to deal with when it is not complicated by a medical regimen that, for the child's benefit, must be strictly followed.

5.2. NONCOMPLIANCE WITH MEDICAL REGIMENS

Rapoff, Lindsley, and Christophersen (1984) asked parents of children with juvenile rheumatoid arthritis to describe the frequency and types of compliance problems they encountered. The parents reported that their children had the most negative reactions—crying, complaining, and noncompliance—to range-of-motion exercises, splint wearing, and medication, in that order.

The authors suggested that higher noncompliance with exercises is due to the pain resulting from following the regimen. Generally, the more effort a child has to exert, the longer he has to put forth that effort, and the more times in a day he has to do something related to his medical regimen, the less likely a child is to comply with the practitioner's recommendations. Whenever possible, redesigning the medical regimen to reduce or eliminate these barriers is advisable.

5.2.1. Tailoring Antecedents to Enhance Compliance

The primary target of medical procedures has been to identify and change the predisposing factors, such as the child's health beliefs, coping style, and overall compliance; the type of preparation for the procedure; the instructions given; and the physical environment. Unfortunately, much of the literature is anecdotal, and changing the factors predictive of noncompliance does not always increase compliance (Rapoff, Lindsley, and Christophersen, 1985).

5.3. PREDISPOSING FACTORS

As a matter of routine, physicians should assess the child's behavior at home as well as the management strategies used by the parents. Identification of general behavior problems indicates a need to provide the parent with information regarding child management or to refer the parent for assistance with the child behavior problems prior to addressing problems of medical noncompliance.

If parents report having difficulties with the child's bedtime, eating habits, aggression, general noncompliance, or high activity levels, for example, the practitioner should recommend that the parent work on general child management strategies (Christophersen, 1988) or, in more severe cases, be referred for professional counseling. Early identification and treatment of such problems may well reduce noncompliance if hospitalization or medical treatment becomes necessary.

If the child presents with behavior problems (independent of any medical procedures), the professional should treat the child, or refer her for treatment, prior to any attempt to treat the medical noncompliance, to avoid confounding behavioral and medical noncompliance. The amount of time spent in dealing with behavioral noncompliance can often significantly reduce the problems that arise when attempting to introduce the medical regimen. Therefore, when implementing a medical regimen, the minimum number of components of the regimen should be introduced while the practitioner works on behavioral compliance. For example, a child who is undergoing treatment for arthritis may need medication, splints, and exercises, but, given that a truly noncompliant child will probably not comply with either the splinting or the exercises, it may be more prudent to wait to introduce these components until the parents have been successful at dealing with the child's behavior noncompliance. Many times, the behavioral procedures can be introduced in a period of 1 to 3 weeks. After the parents have built up their confidence by successfully managing the behavior problems, they are in a much better position to deal with the problems that may stem from the introduction of the splints and the exercises.

Once the practitioner has obtained consistently compliant behavior from the family, simple behavioral strategies such as those described in Handout 3.1 may be all that is needed to obtain medical compliance.

5.3.1. Giving Medication

Similarly, compliance has been enhanced by the use of clear, concise instructions and eye contact preceding an instruction. Handout 5.1 gives an example of a protocol used in our clinic for teaching parents to give medication, using clear instructions to improve compliance.

5.3.2. Pill Swallowing

Blount, Dahlquist, Baer, and Wouri (1984) used small steps to teach children to accept pills, beginning with very small cake sprinkles and gradually increasing the size of the pill until they reached a size larger than the pill they wanted the child to swallow. This is an excellent example of another way to improve compliance: breaking a task down into small steps and teaching each step systematically. Handout 5.2 shows the steps that Blount et al. (1984) recommended. In our experience, the pill-swallowing protocol has often had children swallowing candies that are as large or larger than the pills they will have to take. This gives the child prior experience in swallowing pills and reduces the anxiety that parents may feel when they have no prior experience getting their child to swallow pills.

5.3.3. Helping Children during Procedures

Little has been written about the influence on children of specific auditory, visual, or olfactory stimuli in the physical environment prior to performing a medical procedure. Whether parental presence during procedures is advisable is yet to be established. In spite of equivocal empirical evidence of the advantages and disadvantages of parental presence, however, parents increasingly are being encouraged by hospital personnel to "room in," be present during medical procedures, and participate in the child's medical care while in the hospital (Roskies, Mongeon, and Gagnon-Lefebvre, 1978).

Parental participation may serve an important function for parents, who themselves may feel helpless in a hospital setting. It is advisable to provide specific instructions and feedback to parents wishing to participate in their child's medical care regarding appropriate parental behavior during procedures. Sometimes, when it is possible, it helps to have parents assist in a procedure with a child other than their own prior to trying it with their child. In this way, the parent gets experience with, and, it is hoped, will become more desensitized to, the procedures, thereby reducing their anxiety.

Some parents may prefer not to attend, in which case it is probably advisable to abide by their wishes. If, however, parents will be required to continue treatment at home, gradual, systematic exposure of the parent to the treatment will be necessary. Parental expression of anxiety regarding medical procedures is an indication that the professional should provide parents with information about the illness, the procedures, and the parent's specific role.

Handout 5.3 suggests the ways parents may help their children during medical procedures.

5.3.4. Case Study: Controlling Environmental Factors

In an interesting case study, the crying of a 17-month-old seriously burned child had generalized from treatment situations to social interactions (Shorkey and Taylor, 1973). When gowns of different colors were worn by the staff and the lighting in the room was changed for social interactions and invasive procedures, there was a decrease in crying during social times. Understandably, there was no change in crying during medical treatment. This study suggests that environmental manipulations can help prevent generalization of the aversiveness of some medical procedures to the entire hospital experience. Adaptations of this approach could include undergoing invasive medical procedures only in the treatment room, and only when practitioners are wearing gowns of a particular color.

5.3.5. Tailoring Instructions to Age and Competence Levels

Because children under the age of 6 are at particular risk for noncompliance, instructions to children should be brief and clear and geared to their developmental level.

If the child has a history of behavior problems, parents should be encouraged to learn more effective management strategies that can be continued if the child is hospitalized or requires medical treatment. The child's present coping strategies should be incorporated wherever possible, and the type of instructions prior to a procedure should be adapted to the child's age and previous experience.

While parental presence or participation during procedures may be valuable, parents need to be given clear and systematic instructions and specific feedback regarding appropriate behavior. Also, the professional's decision to involve or not involve a parent should be determined by previous experience with the parent, the parent's expressions of anxiety regarding the procedure, and the future necessity and practicality of parental involvement.

5.4. REDUCING NONCOMPLIANCE WITH MEDICAL REGIMENS

Short-term compliance with medical regimens can be improved greatly by providing clear, written instructions; telephone follow-up; standard patient recording of compliance; and improved physician-patient interactions. Chapter 6 in this book provides examples of these materials.

5.4.1. Environmental Changes

A number of studies have shown that compliance with medical regimens can be improved by environmental changes that cue the parent to comply with the regimen. In addition to simplifying the regimen and gradually implementing it wherever possible, tailoring it to the individual's routine has been shown to improve compliance (Rapoff and Christophersen, 1982).

For example, parents are more likely to remember to administer medication if it coincides with eating meals, leaving for work, or brushing their teeth. In these instances, a reminder on the refrigerator, near the car keys, or by the toothpaste can serve as cues for giving medication.

Successful multicomponent approaches have included such components as a self-monitoring calendar (Finney, Friman, Rapoff, and Christophersen, 1985); telephone reminders (Finney et al., 1985); home visits (Mayo, 1981); self-recording of food intake (Stunkard, 1981); and public posting of number of exercises completed (Waggoner and LeLieuvre, 1981).

The practitioner should spend a little time discussing how the parents are going to implement the treatment recommendations and what kinds of reminders they can use. Discussing, in general, some of the potential problems and how to minimize or alleviate them may substantially reduce noncompliance problems. The practitioner may suggest that parents use yellow "Post-Its" or place the child's medication or splints near his toothbrush as a reminder; such suggestions will show parents that the practitioner is interested in both the medical regimen and how it is implemented. During my discussions with parents, I've sometimes been amazed at the clever suggestions they come up with.

5.5. ROLE OF THE PROFESSIONAL IN ENHANCING COMPLIANCE

The research literature suggests that pediatricians who are warm, give positive feedback, and are in private practice have better success with getting patients to comply with their recommendations (Mattar and Yaffe, 1974).

Other approaches primary-care providers may use to enhance compliance consist of:

- Explaining the regimen clearly and providing written instructions
- Identifying potential barriers and collaborating with the patient to come up with solutions
- Providing a checklist for recording regimen components and discussing where to post the list
- Determining the roles of the parent and child in carrying out the regimen
- Discussing adapting the regimen to the family's routine and using specific environmental cues as reminders in the home
- Discussing child management strategies that enhance compliance, providing management protocols where appropriate
- Planning for follow-up
- Performing medical procedures while giving clear, concise instructions to both the child and the parent
- Introducing invasive instruments and procedures gradually whenever possible
- Considering procedures for reinforcing both child and parent compliance

5.6. CHANGES ON AN INSTITUTIONAL LEVEL

Because children generally perceive hospitals as aversive, hospital administrations should explore ways to lesson the trauma of hospitalization (Cataldo, Bessman, Parker, Pearson, and Rogers, 1979). Efforts have been made in this direction, such as showing preparatory films or giving instruction regarding hospitalization; providing playrooms and child-life staff (professional child-care workers who spend time playing with children during their hospital stay); allowing parents to stay in the child's room and, in some instances, to accompany their children into treatment or induction rooms; and providing social services for families.

Some of these changes have not been empirically evaluated, but practitioners, through their own time and efforts, can often discover which approaches work with which types of families.

Clearly, variables in the physical environment that may prevent noncompliance (such as the setup of waiting rooms, placement of instruments in the treatment room, and clothing worn by the staff) need to be investigated individually in each clinical setting, but this shouldn't prevent practitioners from trying approaches in their own offices.

5.7. CONCLUDING REMARKS

The literature reviewed in this chapter has identified a number of variables that have been correlated with noncompliance in health settings. Children's compliance to medical procedures improves with age, with consistent discipline practices at home, and with predictable variables surrounding the actual procedure (e.g., type of instruction). Identification and initial treatment of children who are generally noncompliant will also help to prevent medical noncompliance.

In spite of the many studies reviewing factors associated with parental non-compliance to medical regimens, there are limitations. Some of these factors—demographics, clinic versus private practice—can serve only as markers for identifying individuals who are at higher risk for noncompliance. Others, although correlated with noncompliance, have not contributed to compliance when eliminated, such as limited knowledge of illness and health beliefs. Still others, like physician-parent relationships, may require substantial changes that the practitioner may not be willing or able to implement. Further, there is not always a direct correspondence between improved compliance and improved medical outcome (Finney et al., 1985). This last finding may have unfortunate implications. If the patient's compliant behavior does not result in medical improvement, there is a higher likelihood of future noncompliance.

For primary-care professionals to be able to use the recommendations in this chapter, they must keep in mind the factors that are known to improve or reduce compliance. Some of these factors, like the use of written handouts and monitoring sheets, can be addressed by keeping a ready supply of handouts in the treatment area where children are seen.

Other factors, such as tailoring of regimens to the parents' lifestyle or adapting instructions to the child's developmental level, cannot be prepared in anticipation of an office visit. By giving clear instructions and approaching the child or parent in an individualized and caring manner, the practitioner can reduce the likelihood of noncompliance.

Finally, more research is needed in this area. In particular, identification and manipulation of specific physical stimuli during medical procedures, further investigation of factors contributing to child compliance with regimens, the impact of coping style on compliance, and parent instruction in child management in medical settings provide exciting areas for future research.

REFERENCES

Blount RL, Dahlquist LM, Baer RA, Wouri D: A brief effective method for teaching children to swallow pills. *Behav Ther* 15:381–387, 1984.

Cataldo MF, Bessman DA, Parker LH, Pearson JER, Rogers MC: Behavioral assessment for pediatric intensive care units. *J Appl Behav Anal* 12(1):83–97, 1979.

Christophersen ER: *Little People: Guidelines for Common Sense Child Rearing*, 3rd ed. Kansas City, MO: Westport Publishers, 1988.

Finney JW, Friman PC, Rapoff MA, Christophersen ER: Improving compliance with antibiotic regimens for otitis media. *Am J Dis Child* 139:89–95, 1985.

Mattar ME, Yaffe SJ: Compliance of pediatric patients with therapeutic regimens. *Postgrad Med* 56(6):181–188, 1974.

Mayo NE: The effect of a home visit on parental compliance with a home program. *Phys Ther* 61(1):27–32, 1981.

Rapoff MA, Christophersen ER: Improving compliance in pediatric practice. *Pediatr Clin N Am* 29(2):339–357, 1982.

Rapoff MA, Lindsley CB, Christophersen ER: Improving compliance with medical regimens: Case study with juvenile rheumatoid arthritis. *Arch Phys Med Rehab* 65(5):267–269, 1984.

Rapoff MA, Lindsley CB, Christophersen ER: Parent perceptions of problems experienced by their children in complying with treatments for juvenile rheumatoid arthritis. *Arch Phys Med Rehab* 66(7):427–429, 1985.

Roskies E, Mongeon M, Gagnon-Lefebvre B: Increasing maternal participation in the hospitalization of young children. *Med Care* 16:765–777, 1978.

Shorkey CT, Taylor JE: Management of maladaptive behavior of a severely burned child. *Child Welfare* 52(8):543–547, 1973.

Stunkard AJ: Adherence to medical treatment: Overview and lessons from behavioral weight control. *J Psychosomat Res* 25(3):187–197, 1981.

Traughber B, Cataldo MF: Behavioral effects of pediatric hospitalization, in Russo DC, Varni JW (eds.), *Behavioral Pediatrics: Research and Practice*. New York: Plenum Press, 1983, pp. 107–131.

Waggoner CD, LeLieuvre RB: A method to increase compliance to exercise regimens in rheumatoid arthritis patients. *J Behav Med* 4(2):191–201, 1981.

Sample Handouts

Tips for Giving Medication

1. Getting ready

   Give medication at the same time every day; work the times into your routine and post reminders (e.g., if giving medication at mealtimes, post a reminder or recording sheet on the refrigerator).

2. Giving medication
   a. Ask your child to come get the medication.
   b. Give him or her small amounts of medication at a time, followed with sips of a chaser of the child's choice (water, milk, soda pop—check with your doctor to make sure the particular liquid can be given with the specific medication).
   c. Praise taking medication without a fuss.
   d. Use time-out immediately (see Handout 2.10) for
      • Refusals or stalling; avoid coaxing
      • Spitting out medication
      • Vomiting (discuss with your doctor whether to give medication again if the child vomits or spits out the medication)
   e. Ignore gagging.

3. Afterward
   a. If the child has taken medication without any problem
      • Praise and give a hug
      • Give 15 minutes of special time to do an activity of his or her choice with the parents
   b. If he or she has had to go to time-out
      • Praise taking the medication
      • Do not comment on time-out or noncompliance
   c. If you have repeated problems with refusals or vomiting, consult your physician.

©Judy Mathews, Linda Ross, and E. Christophersen, 1987.

HANDOUT 5.2

Teaching Pill-Swallowing

1. Model for your child the steps in swallowing a pill

   a. Place pill on the back of your tongue.
   b. Keep the tongue flat.
   c. Take liquid in the mouth.
   d. Tilt the head backward slightly.
   e. Swallow.

2. Gradually increase the size of the pill in the following order:

   a. Oblong, multicolored sprinkle used for cake decoration
   b. Spherical, silver cake decoration
   c. Round, multicolored candy (0.3 cm–0.7 cm diameter)
   d. Red licorice whip cut to 1-cm length
   e. Capsule-shaped candy, multicolored, sold as "Tic Tacs" or "Dynamints"
   f. Normal-sized capsule: the child's actual pill

Have your child practice swallowing each size piece of sprinkle or candy as many times as it takes for him to get accustomed to it. These procedures usually take about 45 minutes to 1 hour but may take you a little longer.

Adapted from "A brief, effective method for teaching children to swallow pills" by R. L. Blount, L. M. Dahlquist, R. A. Baer, and D. Wouri, 1984, *Behavior Therapy*, 15, p. 383.

HANDOUT 5.3

Helping Children to Cope
with Fears during Medical Procedures

1. As a parent, you are your child's most important role model. Be aware of your own fears and how you cope with them. Model your ways of coping. Do not let your child see that you are afraid.

2. Never threaten your child with getting shots or going to the doctor as a punishment.

3. Give the most accurate explanation about what the doctor or dentist visit will include. Have the doctor or dentist explain the procedures to you so that you can explain it to your child in terms your child can understand. If the dentist is going to brush the teeth with the drill and a special toothpaste, tell your child exactly that, including the fact that, although the feeling is new and unusual to him, it will not hurt him.

4. Never lie to your child about whether something will hurt. Be honest, but reassuring and supportive. Tell him how to cope with the pain. If a child has to have a broken arm reduced, after being adequately anesthetized, tell him that he will feel pressure but not pain. Have him concentrate on the pressure and tell you what it feels like.

5. Encourage and reinforce your child for cooperating with examinations, procedures, and taking medication. Any tangible rewards, such as a coloring book, should always be accompanied by physical affection (time-in) and verbally specific praise. Brief time-out (see other handouts) may be necessary for disruptive behavior. Time-out and self-quieting skills will be discussed in detail in the handout on time-out.

SPECIFIC COPING STRATEGIES

Giving Explanations

Give explanations that are appropriate for the child's age and stage of language development. Be aware of how much the child wants and needs to know. Be sure you, as the parent, have had all of your own questions answered satisfactorily.

1. Time the explanations according to the child's age and level of anxiety. Some children need a lot of time to prepare for something fearful, while other children do better with short intervals between explanations and the actual visit/procedure. A good guideline is always to say too little rather than too much. Often, an anxious parent will convey his anxiety to his child by talking endlessly. Try brief reassuring statements and then be quiet while you are holding your child's hand.

2. Listen for the child's questions and concerns and answer them as they occur. Do not give too much information at once.

3. Use visual aids if you have them. Books, pamphlets, coloring books, drawings, puppets, dolls, and videotapes all can serve as visual aids.

4. If there are other children available who have experienced the same procedures and who have coped well, have your child talk to them.

Providing Distractions

Distraction is a way of taking the child's mind off the fearful event and focusing attention on something else in the environment. The following activities create distractions for your child:

• Blowing bubbles
• Reading story books
• Looking at pop-up books
• Telling stories, whether they are familiar or made-up
• Counting items in the room
• Counting to 10, 100, and so on
• Playing Nintendo-style games and other computer games
• Looking at toys
• Watching TV or videotapes
• Listening to audiotapes of music or stories

Relaxation

Relaxation is a simple method of getting your body to be quiet and calm and to counteract your fears.

1. Begin the exercise by having your child take several slow, deep breaths. Quietly tell him to "relax" or "be calm" as he breathes. Plan what you say so that you are talking while your child is exhaling and quiet while he is inhaling. When your talking and your child's breathing are in synchrony, slow down your speech. With practice, you'll probably see that his breathing slows down as you speak more slowly. Don't make big changes; slow down gradually.

2. Your child may close her eyes slightly, if she is comfortable doing so.

3. Demonstrate for your child how to tense various muscle groups, holding them for 5 seconds and then releasing them, to reduce tension. You either may begin at the feet, working up to the head, or may start with the head and work toward the feet. Notice differences between tension and relaxation.

   Alternatively, you may stretch or tense all of the muscles at once, holding for 5 seconds and then releasing. Notice differences between tension and relaxation.

4. If a particular part of the body is already tense or uncomfortable, avoid tensing and concentrate on relaxing and calming there.

Imagination

Children can use their abilities to "make believe," "fantasize," or "imagine" to take their minds off a feared event. By concentrating on something pleasant, fun, and intense, your child can remove himself from the present situation and be in an imagined place.

1. You can help your child use imagination as a coping tool by choosing a particular scene or activity that can be vividly described. For example, describe the colors, people, sounds, smells, temperatures, or tastes associated with a pleasant scene or event. The more real the activity seems to the child, the more imagination the child will be using for coping.

2. Examples of imaginary events children have used successfully to cope with fearful events include:

   - Going to an amusement park like Disneyland
   - Playing a Nintendo-style computer game
   - Playing baseball, soccer, or football
   - Floating or swimming in a pool or ocean
   - Lying on a beach
   - Floating on a cloud over a favorite place
   - Lying in your own bed at home with a favorite blanket or toy

3. Practice using imagination before the fearful events occur so that it will be easier to enter the imagined state quickly when confronted with the doctor visit, the dental chair, or the needle stick.

Self-Talk

When a child is upset or fearful, it is natural for the parent to say comforting, reassuring words. It can also be helpful for the child to learn to say some of these things to herself.

1. Practice saying these phrases before a feared event occurs.

2. Examples of self-talk are:

   "I am doing fine."
   "I can get through this."
   "It is OK to cry when it hurts."
   "This will be over with soon and I can eat lunch."
   "I will feel lots better when the doctor is finished."

©Linda V. Ross, Ph.D., 1988.

Chapter **6**

Improving Compliance with Medical Regimens

Since Haynes, Taylor, and Sackett (1979) published their classic text on medical compliance, physicians have become increasingly aware that patients who fail to improve medically may not have been sufficiently compliant to realize the benefits of treatment. For instance, at least one-third of all patients fail to comply adequately with such short-term treatment regimens as a 10-day course of antibiotics (Becker and Maiman, 1975). Compliance with chronic disease regimens is reportedly even worse (Gordis, Markowitz, and Lilienfeld, 1969).

Compliance problems have been documented with virtually every type and kind of medical regimen. Physicians and other health-care providers, it has been shown, have no reliable methods of estimating which patients will be noncompliant. In fact, health-care providers' estimates of compliance are no better than chance (Rapoff and Christophersen, 1982).

Chapter 3 presented a broad approach to obtaining general behavioral compliance. Material in this chapter assumes that the practitioner has discussed general compliance issues with the parents and received assurance that the parents are able to obtain reasonable compliance levels from their children. If this assumption is not valid, the health-care practitioner should have the parents work on general behavioral compliance prior to attempting to obtain patient compliance with a difficult, painful, or inconvenient regimen.

6.1. TECHNIQUES FOR IMPROVING COMPLIANCE WITH MEDICAL REGIMENS

Although acute and chronic disease regimens are frequently discussed separately, most of the strategies for acute regimens are applicable to chronic regimens. Short-term compliance with medical regimens can be improved by providing clear written instructions, by using telephone follow-up, by having patients (or parents) record symptoms on standardized sheets, and by promoting positive physician-patient interactions.

6.2. STEPS TO FOLLOW IN PROVIDING PARENT/PATIENT EDUCATION

A necessary basis for compliance is the patient's or parent's understanding and recall of factual information provided by the health-care practitioner. Parent/patient comprehension and recall of medical information can be enhanced by using efficient and understandable verbal presentations and by providing written handouts to patients and parents.

Ley (1977) offered a number of suggestions for health-care providers to use when communicating information to their patients. The following recommendations are based on Ley's work.

1. *When providing patients with instructions and advice, stress how important the advice is.* For example, tell mothers why they should not administer aspirin to a young child with a fever.

2. *Point out the advantages of complying with your recommendations, as well as the disadvantages of failing to comply with them.* For example, in the research literature on encouraging parents to obtain and correctly use automobile child-restraint seats, Treiber (1986) found that pointing out the advantages, as well as the disadvantages, worked much better than either just a positive or just a negative approach. The advantages of using automobile child-restraint seats include a child who behaves better, is less distracting, has less motion sickness, sleeps better, and distracts the driver less. The disadvantages include the risk of injury, disability, and death.

3. *Use short words and short sentences* Avoid medical jargon. For example, talk about "ear infections," not otitis media. Sometimes there has to be a conversation with a parent just to determine whether you are both referring to the same thing.

4. *Use explicit categorization where possible.* Tell the parent you are going to explain what is wrong with his child and what tests and treatment will be needed. Then, proceed with your instructions in a stepwise fashion.

5. *Repeat information, where feasible, for emphasis.* Often, it's a good idea to ask the parent to repeat back to you the important steps in the treatment regimen.

6. *When giving advice, make it as specific, detailed, and concrete as possible.* Whenever you find yourself giving the same advice repeatedly, consider making up a written handout to supplement, not take the place of, what you have to say. This book provides many examples of commonly used patient information handouts.

7. *Find out what the patient's worries are.* Do not confine yourself merely to gathering objective medical information. A good way to end an office visit is to ask the patient if there is anything she wanted to ask you but didn't have the opportunity to do so.

8. *Find out what the patient's expectations are. If they cannot be met, explain why.* Sometimes patients do not want medication as much as they want an explanation. And sometimes they don't want an explanation; they want medication.

9. *Provide information about the diagnosis and cause of the illness.* Written handouts from professional associations, drug companies, and infant formula manufacturers can be made available for illnesses and conditions commonly seen in the office. Providing parents with a written description of their child's diagnosis and treatment can help the health-care practitioner verbally communicate with parents. In addition, the handout provides parents with guidelines to follow after they have left the practitioner's office.

10. *Adopt a friendly, businesslike attitude.* Many parents simply want to know that you care. They don't expect you to "sit and chat," nor do they expect you to take an inordinate amount of time with them.

11. *Spend some time conversing about nonmedical topics.* Personalize your discussion. For example, if you know that one of the baby's parents recently started a new business, ask the parent how the new business is going. I usually make a small notation in a patient's chart about what the parents do for a living or what interests them. These types of interactions are likely to be perceived by patients as supportive and informative. This form of counseling will not add appreciably to the length of the office visit.

6.3. WRITTEN INSTRUCTIONS

Although it is sometimes hard for practitioners to appreciate, because we are in the office every day, many parents are nervous about their doctor's appointment. Notice, sometime, how many parents have cold hands when you shake hands with them. Regardless of how thoroughly you explain something to them, they may still have difficulty remembering everything you told them. For the kinds of problems you see routinely, it's a good idea to either locate written instructions or write your own instructions for parents that summarize your treatment recommendations.

Handouts 6.1 and 6.2 are examples of written instructions for management of diarrhea and strep throat. When you use written recommendations, I recommend you explain your treatment regimen to the parents first, ask them if they have any questions, then provide them with the written summary of what you said. With handouts of this type, parents have something to refer to after they have left the health-care practitioner's office. The handout serves to refresh the parents' memory of what the practitioner said during the office visit.

6.4. SYMPTOM RECORDINGS

Patients can be asked to record their symptoms on a standardized recording sheet (see Handout 6.3). Recording sheets of this type serve as reminders for patients to follow the treatment regimen, and also allow the health-care practitioner to track the patient's progress since the last office visit. Symptom recording sheets greatly facilitate the transmission of information from the family to the health-care practitioner.

Symptom sheets are more accurate than a parent's description of the child's progress because symptoms are recorded at the time of occurrence, or at least a couple of times between office visits, rather than recalled from the parent's memory weeks or months after the occurrence. The practitioner will be able to scan over 3 or 4 months of recordings in a matter of seconds and be able to tell what the parents were doing and how the child's symptoms changed.

A study of compliance with an antibiotic regimen for children diagnosed with acute otitis media demonstrated that parents who were provided a special compliance improvement package were significantly more likely to follow their health-care provider's recommendations, as measured by the levels of antibiotic in the child's urine (Finney, Friman, Rapoff, and Christophersen, 1985).

In the 1985 study, home visits were made to collect urine specimens, to measure remaining medication, and to review the parents' diaries of medication use. Results revealed that only 49% of the control group (no special procedures to improve compliance) complied with the antibiotic regimen; 82% of the experimental group was compliant. The study clearly demonstrated the advantages of devoting a few minutes to compliance issues when treating a child for otitis media. Numerous studies have appeared in the pediatric literature documenting similar approaches with similar outcomes (Colcher and Bass, 1972; Linkewich, Catalano, and Flack, 1974).

The intervention package, which required only a few minutes to complete, consisted of a written handout on otitis media (Handout 6.4) and a recording sheet (Handout 6.5) on which the parent could write down the day and time each dosage of the medication was administered. The written handout described otitis media, its associated symptoms, and the importance of continuing medication until all of the prescribed antibiotic was administered. The written recording sheet provides a simple format for the parent to record administration of the medication.

6.5. INCREASED FOLLOW-UP

To reduce the possibility of poor compliance, the physician's office nurse or other personnel can telephone the parents, after the first few days of the therapeutic regimen, to encourage adherence to the prescribed course. The telephone contact should not put parents on the defensive by suggesting poor compliance. Rather, the parents can be asked about the child's state of health and whether they have any questions. Within this context, parents can be encouraged to continue therapy even though the child is asymptomatic. This follow-up call can usually be limited to 2 or 3 minutes.

6.6. CHRONIC DISEASE REGIMENS

Many of the strategies that maximize compliance with acute disease regimens are also effective with chronic disease regimens. However, additional interventions are often necessitated by the added complexity and lifestyle intrusions of chronic disease regimens (Rapoff and Christophersen, 1982). Much of the research on compliance has focused on assessing levels of compliance among different disease regimens; there has been less emphasis on how the busy practitioner might put the procedures into practice. The suggestions for improving compliance in this chapter require little additional time to implement but have the potential for increasing the level of compliance. The health-care practitioner who is cognizant of the varied problems that noncompliance may cause, and shares this information with patients, may maximize compliance. Handout 6.6 summarizes the factors that have been shown to increase compliance with chronic disease regimens. These suggested factors each will be described in more detail.

6.6.1. Regimen Checklists Record Changes in the Medical Regimen

Some health-care professionals have found that a summary sheet in the front of a patient's chart, indicating changes in the medical regimen and the date they were made, makes it easier to keep track of the patient's progress and the frequency of changes in the patient's regimen. The regimen checklist used by the Pediatric Endocrinology Section at the University of Kansas Medical Center (Rapoff and Christophersen, 1982), shown in Handout 6.7, has proved valuable in this regard.

On this checklist, the provider indicates the date when changes are made in the regimen, including the type and amount of insulin, how often it is administered, and how often blood sugars should be measured. When the checklist is used in conjunction with the symptom recording sheet described below, the provider can, in a matter of seconds, see a summary of the child's regimen and symptoms. The regimen checklist lets the provider know whether the last change in the regimen was made 1 month ago or 2 years ago. Sometimes just knowing that the regimen has been changed repeatedly over the past 6 months will alert the provider to review the patient's regimen more carefully.

A similar checklist (Handout 6.8) has been used in a Pediatric Arthritis Clinic at the University of Kansas Medical Center (Rapoff, Lindsley, and Christophersen, 1984). The checklist increases the ease with which the health-care provider can track changes in the patient's medical regimen. Rather than reviewing a narrative in the patient's chart, often complicated by multiple service notes by various medical professionals, including medical students, residents, fellows, and attending physicians at teaching hospitals, the health-care practitioner can quickly determine how many, what types, and over what period of time changes have been made.

6.6.2. Complex Educational Strategies

Whenever a patient or his parents need to learn a complex procedure, such as exercises for arthritis patients or checking hemoglobin A1c levels of diabetics, actual rehearsals with the physician or nurse observing and providing feedback is a much better teaching strategy than doing a simple demonstration or providing the patient with a written handout. One of the main reasons that dummies have been developed as an aid in the education of medical students is that it is simply not possible to guarantee that the appropriate patient population will be available when medical students are ready to practice a given procedure. In cases like the dummy used for teaching CPR (Annie), the dummy can be repeatedly resuscitated without a concern for damaging her ribs or wearing her out. In later versions of Annie, a recording device was installed inside the chest to provide feedback on how much pressure was actually administered to Annie's chest. This feedback, used by a competent instructor, can facilitate the process of learning a procedure. In fact, such "dummies" are becoming much more common in medical education. Such simulation devices are as useful for educating patients about medical procedures as they are for medical students. Ideally, patients should be provided with:

- A demonstration
- A verbal explanation
- An opportunity to rehearse, with observation and feedback
- A written description

The patient or her parents should rehearse the procedure several times, preferably at more than one office visit. For example, an insulin-dependent juvenile diabetic will generally be kept on a medical regimen for a long time. It is much more efficient initially, to devote time to train the parents or patient properly than to deal later with deciding whether the child is noncompliant or requires a different treatment regimen (Barnard, Moore, Russo, and Christophersen, 1984).

6.6.3. Gradual Implementation of Complex Regimens

Whenever feasible, regimens containing several components should be implemented gradually or in stages. Often there is a temptation to try to teach the patient everything at once. The patient may get "information overload," remembering little of what he or she has been told. Scheduling several appointments, during which components of the multifaceted regimen can be more thoroughly explained and rehearsed, usually makes the entire process easier on the family, as well as on the health-care provider. Barnard, Christophersen, and Moore (1984) described the following procedure for insulin-dependent juvenile diabetics. The health-care provider, in addition to traditional 3- or 4-month return visits, required patients to return monthly, solely to have their glycosylated hemoglobin assessed. During the first visit, the patient/parent was provided with a graphical representation of the patient's glycosylated hemoglobin over the past 6 to 12 months. After results were obtained from the monthly assay, the health-care provider would telephone the patient to report the most recent glycosylated hemoglobin and to tell the patient to add the newest data to his or her chart. In our experience, many juvenile diabetics may be very compliant for 3 to 4 weeks after an office visit, but their compliance slips after that. By the time the patient returned after a 3- to 4-month interval, his glycosylated hemoglobin was the same as it had been at the last visit, suggesting that the patient had not been trying harder to follow the medical regimen, although, in fact, he had tried for a month or so, then had fallen back into his old habits. Using the strategy of brief returns at 1-month intervals to obtain the glycosylated hemoglobin assay, the patient receives more frequent feedback. Most of the patients liked the fact that they were doing better at following the medical regimen and were encouraged by noting the gradual improvement in their glycosylated hemoglobin that resulted from just 3 to 4 weeks of compliance. Handout 6.9 shows the kind of form given to the patients to follow their glycosylated hemoglobin graphically.

6.6.4. Tailoring the Regimen

There is a temptation to recommend that the patient follow an "ideal" schedule. However, it is much more realistic to plan a schedule around the patient's existing lifestyle. Most medical regimens for chronic illness may be adapted to meet the personal habits and style of a patient and his or her family.

For example, a number of years ago, when I met with a group of parents who all had a child with cystic fibrosis, one mother asked me if it was all right to do the postural drainage exercises while her child watched a favorite television program. Before answering her question, I asked the entire group how many of them did the exercises while their child watched television. Every parent put his or her hand up. The policy of doing the exercises in front of the television set made good sense. Now the cystic fibrosis clinic personnel recommend that the parents find some type of distracting activity, like watching television, for their child to do during the postural drainage exercises. The television program serves to distract the child, making the procedure easier for both parent and child. Similarly, when a management plan for constipation or encopresis is formulated, the treatment usually can be performed either in the morning or in the evening. For a family who has a much busier schedule in the morning, common sense dictates that the provider recommend that the treatment plan be implemented during the evening hours. The more a family is required to adjust their lifestyle in order to follow a treatment regimen, the greater the probability is that they will become less compliant over time.

6.6.5. Monitoring Compliance and Symptoms of Disease

Traditional questions asked during a routine office visit, such as, "How has your child been doing over the past 3 months?" are usually answered by most parents with little useful information. They say something like, "Oh, pretty good." Recommending that the parents keep symptom rating scales or diaries of their child's symptoms often makes it easier to teach them about their child's disease. The diary also provides the health-care provider with more detailed information about the patient's progress. Record sheets can be reviewed with the patient during scheduled visits. Handout 6.10 is an example of a recording sheet for encopretics (Christophersen and Berman, 1978).

When a patient returns for an office visit with 2 or 3 months of symptom recordings, the health-care provider may need only a few seconds to scan the symptom recording sheets and review how the child has been doing in order to determine any adjustments that may need to be made in the treatment protocol. With a symptom recording sheet, it is often possible for the health-care provider to identify changes required in the treatment protocol based on the child's response to the prior treatment recommendations. At the end of an office appointment, we usually photocopy the symptom recording sheets for our files and return the originals to the parent.

6.7. PARENTAL MANAGEMENT OF COMPLIANCE

Many children and the majority of adolescents are not capable of managing the entire responsibility for their own chronic disease regimen. If the child initially assumes the responsibility for managing her medical regimen, but is unsuccessful, she may encounter parental friction when parents attempt to assume management. In many families, the child starts out intending to accept responsibility for his medical regimen only to find out that he doesn't do very well. The parents, in turn, will often get angry with the child, partly because the child didn't follow the regimen correctly and partly because they fear that not following the regimen correctly can have negative consequences. Because children and adolescents often are not capable of assuming responsibility for their own treatment (Rapoff, Lindsley, and Christophersen, 1985), the parent should supervise the medical regimen initially and gradually shift the responsibility to the child over a period of years, as the child demonstrates the capability of handling it.

6.8. ROLE OF THE MEDICAL PROFESSIONAL IN ENHANCING COMPLIANCE

Research literature suggests that private-practice providers who are warm and give positive feedback have better success with patient compliance (Mathews and Christophersen, 1989). Obviously, although it is not always possible for patients to see the same practitioner, this point should be kept in mind when scheduling patients for return appointments.

In addition to the strategies discussed above, the practitioner may use other strategies to enhance compliance, including the following:

1. Explore the child's and parents' health beliefs and provide alternative information if these beliefs are predictive of noncompliance. For example, if you suggest the parents try medication on a child with a short attention span, they might appear to agree with you in the office, leave with a prescription, but never get it filled because they don't believe in medicating their child.

   If you are able to identify that the parents would consider the use of medication only as a last resort, you may have to come up with suitable alternatives. Thus, you might recommend some behavioral and organizational strategies, and tell the parents you are willing to start here, but you will feel compelled to readdress the issue of medication if the child does not improve with the strategies you've recommended.

2. Identify potential barriers and collaborate with the patient in coming up with solutions. For example, if you recommend that the parents wait to begin toilet training, you might inquire whether this might be a problem with the day-care center she attends. If the parents say the day-care center insists all children be potty trained before they are allowed in the "upper" group, you may have to discuss the feasibility of changing to another day-care center.

3. Provide a checklist for recording regimen components, and discuss where to post the list (see Handout 6.5 for an example of a monitoring sheet).

4. Determine the roles of the parents and child in carrying out the regimen. Most children under 12 years of age simply are not dependable enough to be given responsibility for taking their own medication. It is preferable to get some agreement with the parents before they entrust the child with this responsibility.

5. Discuss adapting the regimen to the family's routine and using specific environmental cues as reminders in the home. Recommending, for example, that parents perform postural drainage on a child with cystic fibrosis while the child watches a favorite television show may make the regimen easier for everyone involved.

6. Discuss child management strategies that enhance compliance and provide management protocols where appropriate. Chapter 3, "Behavioral Problems," discusses this issue at length.

7. Plan for follow-up and explain to the parent the importance of follow-up. Follow-up can be in the form of routine office visits, written reports, or phone calls from the parents. An answering machine that takes messages around the clock can be an excellent way for parents to leave progress reports without taking up your receptionist's valuable time in the office.

8. When performing a medical procedure, give clear, concise instructions to both the child and the parent. Many offices now provide patients with a written booklet describing what procedures are routinely performed, with some detail depending on the specific procedure. These booklets are usually available to all patients in the waiting room but are also offered to each patient when appropriate. Some patients like to have the practitioner explain step by step what she is doing; others would rather not know. It is best to ask the patient ahead of time what his preference is.

9. Consider procedures for reinforcing compliance by both child and parent. Most offices already have stickers and small toys for children. A kind word to a parent who has worked hard under difficult circumstances is often the most reinforcing thing a practitioner can provide. With some of my more difficult cases, I have arranged for different types of reinforcers—everything from a visit by a famous baseball player for a critically ill child, to an Oakland Raiders pennant for an adolescent who was starting to manage his anger in more appropriate ways.

6.9. CONCLUDING REMARKS

Over the past 10 to 15 years, a good deal of information has become available on improving compliance with medical procedures. The days of simply telling a patient what to do and expecting maximal compliance are long past.

Generally, a relatively small amount of time spent reviewing office practices and procedures can result in increased patient compliance at little additional cost to the practitioner. Patients who comply with their treatment regimen usually can reduce their costs for medical care, as well as the frustration that both the provider and the parent feel when the regimen seems to be producing less-than-desirable results.

If patients have questions or reservations about a treatment regimen, they should be encouraged to discuss them with their provider during the appointment when the recommendations were made. These kinds of conversations between practitioners and patients usually take up less of the practitioner's time in the long run. Even if the parents' questions about the regimen don't surface until they have returned home, it is far better to phone the provider than simply not to comply with the regimen.

The health-care practitioner who takes into account the human factors as well as the medical regimen can find that his or her practice is much more rewarding. It is very frustrating to repeatedly remind patients and their parents that they are not following a regimen correctly. It takes far less effort to implement complex medical regimens correctly in the first place than it does to constantly be making corrections. The provider working cooperatively with the parents and the patient makes an excellent team.

REFERENCES

Barnard MU, Christophersen ER, Moore WV: Glycosylated hemoglobin feedback profile as one behavioral strategy in Type I diabetes. *Res Abstr Diabetes*, 1984.

Barnard MU, Moore WV, Russo L, Christophersen ER: Pseudo-noncompliance in insulin dependent diabetes mellitus. *Program and Abstracts of the 24th Annual Meeting of the Ambulatory Pediatric Association*, 47, 1984.

Becker MH, Maiman LA: Sociobehavioral determinants of compliance with health and medical care recommendations. *Med Care* 13:10–24, 1975.

Christophersen ER, Berman R: Encopresis treatment. *Issues Comprehensive Pediatr Nurs* 3(4):51–66, 1978.

Colcher IS, Bass JW: Penicillin treatment of streptococcal pharyngitis: A comparison of schedules and the role of specific counseling. *JAMA* 222:657–659, 1972.

Finney JW, Friman PC, Rapoff MA, Christophersen ER: Improving compliance with antibiotic regimens for otitis media. *Am J Dis Child* 139:89–95, 1985.

Gordis L, Markowitz, M, Lilienfeld AM: Why patients don't follow medical advice: A study of children on long-term antistreptococcal prophylaxis. *J Pediatr* 75:959–968, 1969.

Haynes RB, Taylor DW, Sackett DL: *Compliance in Health Care*. Baltimore: Johns Hopkins University Press, 1979.

Ley P: Psychological studies of doctor-patient communication, in Rachman S (ed.), *Contributions to Medical Psychology*, Vol. I. New York: Pergamon Press, 1977.

Linkewich JA, Catalano RC, Flack HL: The effect of packaging and instruction on outpatient compliance with medication regimens. *Drug Intelligence Clin Pharmacol* 8:10–15, 1974.

Mathews JR, Christophersen ER: Enhancing pediatric compliance in primary care. *Developmental-Behavioral Disorders: Selected Topics* 2:193–212, 1989.

Rapoff MA, Christophersen ER: Improving compliance in pediatric practice. *Pediatr Clin N Am* 29:339–357, 1982.

Rapoff MA, Lindsley CB, Christophersen ER: Improving compliance with medical regimens: A case study with juvenile rheumatoid arthritis. *Arch Phys Med Rehab* 65:267–269, 1984.

Rapoff MA, Lindsley CB, Christophersen ER: Parent perceptions of problems experienced by their children in complying with treatments for juvenile rheumatoid arthritis. *Arch Phys Med Rehab* 66:427–429, 1985.

Treiber FA: A comparison of the positive and negative consequences approaches upon car restraint usage. *J Pediatr Psychol* 11:15–24, 1986.

Sample Handouts

Management of Diarrhea

Diarrhea often occurs in children and may be due to a viral or bacterial infection. If diarrhea continues without treatment, dehydration may result. Signs of dehydration are decreased urine output, dry mouth, an absence of tears, a sunken soft spot in infants, and a sunken appearance to the eyes. The goal of therapy is to prevent dehydration.

The best treatment for diarrhea is as follows:

1. Give your child clear liquids for 24 hours or until stools decrease in number. Clear liquids are 7-Up; ginger ale; Jell-O water (one package per quart of water); Pedialyte; Lytren; weak, sweetened tea; and Popsicles. Give no juice, milk or milk products, raw fruits or vegetables, spices, or any foods that cause diarrhea. There is no reason to stop breast-feeding an infant with diarrhea; just give him extra water between breast feedings.

2. If the diarrhea has improved (the number of stools has decreased) after 24 hours, start the following solid foods: canned applesauce, fresh bananas, dry toast, boiled or baked potato (without butter), carrots, rice, or rice cereal (without milk). Avoid milk products until your child's stools become more firm. For formula-fed infants, use the formula half-strength for 24 hours, then advance slowly to the regular concentration.

3. Gradually advance the diet back to normal over the next few days.

4. Call your health-care provider if the diarrhea continues more than 3 days, if the child under 2 years of age has more than 10 stools per day, if the child older than 2 years has 15 stools per day, or if any blood, pus, or mucus appears more than once in the stools.

5. Do not use constipating medicines such as Kaopectate or Pepto Bismol.

©Bruce Lieberman and Susan Gifford Lieberman, 1981.

Management of Strep Throat

Strep throat is an infection in the throat that may cause high fever, difficulty in swallowing, headaches, tiredness and weakness, loss of appetite, and sometimes nausea and vomiting. Usually your child will have swollen glands in the neck, and the throat and tonsils will be very red and have pus on them.

If the infection is not treated with antibiotics, your child can develop more serious conditions such as rheumatic fever or kidney disease.

We have done a throat culture, which will tell us whether the germ causing your child's sore throat is strep. If it is, *your child must take 10 days of antibiotics to cure this condition. Anything less will not cure your child.*

We have prescribed an antibiotic for your child; if taken as directed, it will be effective in curing your child's strep throat. If her culture comes back from the laboratory positive for strep, she must take this antibiotic for 10 full days. Continue giving the antibiotic even though your child may feel better after taking the medicine for 2 or 3 days.

When your child has completed the medicine, wait 4 days and come back to the office for another culture to make sure the strep is gone. Strep rarely survives a 10-day course of antibiotics, but if this happens, further treatment is needed. That is why it is important that we see your child and do another culture after the medicine has been finished.

When you come back to the office, please bring the container your child's medicine was in and your medicine recording sheet. Even if there is still medicine in the bottle, or you forgot to mark your sheet every time your child took his medicine, you should bring back both the container and the recording sheet.

©Janice Abernathy and Carl Myers, 1980.

HANDOUT 6.3

Symptom Recording Sheet

Child's Name _____ Month/Year _____

Date	Morning Stiffness	Fever	Pain Complaints	Rash	Activity	Disposi- tion
1						
2						
3						
4						
5						
6						
7						
8						
9						
10						
11						
12						
13						
14						
15						
16						
17						
18						
19						
20						
21						
22						
23						
24						
25						
26						
27						
28						

Date	Morning Stiffness	Fever	Pain Complaints	Rash	Activity	Disposition
29						
30						
31						

KEY:

Morning Stiffness: 0 = no stiffness; 1 = mild stiffness; 2 = moderate stiffness, dressing and moving with difficulty; 3 = severe stiffness, dressing and moving with great difficulty.

Fever: N = none; if present, please write down specific temperature.

Pain complaints: 0 = no complaints; 1 = occasional complaints; 2 = frequent complaints; 3 = complaints frequent and throughout day.

Rash: N = none; 1 = present (please note area rash appeared, for example, "chest").

Activity: 0 = normal activity; 1 = activity somewhat limited; 2 = very little activity, resting often.

Disposition: 0 = pleasant; 1 = neutral; 2 = negative.

©Michael A. Rapoff and Carol B. Lindsley, 1981.

Management of Otitis

The doctor examined your child and found that he has an ear infection—this is called *otitis*. Children who have an ear infection may:

• Complain of an earache
• Rub or tug at their ears
• Be fussy and irritable
• Have a runny nose and cough
• Have a fever
• Have diarrhea
• Not eat very well
• Not sleep very well

Or your child may not show these signs or symptoms. It is very important that you give your child the medicine the doctor prescribed so that your child's ear infection will go away. You *must* give your child the medicine for _____ days to cure the ear infection or the ear infection may come back.

Don't stop giving the medicine to your child because she feels better. Although your child doesn't act sick, she needs the medicine to stay well.

Medication Recording Sheet

Medicine record for _____

Please write in the time you give your child the medicine(s) each day. If you forget a dose, put an "X" in the space. Bring this record and the medicine bottle with you when you return for your child's clinic appointment.

Medicine: _____   Medicine: _____   Medicine: _____

Amount/Dose: _____   Amount/Dose: _____   Amount/Dose: _____

Number Doses/Day: __   Number Doses/Day: __   Number Doses/Day: __

March 1994

Sun	Mon	Tues	Wed	Thurs	Fri	Sat
	1	2	3	4	5	6
7	8	9	10	11	12	13

Protocol for Maximizing Patient Compliance with Chronic Disease Regimens

1. Use regimen checklists for each patient to note the current regimen, as well as any previous or current changes in the regimen.

2. Model and have patients/parents rehearse prescribed regimen components. Give corrective feedback as needed and provide written handouts describing the regimen requirements.

3. Gradually implement complex regimens. Introduce regimen components in a step-by-step fashion as the patient/parent masters prior components ordered in terms of difficulty.

4. Tailor the regimen to the patient's/parents' lifestyle and routine.

5. Provide increased supervision by phone and at return clinic visits.

6. Have patients/parents monitor compliance and disease symptoms using standard recording forms.

7. Teach parents behavior management techniques that can be used to manage general as well as medical compliance problems.

Reprinted with permission from Barnard, M. U. (1985). Glycosylated hemoglobin feedback profile as one behavioral strategy for improving adherence to long-term regimens: Insulin dependent diabetes mellitus. *Dissertation Abstracts International, 47,* 840. University Microfilms No. ADG86-08373.

HANDOUT 6.7

Diabetes Regimen Checklist

Patient's Name _____ Hospital Number _____

	Date	Date	Date	Date	Date
INSULIN					
Type(s)					
Mixture A.M./P.M. Ratio					
Number of Shots					
Rotation					
URINE TESTS					
Types of Test for Sugar and Acetone					
Number Times/Day					
Keep Records					
GHb (A_{1c})					
Blood Glucose					
DIET					
Calories					
Number of Meals					
Number of Snacks					
EXERCISE					
Planned					

Note: Please note changes in prescribed regimen in successive rows for each regimen requirement. In those where there is no change, mark same.

Reprinted with permission from Barnard, M. U. (1985). Glycosylated hemoglobin feedback profile as one behavioral strategy for improving adherence to long-term regimens: Insulin dependent diabetes mellitus. *Dissertation Abstracts International*, 47, 840. University Microfilms No. ADG86-08373.

HANDOUT 6.8

Treatment Regimen Chart

Name _____ Dates _____

	Sun	Mon	Tues	Wed	Thurs	Fri	Sat
Medications							
Exercises							
Splints							

©Michael Rapoff, Ph.D., 1992.

HANDOUT 6.9

HbA$_{1c}$ Chart for Insulin-Dependent Diabetics

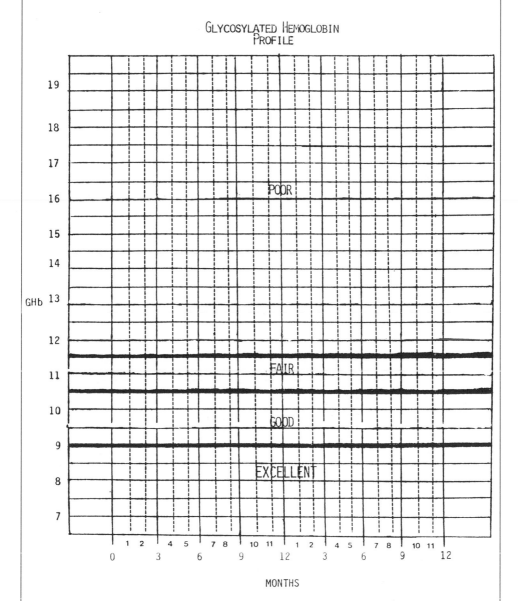

Reprinted with permission from Barnard, M. U. (1985). Glycosylated hemoglobin feedback profile as one behavioral strategy for improving adherence to long-term regimens: Insulin dependent diabetes mellitus. *Dissertation Abstracts International, 47,* 840. University Microfilms No. ADG86-08373.

HANDOUT 6.10

Encopresis Recording Sheet

	Mineral Oil	No. of Suppositories	No. of Enemas	No. of Soilings	No. of Bowel Movements	Size/Consistency	Diet (No. of Servings)	Water (No. of Glasses)	Activity	Time	Comments:
1											
2											
3											
4											
5											
6											
7											
8											
9											
10											
11											
12											
13											
14											
15											
16											
17											
18											
19											
20											
21											

Patient _____

Month _____

	Mineral Oil	No. of Suppositories	No. of Enemas	No. of Soilings	No. of Bowel Movements	Size/Consistency	Diet (No. of Servings)	Water (No. of Glasses)	Activity	Time	
22											
23											
24											
25											
26											
27											
27											
29											
30											
31											

KEY:

Mineral Oil:	Number of tablespoons
Number of Bowel Movements:	In toilet
Size and Consistency:	Approx. no. of cups; H = Hard, S = Soft Formed, D = Diarrhea
Diet:	3 = 3 meals with high-fiber foods; 2 = 2 meals; 1 = 1 meal; 0 = 0 meals
Water:	No. of glasses (6–8 oz.) of water or juices per day
Activity:	3 = very active; 2 = moderately active; 1 = little activity
Time:	Indicates how much time parent spent with child for each BM in toilet (1 BM = 15 minutes; 2 BMs = 30 minutes, etc.)

MEDICAL/BEHAVIORAL PROBLEMS

The problems categorized in Part II as medical/behavioral are those problems that have both a medical and a behavioral component. When parents deal with these types of problems, there is often a physiological component, however small, that enters into the problem. For example, a parent can put a child to bed but cannot make the child sleep. A parent can prepare a meal and place it in front of the child but cannot make the child swallow it. Or a parent can place a child on a toilet but cannot make the child urinate or defecate.

These types of problems often require more skill on the parents' part, because the noncompliance these children exhibit must be dealt with. My experience is that it is far easier, and usually more efficient, to teach parents how to deal with simple noncompliance than it is to teach them to deal with the combination of noncompliance and sleeping, eating, or toileting problems. If the noncompliance is dealt with first, successfully, then parents have the advantage of already having at least some of the skills for encouraging compliance from their child.

Attention Deficit Hyperactivity Disorder also usually has both a compliance component and an organic component. But, unlike sleeping, eating, and toileting problems, it is not usually the case that the behavioral compliance should be dealt with first. Rather, if a child presents with the symptoms of Attention Deficit, he may well learn more from behavior management strategies after he has been placed on a therapeutic dosage of a stimulant medication. What started out as a controversy between behavioral and pharmacological management has gradually evolved into a cooperative effort that often includes both approaches.

Habit disorders, although very common, have probably had the least amount of research time and effort devoted to them. While habits such as thumb sucking and nail biting are extremely common, research on effective treatment programs is not. The work of Azrin and his colleagues is discussed, and recommendations are made for incorporating the management of habit disorders into an office practice.

Each of the chapters in this part includes suggestions on initial evaluation, including intake forms and assessment tools to assist in the gathering of an adequate history prior to any treatment attempts.

Each chapter also includes examples of written treatment protocols that can be used by the practitioner, after the family has had the treatment recommendations explained to them in detail and after they have had adequate time to have their questions answered.

Chapter 7

Techniques for Treating Sleep Onset and Eating Problems

Many problems commonly seen in primary-care settings involve the child's physiology as well as his behavior. The most frequently encountered are problems with eating, sleeping, and toileting. The primary-care provider usually is in the best position to make diagnostic decisions and treatment recommendations for biobehavioral problems, following a thorough assessment of the parents' ability to obtain general behavioral compliance. (See Chapter 8 for a discussion of toileting problems and their treatment.)

7.1. PREVENTING SLEEP PROBLEMS

Problems with children's sleep are quite common and familiar to most pediatric health-care providers. Between birth and about 8 to 12 weeks of age, newborns often fall asleep while nursing. After the first 3 months, babies usually are able to remain awake at the end of a feeding. During this first 3 months, many parents place their sleeping infant in her crib, assuming that they have a "good" baby—a baby who goes to sleep without fussing. However, the time will come when the baby can no longer be placed in the crib asleep. The parents carry the drowsy infant, as carefully as possible, to the crib, but he wakes up and cries when placed in the crib, which results in the parents picking him up again, and so on.

The issue of sleep onset is best dealt with preventively. To facilitate sleep onset, babies should be placed in their crib or bassinet awake, but drowsy, so that they will come to associate the crib or bassinet, or some item or activity in their crib or bassinet, with relaxing and drifting off to sleep. In this way, babies learn "self-transitions" or "sleep-onset" skills they can use every day to assist them in falling asleep. If the child learns to rock herself, suck on her thumb, or hold her blanket a certain way, these transition behaviors will become associated with going to sleep. More important, these sleep onset skills do not require the presence of an adult.

Conversely, the parent who helps the baby go to sleep by rocking, nursing, or lying down next to him is teaching the child sleep onset or transition skills that require the presence of an adult; ultimately, this may create sleep problems.

Anders, Halpern, and Hua (1992) have documented that children who receive assistance with sleep onset at bedtime need the same type of assistance if they awaken in the middle of the night. If, for example, a child is always rocked to sleep, the child will have difficulty falling back to sleep without rocking; thus, the child will cry out for assistance from the parent. The parents thought they had a good baby, a baby who went to sleep easily, when in fact they were actually creating a problem and didn't even know it.

Let's look at two contrasting scenarios.

One mother always nurses her infant to sleep, for each nap during the day and when putting the infant down for the night. When her infant awakens in the middle of the night, she must be nursed in order to get back to sleep.

A second mother always nurses her infant before naps and before bedtime but, after 12 weeks of age, she begins to make sure she places her infant in his crib awake but tired. Sometimes she has to work to get him awake but, realizing the importance of sleep-onset skills, the mother is willing to put forth this additional effort. While the infant almost always stays awake for a little while—a couple of minutes, sometimes cooing or babbling and sometimes fussing or crying—he always manages to fall asleep on his own. The second infant has been encouraged to develop his own sleep-onset skills such that, if he awakens during the night, he has the skills to get back to sleep on his own.

7.1.1. Consistent Sleeping and Waking Schedules

In my experience, children who are put to bed for the night at about the same time every night and awakened at about the same time every morning are easier to get up. They're also more pleasant during the day, and they act as though they feel better.

The only logical reason for parents letting their children sleep later on weekends is that the parents want to sleep later on weekends. If, in fact, the parents and their children awakened at the same time every day, month after month, everyone in the family would probably feel much better, have an easier time with sleep onset, and wake up much more easily. There is little, if anything, to be gained by varying sleep schedules from day to day. Adults who have traveled across multiple time zones well know the feeling of "jet lag." Why subject a child to "home jet lag" when it isn't necessary and when there is no advantage to doing so?

7.1.2. Morning Routines

Before about 3 months of age, infants typically wake from a nap or from a night's sleep and start crying immediately. Between birth and about 3 months of age, there isn't much a parent can do about this awakening procedure. After an infant reaches about 3 months of age, she will wake and make cooing or babbling noises before she starts to fuss or cry. If the parents discipline themselves to go into the infant's room and get her up while she is making these cute noises and before she starts to cry, she will learn to awaken and make cute noises, knowing that an adult will be in to assist her shortly. Contrast this with the parents who always wait until their infant is crying before going into his room to get him up for the day. This second infant is learning that he must cry if he is to receive any assistance from an adult.

7.1.3. Day Naps

One of the biggest temptations for new parents is to allow a sleeping baby, during the day, to continue sleeping until she wakes up on her own. Unfortunately, since babies need only about 16 hours of sleep out of every 24 hours, if they get much of this sleep during the day, they probably will not sleep well at night. For this reason, I recommend, as do other authors (Schmitt, 1991), that under normal circumstances, babies not be allowed to sleep more than 3 hours at a time during the day. That is, if a baby is put down for a nap at 9 A.M. and is still sleeping at noon, I recommend the parent gently awaken the infant.

7.1.4. Intervals between Feedings

Under normal circumstances, I recommend infants not be nursed more frequently than every 3 hours during the day. Schmitt (1991) agrees with this recommendation.

One of the most frequent correlates of night awakenings is what Schmitt calls a "trained night feeder." This refers to a baby who is fed every 2 hours or so during the day.

7.1.5. Carrying Quiet Babies

Schmitt (1991) also recommends that babies be carried for about 3 hours each day—when they are not fussing. While this may be a difficult practice to initiate, because babies do fuss a lot during the first 6 weeks of life, it is important that babies learn how much comfort comes from their parents or caregiver.

7.1.6. Routine Exercise

Most children and their parents don't get enough vigorous exercise. I think that some parents have never established a routine of exercising regularly because they never exercised when they were children and adolescents. If parents make exercise a part of their children's day, beginning during infancy or the toddler years and continuing through adolescence, the children will grow up with exercise as a part of their lives. Three-wheeled strollers are specifically designed for parents who jog, so they can take their children along with them. Long walks through shopping centers on a routine basis can acclimate a child to walking without her ever knowing it is a natural form of exercise.

Regardless of the parents' schedule, either they should organize their child's day to promote good sleep habits or they should require that the child's day-care provider promote these habits. Many day-care centers are now cognizant of good nutrition and the need for exercise. Parents need to ask about these practices before they enroll their child in a day-care center.

7.1.7. Self-Quieting Skills

Brazelton introduced the concept of "self-quieting skills" in 1973. Christophersen (1990) expanded the concept to include teaching self-quieting skills to infants and toddlers.

Most adults who fall asleep easily at bedtime have several characteristics in common:

- They usually fall asleep the same way each evening.
- They usually sleep on the same side of the bed, in the same basic position, every night.
- They have the ability to relax enough to drift off to sleep, which is perhaps as important as any other characteristic.

Infants and toddlers can learn to self-quiet so that they can fall asleep easily almost every night. A comprehensive discussion of self-quieting skills is contained in Chapter 2, including how to encourage the development of self-quieting skills in your infant or toddler.

For children who have trouble relaxing at bedtime, I recommend a procedure called "day correction of sleep problems," which is discussed in the next section.

7.2. MANAGEMENT OF SLEEP PROBLEMS

Prior to recommending any procedure for dealing with sleep problems, a comprehensive history should be taken. Handout 7.1 is the Sleep Intake Form used in our office. The purpose of the Sleep Intake Form is to identify strategies the parents have used in the past, particularly those that created or exacerbated the sleep problems.

The use of such problem-specific intake forms ensures that the same data are collected on each patient, regardless of how hectic the office schedule is on any particular day. The forms also provide a database for the practitioner, in terms of routinely gathering information on the way parents in his or her practice handle their infants' naps and bedtimes.

Because we usually are able to allow the parents adequate time to complete the form (by mailing it out when the parent schedules the appointment), the parents can think about the answers prior to completing the form. With sleep problems as common as they are, and the form as easy to complete as it is, every parent can be asked to complete the form prior to the checkup for their 2-month old infant.

7.2.1. Treatment Options for Sleep Onset

Historically, most of the treatment options for sleep onset have ignored what parents were doing during the day, and treatment options for dealing with night awakening often have not addressed how the child was being put to sleep for the night. Recent research literature has examined planned ignoring, scheduled awakening (Rickert and Johnson, 1988), positive bedtime routines (Adams and Rickert, 1989), and a combination of medication and planned ignoring (France, Blampied, and Wilkinson, 1991). Each has reported some success with the majority of infants.

7.2.1a. Planned Ignoring or Extinction

The terms "planned ignoring" and "extinction" refer to the parents placing a child in bed for the night and walking out, or ignoring the child if he wakens during the night and cries out to his parents. Although Rickert and Johnson (1988) found that planned ignoring was more effective than scheduled awakening for children who awakened during the night and could not go back to sleep by themselves, they reported that parents did not like to use the planned ignoring procedures. Planned ignoring, which has also been called extinction and "letting them cry it out," has been recommended by various professionals for a long time. At the end of 4 weeks of treatment, Rickert and Johnson (1988) reported an average of three night awakenings per week.

7.2.1b. Graduated Extinction

Graduated extinction is a variation of planned ignoring or extinction. The major difference is that the parents, instead of abruptly beginning the procedure of placing their child in bed and leaving him there for the entire night, go in after increasingly longer and longer periods of time. Thus, they may go back into the child's room at 5-minute intervals, then 10-minute intervals, then 15-minute intervals. Using graduated extinction, Adams and Rickert (1989) reported that, after 4 weeks of treatment, the typical family had an average of 1.5 night awakenings per week. The graduated extinction procedure is similar to what Ferber (1985) recommended.

If the parents can follow through with the planned ignoring, and if what they are doing during the day does not act directly against what they are doing with the night awakenings (see section below on "Day Correction of Sleep Problems"), the child will usually learn to sleep through the night.

7.2.1c. Scheduled Awakening

Scheduled awakening refers to a procedure in which the parents are instructed to set their own alarm clock so that they can go into their child's room and awaken him prior to the time that he normally awakens in the middle of the night. At the end of 4 weeks of treatment, Rickert and Johnson (1988) reported an average of eight night awakenings per week. While planned ignoring works better than scheduled awakening, according to Rickert and Johnson (1988), parents prefer to use the scheduled awakening procedures.

7.2.1d. Positive Routines

Adams and Rickert (1989) also evaluated a procedure called "positive routines." With positive routines, parents are instructed to select several quiet activities to do with their child in the 20 minutes immediately prior to bedtime. At the end of the 20 minutes, the parents would refuse to interact with the child (similar to planned ignoring except for the 20 minutes of pleasant activities preceding bedtime). Adams and Rickert reported that, after 4 weeks of treatment, the average child was exhibiting bedtime tantrums 1.5 times per week.

7.2.1e. Medication and Extinction Combined

France et al. (1991) reported on the use of medication during the initial introduction of planned ignoring or extinction in an effort to lessen the fussing at bedtime that many parents find so objectionable. They medicated children (with trimeprazine) and instructed the parents to put the children to bed and not go back into the child's room. The medication was decreased each evening for 10 nights until no medication was used prior to bedtime. The children in the extinction plus medication group showed an immediate decrease to an average of 0.5 awakenings per night. The children in both the extinction alone and the extinction plus medication group had an average of 0.5 awakenings per night by the end of the second week of treatment. In the extinction plus medication group, there was a sharp increase in night awakenings following the discontinuation of the medication on the 10th night.

7.2.1f. The Breast-Fed Infant

Pinilla and Birch (1993) demonstrated that infants who were exclusively breast-fed could be taught to sleep through the night during the first 8 weeks of life. The mothers were taught to gradually lengthen the intervals between middle-of-the-night feedings by carrying out alternative caregiving activities such as diapering, reswaddling, and walking.

7.2.2. Day Correction of Sleep Problems

Research by Rapoff, Christophersen, and Rapoff (1982), Adair, Zuckerman, Bauchner, Philipp, and Levenson (1992), and Anders, Halpern, and Hua (1992) has shown that problems with sleep onset are correlated with what the child's parents are doing with their child when he is put down for the night. For this reason, we have developed and evaluated a treatment program that begins by changing what the parents are doing during the day as well as at bedtime (Christophersen, 1990).

Children need three important conditions to fall asleep alone at night. First, *they must be tired*. The easiest way to ensure a child will be tired when she goes to bed is by providing opportunities during the day for vigorous exercise that requires a good deal of energy. Second, *they must be quiet*. We recommend parents close an infant's door and keep it closed throughout the night. This will keep the infant's room quiet without the entire household having to be quiet. Parents can turn on the furnace or air-conditioning fan for the first few days and nights as a masking noise. Third, *they must be relaxed*. The only way children can relax is if they have learned, or been taught, self-quieting skills. While older children (at least 6 years of age) can actually be taught relaxation procedures, infants and toddlers need to practice self-quieting skills in order to learn them. The baby who goes to sleep with assistance from one of his parents (through nursing, rocking, or holding) learns only adult-dependent sleep-onset skills: The adult must be present in order for the child to fall asleep. The baby or toddler who goes to sleep alone (with a Care Bear, with his favorite blanket, or by sucking his thumb) learns valuable self-quieting behaviors that can be used for many years to come. When these three conditions have been met, children who have adequate self-quieting skills will be able to fall asleep easily.

Children who go to bed easily and sleep through the night uninterrupted get a much better night's sleep than children who wake up several times during the night. As a result, they feel better during the day—just like adults feel better the day after they've had a good night's sleep.

Handout 7.2 for parents summarizes the recommendations for what we have termed "day correction of sleep problems." The essence of these recommendations is that parents should provide many opportunities for their children to learn self-quieting skills during the day, prior to any attempt to directly address sleep onset.

In Edwards's study (1992), half of the young children's problems with sleep onset were resolved by teaching them self-quieting skills during the day—without actually treating the child at the time of sleep onset. The other half of the children's problems with sleep onset were resolved within 1 week after the parents began "planned ignoring" at bedtime and in the middle of the night. Perhaps the most interesting finding in the Edwards study was that the parents actually liked using the procedures. This contrasts sharply with Rickert and Johnson's (1988) study, which showed that traditional planned ignoring took a full month to reach less than 90% effectiveness and the parents reported disliking the treatment procedures. Rickert and Johnson's study showed that, although planned ignoring was the most effective procedure that they investigated, the parents disliked it because they had to listen to their child cry, sometimes for long periods of time, at bedtime and/or in the middle of the night. With our day correction procedure, the child learns self-quieting skills during the day, which means that the parents have much less fussing to cope with at bedtime. In fact, several of the parents in our study reported, after the study was over, that they were dreading the time when they had to put their child to bed, leave the room, and listen to their child cry, only to find out that the child simply didn't fuss that much.

A recent study by Adair et al. (1992) produced similar findings with similar intervention procedures (facilitating sleep onset without the parent present).

7.3. PREVENTING EATING PROBLEMS

The vast majority of eating problems in young children are the result of parents' simply not knowing enough about how eating behaviors develop—not from an organic problem in the child (O'Brien, Repp, Williams, and Christophersen, 1991).

As many as 45% of normally developing children have mealtime problems (Bentovim, 1970). Only recently has much research been published on the development of eating behaviors with normal infants and toddlers. Several recommendations, if implemented with the infant, may help prevent eating problems later on in life. If implemented for a toddler, the recommendations may resolve existing problems.

Most adults will notice their appetites are greater when they have done a lot of physical work; children are the same way. The same exercise that benefits children at bedtime also can give them better appetites.

Like sleeping, eating seems to be greatly facilitated by placing the child on a consistent schedule and keeping her on it. Putting a child to bed at about the same time every night and waking her about the same time each morning can contribute to making a child a good eater.

Until they are eating well, children should be offered meals at consistent times, given regular exercise, and given little by mouth (except perhaps water) between meals. They never should be coerced or forced to eat a particular food. Distractions during meals, like television or commotion at or near the dinner table, negatively affect children's eating.

Finney (1986) has provided an excellent review of the research literature on common feeding problems in young children. Handout 7.3 lists his recommendations for introducing solid foods to babies between the age of 2 months and 4 months. This handout is intended to be distributed to parents at the 2-month office visit. These recommendations come from a professional who has extensive experience treating children with eating disorders, and the recommendations merit consideration for adaptation in primary-care settings. Parents who follow these recommendations will, generally, not need significant changes in mealtime until their child is older and they are faced with introducing much greater varieties and textures in food.

A second Finney handout, Handout 7.4, provides mealtime suggestions for parents of 15- to 18-month-old children.

7.4. EARLY DETECTION OF EATING PROBLEMS

The present author (Christophersen, 1982) suggested using a series of questions during well-child visits to determine whether parents have mealtime problems:

1. What are your child's favorite foods?
2. What are some foods your child doesn't like?
3. How long does a meal typically take?
4. How many times does your child disrupt a meal?
5. What kinds of snacks does your child prefer?
6. How often does your child get snacks?

These questions enable the pediatrician to solicit information from the parents to determine whether the child is starting to develop mealtime problems.

The time-honored tradition of asking parents if they have any mealtime problems or questions assumes parents know how to identify such problems. If the pediatrician needs more information about a child's behavior during mealtimes, Handouts 7.5 and 7.6 will elicit a good deal of information regarding the child's eating behavior.

If the answers to the feeding intake suggest that the parents are using troublesome strategies at mealtime, the pediatrician may need to schedule the parents for more time to discuss the parents' feeding practices or, alternatively, to refer the family to a professional experienced in dealing with mealtime problems.

7.5. BEHAVIOR PROBLEMS AT MEALTIME

Behavior problems at mealtimes often can be handled with relatively simple solutions, primarily because, as O'Brien et al. (1991) point out, the majority of mealtime behavior problems stem from parental mismanagement. That is, the way parents approach mealtime can actually contribute to problems at mealtime. In the vast majority of children who present with mealtime problems, the parents aren't able to demonstrate behavioral compliance with other requests or demands. Mealtime problems, then, are simply an extension of the child's noncompliance.

Handouts 7.7 and 7.8 are designed to help parents handle the two most commonly encountered mealtime problems: behavioral problems and poking and stalling.

Children who present with serious eating problems should be referred to a medical center that has a treatment program that specializes in children with eating disorders. Inquire carefully about the background and training of professionals before referring a young child with eating problems to them. Major problems at mealtime require a professional with extensive prior training in the treatment of pediatric eating disorders. Often, referral to a major teaching program hundreds of miles away is preferable to referral to a local practitioner who is not properly trained, simply because major tertiary-care centers are more likely to have individuals on staff who are experienced in dealing with eating disorders.

7.6. IMPROVING THE APPETITE OF INFANTS

When children below the age of 30 months are seen with weights and heights below the fifth percentile but no demonstrable organicity, they typically also present with a lack of appetite.

Initially, as with the vast majority of biobehavioral problems, parents should be given general compliance training for approximately 1 month, or until they demonstrate to the primary-care provider that they can routinely obtain compliance with the normal day-to-day requests of their children.

If the parents cannot obtain general compliance, treatment of the eating problems should be discontinued until the parents can demonstrate their child's compliance with reasonable day-to-day commands. While the parents are practicing how to obtain general compliance with their children, the child with eating problems can be placed on a protocol for increasing his appetite.

7.6.1. Increasing the Appetite

Some children get accustomed to eating very little food and place severe restrictions on the types and textures of foods they will eat. Typically, these children do not have much of an appetite. The following recommendations are designed to improve the child's appetite while removing pressure from parents who are trying to get the child to eat more. Normally, the protocol should be followed for at least 1 month.

7.6.1a. Scheduled Mealtimes

The child should be given four liquid meals per day, spaced equally throughout the waking hours. Meals should consist of a balanced liquid diet, such as Ensure, for children 2 to 6 years of age; PediaSure, for children 1 to 3 years old; and Isomil, a soy-based formula for babies who cannot tolerate milk products.

At each meal, offer the child the contents of one full can. If she will drink more, give her more. Meals should be given at about the same time each day.

7.6.1b. Intake Records

Parents and caregivers should keep track, in writing, of how many ounces the child consumes at each meal. A written diary should be kept of every food the child swallows so that the exact number of calories consumed can be computed. The primary-care practitioner must be able to document that the child has had enough daily calories to gain weight.

7.6.1c. Weight

The child should be weighed monthly and his weight recorded, preferably on the same professional scale. Weighing more often is unnecessary and can lead to more frustration on the parents' part.

7.6.1d. Eating between Meals

The less the child eats between meals, the better. Under no circumstances should the child be given anything by mouth within 90 minutes of the next scheduled meal. Parents and caregivers must resist the temptation of giving food between meals.

7.6.1e. Exercise

Children need good, sustained, vigorous exercise every day. In bad weather, this can consist of a long walk in a shopping mall. In good weather, children should be taken for long walks outside. The optimum is about 20 minutes of sustained exercise.

7.6.1f. Mealtimes

Mealtimes should be pleasant. The parent or caregiver should sit with the child and eat as though it is a normal meal. There should be no nagging, coaxing, or the like.

7.6.1g. Length of Meals

After about 20 minutes, the meal should be terminated without any fanfare. Parents or caregivers should clear the table in much the same manner they would for a normal meal the family had completed.

By following this protocol, the parent or caregiver is able to document whether the child has ingested enough calories to gain weight. This protocol also removes most of the pressure parents may have been feeling about getting their child to eat. The liquid meals are nutritionally balanced and include all of the ingredients currently known to be necessary for a child.

Any decisions regarding modifications in the protocol must await adequate weight gain for at least 1 month, possibly longer. If the child is given an adequate number of calories to gain weight, and does gain weight, it is less likely a medical problem is responsible for the child's inability to gain weight. Conversely, if the child is given enough calories to virtually guarantee adequate weight gain, but does not gain weight, the search for organic causes can be resumed with confidence.

7.7 CONCLUDING REMARKS

When problems related to sleeping and eating are diagnosed and treated, the physical components of these problems cannot and should not be overlooked. The practitioner should always begin with a thorough history and physical examination to rule out organicity. When the initial evaluation suggests there is no relevant organicity, the practitioner should proceed with behavioral intervention. General compliance training should always precede attempts to deal with the specific problem. A number of treatment procedures are now available that have been in use for a long time and that have a sound scientific basis.

REFERENCES

Adair R, Zuckerman B, Bauchner H, Philipp B, Levenson S: Reducing night waking in infancy: A primary care intervention. *Pediatrics* 89:585–588, 1992.

Adams LA, Rickert VI: Reducing bedtime tantrums: Comparison between positive routines and graduated extinction. *Pediatrics* 84:756–761, 1989.

Anders TF, Halpern LF, Hua J: Sleeping through the night: A developmental perspective. *Pediatrics* 90(4):554–560, 1992.

Bentovim A: The clinical approach to feeding disorders of childhood. *J Psychosom Res* 14:267–276, 1970.

Brazelton TB: *Neonatal Behavioral Assessment Scale*. Philadelphia: Lippincott, 1973.

Christophersen ER: Incorporating behavioral pediatrics into primary care. *Pediatr Clin N Am* 29(2):261–296, 1982.

Christophersen ER: *Beyond Discipline: Parenting That Lasts a Lifetime*, Kansas City, MO: Westport Publishers, 1990.

Edwards KJ: Assisting young children with sleep onset by changing what the parents are doing during the day. Unpublished manuscript, 1992.

Ferber R: *Solve Your Child's Sleep Problems*. New York: Simon and Schuster, 1985.

Finney JW: Preventing common feeding problems in infants and young children. *Pediatr Clin N Am* 33:775–788, 1986.

France KG, Blampied NM, Wilkinson P: Treatment of infant sleep disturbance by Trimeprazine in combination with extinction. *J Dev Behav Pediatr* 12:308–314, 1991.

O'Brien S, Repp AC, Williams GE, Christophersen ER: Pediatric feeding disorders. *Behav Modif* 15:394–418, 1991.

Pinilla T, Birch L: Help me make it through the night: Behavioral entrainment of breast-fed infants' sleep patterns. *Pediatrics* 91:436–444, 1993.

Rapoff MA, Christophersen ER, Rapoff KE: The management of common childhood bedtime problems by pediatric nurse practitioners. *J Pediatr Psychol* 7(2):179–196, 1982.

Rickert VI, Johnson M: Reducing nocturnal awakening and crying episodes in infants and young children: A comparison between scheduled awakenings and systematic ignoring. *Pediatrics* 81:203–211, 1988.

Schmitt BD: *Your Child's Health*. New York: Bantam Books, 1991.

Sample Handouts

Intake for Children with Sleep Problems

Child's Name _____ Date of Birth _____

Mother's Name _____ Age _____

Father's Name _____ Age _____

Street _____ City/State _____ Zip _____

Home Phone _____ Office Phone _____

What is the present problem? _____

Breast-Fed _____   Bottle-Fed _____   Solids _____

Where did child sleep as a newborn? _____

Where does child sleep now? _____

Number of night feedings as newborn _____

Age when slept through the night first time _____

Length and time of morning nap _____

Length and time of afternoon nap _____

Time put down for the night _____

Where put down for the night _____

Number of night awakenings _____

How does child fall asleep for naps? _____

How does child fall asleep for night? _____

Is sleep any different for sitters/relatives? _____

What have you tried before? _____

    Breast-feeding   _____   Rocking   _____

    Crying to sleep   _____   Lying down with child _____

    Alone with bottle _____   On sofa/parent's bed   _____

    Medication   _____   Other devices   _____

From whom have you sought help before? _____

When did present problem start? _____

What do you think is going on? _____

Other children and their ages _____

HANDOUT 7.2

Day Correction of Bedtime Problems

There are three important components to getting a child to go to sleep alone at night. The child must be:

1. Tired.   2. Quiet.   3. Relaxed.

When these three components are in place, children who have adequate "self-transition" behaviors will be able to go to sleep rather easily.

Tired. The easiest way to make sure your child will be tired when she goes to bed is by giving her an adequate amount of exercise during the day—vigorous exercise that requires a good deal of energy. For an infant, this might include several long periods of time when he is on the floor and can see what you are doing, but he must hold his head up in order to really see much. For almost any child, 20 minutes of good exercise each day is usually adequate.

Quiet. You can elect to either quiet down the entire house or quiet down your child's room. Quieting down the child's room by closing the door and keeping it closed is probably easiest. You might need to turn on the furnace or air conditioning fan as a masking noise for the first few days and nights.

Relaxed. Children can relax only if they have learned, or been taught, self-quieting skills. Self-quieting skills refer to a child's ability to calm himself, with no help from an adult, when he is unhappy or angry. While older children (above at least 6 years of age) can actually be taught relaxation procedures, infants and toddlers need to practice self-quieting in order to learn it. Perhaps the easiest way to teach self-quieting, during the day, is through the frequent use of time-outs (either in the playpen for babies or in the chair for toddlers).

Self-transition behaviors. The baby who goes to sleep with help from one of her parents by nursing, rocking, or holding learns only adult-transition behaviors and needs an adult present in order to fall asleep. The baby or toddler who goes to sleep alone cuddling a Care Bear, holding his favorite blanket, or sucking his thumb learns valuable self-transition behaviors that can be used for many years to come.

How they feel. Children who go to bed easily and sleep through the night uninterrupted get a very good night's sleep. They will feel better during the day—just like you feel better during the day after you've had a good night's sleep. It may take from several days to 1 week to teach a child the skills she needs for going to sleep alone, but this is one behavior she'll be able to use for years to come.

The three components described here have the added advantage that they can be taught during the day, which removes many of the fears parents have about handling behavioral problems encountered at bedtime.

Edward R. Christophersen, *Beyond Discipline: Parenting That Lasts a Lifetime.* Kansas City, MO: Westport Publishers. ©Edward R. Christophersen, 1992.

Introducing Solid Foods to Infants

1. *Feed only breast milk or infant formula to infants under the age of 4 months.*

2. *From 4 to 6 months of age, begin to introduce solid foods*, starting with iron-fortified infant cereal. At first, solids are started simply to give your baby practice with new tastes, new textures, and a new way of eating. Your baby will continue to get all the food he needs from breast- or bottle-feedings.

3. *In the beginning, do not expect your baby to swallow much cereal.* Your baby will take bites, but her tongue movements will push the food out of her mouth. That's normal. It takes a while for your baby to learn to keep the bites in her mouth.

4. *Start with one new food at a time.* Feed your baby the new food a few times over 3 or 4 days, before starting another new food, to make sure your baby doesn't have an allergic reaction. Vomiting, diarrhea, a skin rash, or gas is a sign that the food does not agree with your baby. If your baby has a reaction, do not serve that food again for a few months.

5. *Be relaxed about the first few weeks of introducing solid foods.* In the first few weeks it is not important how much cereal or fruit your baby eats. Your baby needs time to adjust to the new tastes, textures, and way of eating that solid foods require.

6. *Do not rush through mealtimes.* If you rush, meals will not be pleasant for you or your baby.

7. *Talk, sing, make faces, and touch your baby during meals.* Meals should be fun times for you and your baby.

8. *Expect your baby to be distracted during meals.* She is likely to turn her head when there are noises, when people talk, or when the telephone rings. Wait until your baby turns back before you offer another bite, or talk to your baby to get her attention.

9. *Keep mealtimes safe.* Use straps to keep your baby in an infant seat or high chair. Do not put an infant seat on a table, but rather sit on the floor to feed your baby so that there is no chance for him to fall. Never leave a baby alone in a room while he is eating.

10. *Get a bib that is plastic-backed.* Bibs with sleeves help keep shirt sleeves clean, but expect your baby to learn quickly how to get food on clothing even with a bib.

11. *Expect every meal to result in a mess.* There will be food on the baby, on you, and on the floor. When your baby begins to hold a cup, grab the spoon, and practice with finger foods, the mess will be worse.

12. *Most babies from 6 to 9 months of age want to hold a cup and finger foods.* After your baby has eaten the main foods for each meal, give her practice with a cup and finger foods toward the end of each meal. When your baby begins to hold a cup and finger foods, she will spill liquids and smear food all over her face and arms, the table or high chair, and the floor. Dropping cups, spoons, and food becomes a favorite game for most babies.

13. *Put a small blanket, a sheet, a drop cloth, or newspapers under your baby's high chair* if you prefer washing those rather than the floor. A small portable vacuum can be useful for quick cleanups.

14. *Babies often gag when new foods are introduced.* New tastes and textures can make your baby gag. If the food is lumpy, make the lumps smoother and try a few more bites. If the food has a new taste, combine a few bites with a favorite food to get your baby used to the taste. Babies sometimes gag toward the end of the meal; this usually means your baby is not hungry and the meal should be over.

15. *Babies sometimes spit up or vomit at meals* if they eat too fast or eat too much. Clean up spit-up and vomiting matter-of-factly. If your baby doesn't seem to be sick and still seems hungry, offer a few bites more.

16. *When your baby consistently refuses to eat a food, wait* for about 2 weeks before offering that food again. For example, if you offer carrots and your child spits out every bite, wait 2 weeks before offering carrots again. If she still refuses, try putting a small bite of carrots with a bite of her favorite food, gradually adding more carrot and less of the favorite food. Don't expect your baby to eat all foods, however. As long as she eats a few selections from the major food groups (cereal, fruit, vegetable, and meat), your baby can have a balanced diet.

17. *Snacks can fill up babies.* Keep between-meal snacks to a minimum. Give water and juice between meals and bottle-feedings to satisfy thirst, especially in hot weather, but don't go overboard. On days when your baby doesn't eat well, review the snacks he received; too many snacks may result in poor eating at meals.

18. *When your baby cries or turns away from you, turn away* briefly from your baby for 10 to 15 seconds, then offer him another bite of food. Babies often cry at the beginning of a meal when they are very hungry. Several bites of food should calm them down.

19. *End a meal if your child gets really fussy* or just wants to play with the food. When your baby starts to fuss or play, it probably means she has had enough to eat. Don't let a big battle start because your child doesn't want to eat or you don't want to waste food. Your child will be ready to eat better at the next meal.

20. *Talk to your child frequently.* Play a game—airplane is a favorite—when giving bites to keep the meal interesting and fun. Make funny faces and noises. Use touch to let your child know that mealtime is a special time. Remember that mealtimes can be a pleasant time to nurture and interact with your child. There are many opportunities for parent and child battles; don't make mealtimes "battle times."

©Jack W. Finney, 1986.

HANDOUT 7.4

Suggestions for Feeding Children Aged 15 to 18 Months

Mealtime should be a pleasant family time. Yet, most parents have problems at one time or another with their child's mealtime behavior. Perhaps your child:

- Frequently leaves the table.
- Throws food.
- Does not use eating utensils.
- Watches TV instead of eating.
- Refuses to eat, then constantly demands snacks.
- Eats very slowly.
- Is a picky eater.
- Cries or throws a tantrum during meals.
- Rushes through the meal.

Mealtime is the time to teach your child the kind of manners and behavior you want him to exhibit when eating. Your child should learn one set of manners that are appropriate at all meals—whether eating at home, with company, at a restaurant, or at someone else's house.

The following guidelines will help you teach your child appropriate mealtime behavior. If you follow the guidelines consistently, mealtime will no longer be a problem. You and your child will enjoy mealtime and will be able to look forward to it as a special time you have together.

GUIDELINES FOR IMPROVING MEALTIME BEHAVIOR

1. *Establish sit-down, family-style meals*, where everyone sits down together to eat. Turn off the television.

2. *Set a reasonable time limit for each meal* (for example, from 15 to 25 minutes). Try using a portable kitchen timer to indicate when the meal is over.

3. *Establish a set of mealtime rules for your child*. Some examples are:

   - You must remain seated.
   - You are to use your silverware, not your fingers.
   - Don't throw food.
   - Close your mouth when you chew.

185

The rules should be reasonable and be based on the age of your child. Don't expect a young child to learn all the rules quickly. Start with two or three rules. After your child has learned to follow them, add a few more rules at a time, until gradually you have introduced all the rules.

4. *Tell your child the rules* (using a nice tone of voice) once at the beginning of each meal until the child has learned to follow them consistently. Do not nag your child about the rules.

5. *Give your child small portions of preferred foods*—an amount you are sure the child will eat. You can always give more. At first, give a small amount that your child must eat to succeed, then praise your child for eating it. Gradually increase the quantity you require the child to eat and the types of food you want the child to try. Do not make your child "clean the plate."

6. *Do not carry on conversations with another adult* for longer than a few minutes at a time. Include your child in conversations and talk about things you know interest your child. Make sure you do not nag, threaten, or warn during mealtimes. Use mealtime as an opportunity to praise your child for appropriate behaviors throughout the day and to teach your child how to behave in a social situation.

7. *Be sure to praise your child for appropriate behaviors* such as using utensils, sitting quietly, and talking nicely whenever they occur throughout the meal. You cannot praise too often. Praise is how you teach your child what behavior pleases you.

8. *If your child breaks a rule, have the child practice the correct behavior.* The third time your child breaks any rule, use discipline. Time-out is one good way to teach your child the rules at meals. Put your child in time-out for misbehaviors as many times as necessary until the time limit for the meal is up.

9. *When the time for the meal is up, clear the table,* regardless of whether your child is finished. Do not say anything to your child beyond announcing that the meal is over. Once your child usually stays at the table and finishes meals on time, you can stop using the timer.

10. *If your child did not finish the last meal,* either because he refused to eat or because he was in time-out and ran out of time, do not offer dessert and do not allow your child to eat or drink anything except water until the next meal. If your child whines and constantly asks for snacks, place the child in time-out.

11. *Even under normal circumstances, limit snacks.* If you allow your child to fill up on snacks, the child will not be as hungry at mealtimes. Give snacks that have nutritional value, such as carrot sticks, raisins, and fruit, rather than junk food like potato chips, corn chips, and cookies. You will also be teaching your child good eating habits.

12. *When your child has learned to follow your mealtime rules consistently,* you no longer need to go over them at the beginning of each meal. However, it is still a good idea to review the rules from time to time. The best way to do this is to "catch 'em being good": Remind your child of a rule by praising the child for following it.

SUMMARY

1. Set a reasonable time limit for the meal.
2. Establish mealtime rules.
3. Give small portions.
4. Include your child in the conversation.
5. Provide frequent, gentle, nonverbal physical contact, with occasional verbal praise.
6. Use time-out after the third time your child breaks a rule.
7. End the meal when the time is up.
8. Do not give your child dessert, snacks, or drinks, except water, if she did not finish the last meal.
9. Limit snacks.
10. "Catch 'em being good."

©Jack W. Finney, 1986.

HANDOUT 7.5

Behavioral Pediatrics Feeding Intake Form

Interviewed by: _____

Date of Evaluation: _____ CMH No.: _____

Child's Name: _____

Parent's Name: _____

Date of Birth: _____

Telephone No. Home (   ) _____ Work (   ) _____

Address: _____

City/State _____

Zip Code _____

Child's Weight _____ Height _____ Head Circumference _____

Height/Weight Percentile _____

Family history of small stature? _____

Present medications taking _____

Medications taken during the last year _____

_____

Allergies _____

Vitamins _____

Caloric supplements _____

Diet restrictions _____

Presenting problem _____

_____

Referred by _____

Child has been seen in the last 6 months by (circle all appropriate)

    Medical Doctor   Occupational Therapist   Physical Therapist

    Nutritionist   Speech Therapist   Psychologist

PLEASE CIRCLE ALL APPROPRIATE ANSWERS

Mental Development: Normal   Delayed
    Describe any mental delays _____
Physical Development: Normal   Delayed
    Describe any physical delays _____
Physical Problem: CP   Cardiac   Cancer   Metabolic   Other
    Describe any physical problems _____

Oral/Motor Development:
    Tongue thrust   Poor suck   Drools   Hypersensitivity
Child is fed in:
    Lap   Infant seat   Highchair   Bed   Chair at table   Booster seat
Child drinks from:
    Bottle   Training cup   Straw   Cup/Glass
Child is fed by:
    IV   CT   NG tube   Breast
Who feeds the child?
    Parent   Nurse   Self   Other _____
Child will accept the following texture of foods:
    Strained   Junior   Blenderized   Mashed   Chopped   Regular
At mealtime, child:
    Drools   Refuses   Won't swallow food   Gags   Vomits
    Cries   Spits food   Throws food   Steals food   Messy eater
    Other _____
How do you get bites accepted?
    Praise   Ignore   Distract   Reason   Force   Threaten
    Mix or coat foods   Other _____
Child's activity level is:
    None   Low   Average   Active   Overactive
Child's appetite is:
    Poor   Fair   Good   Average   Excellent   Eats too much

PLEASE ANSWER THE FOLLOWING QUESTIONS

Generally, meals last for how long? Breakfast _____ Lunch _____ Dinner _____

    Snacks _____

Typical meal times are: Breakfast _____ Lunch _____ Dinner _____ Snack _____

Who typically prepares/feeds the meal? Breakfast _____ Lunch _____

    Dinner _____ Snacks _____

Is TV on during the meal? Yes _____ No _____

Does your child play with toys during meals? Yes _____ No _____

    Which ones? _____

List preferred foods your child will eat:

    Meats _____

    Vegetables _____

    Starches _____

    Fruits _____

    Sweets _____

    Liquids _____

    Other _____

List foods your child will not eat:

    Meats _____

    Vegetables _____

    Starches _____

    Fruits _____

    Sweets _____

    Liquids _____

    Other _____

How often are nonpreferred foods served? _____

What food/liquids does your child receive between meals? _____

_____

Describe a typical meal for the day:

    Breakfast _____

    Lunch _____

    Dinner _____

    Snacks _____

Is there a sequence in which foods are presented (e.g., liquids are always served first)? _____

_____

Bedtime _____ Wake-up time _____ Naptime _____

Activities your child likes to do _____

_____

HANDOUT 7.6

Behavioral Pediatrics Feeding Assessment

Name: _____ Date: _____

Directions: Below is a series of phrases that describe children's eating and parental behaviors. Please (1) circle the number describing how often the behavior occurs with your child and (2) circle "Yes" or "No" to indicate whether the behavior is currently a problem for you.

Child	Never		Sometimes		Always	Problem for You?	
1. Has a poor appetite	1	2	3	4	5	Yes	No
2. Refuses strained baby foods	1	2	3	4	5	Yes	No
3. Refuses junior baby foods	1	2	3	4	5	Yes	No
4. Refuses toddler baby foods	1	2	3	4	5	Yes	No
5. Refuses ground table foods	1	2	3	4	5	Yes	No
6. Refuses regular table foods	1	2	3	4	5	Yes	No
7. Won't chew foods	1	2	3	4	5	Yes	No
8. Has strong likes or dislikes	1	2	3	4	5	Yes	No
9. Throws foods or mealtime objects	1	2	3	4	5	Yes	No
10. Refuses to self-feed	1	2	3	4	5	Yes	No
11. Refuses medications	1	2	3	4	5	Yes	No
12. Refuses vitamins	1	2	3	4	5	Yes	No
13. Eats longer than 20 minutes	1	2	3	4	5	Yes	No
14. Goes to sleep by breast/bottle	1	2	3	4	5	Yes	No
15. Spits out food	1	2	3	4	5	Yes	No
16. Holds food in mouth	1	2	3	4	5	Yes	No
17. Gags or coughs during meals	1	2	3	4	5	Yes	No
18. Doesn't eat meats	1	2	3	4	5	Yes	No
19. Doesn't eat vegetables	1	2	3	4	5	Yes	No
20. Doesn't eat starches	1	2	3	4	5	Yes	No
21. Doesn't eat fruits	1	2	3	4	5	Yes	No
22. Refuses liquids	1	2	3	4	5	Yes	No
23. Drinks limited types of liquids	1	2	3	4	5	Yes	No
24. Tantrums at feeding time	1	2	3	4	5	Yes	No
25. Cries at feeding time	1	2	3	4	5	Yes	No
26. Drools	1	2	3	4	5	Yes	No
27. Has nausea	1	2	3	4	5	Yes	No
28. Vomits or ruminates	1	2	3	4	5	Yes	No
29. Plays with food at table	1	2	3	4	5	Yes	No
30. Gets up from table during meal	1	2	3	4	5	Yes	No
31. Nags for or sneaks snacks	1	2	3	4	5	Yes	No
32. Has a weight problem	1	2	3	4	5	Yes	No
33. Is noncompliant outside meals	1	2	3	4	5	Yes	No

Parent

	Never		Sometimes		Always	Problem for You?	
34. Frustrated with feedings	1	2	3	4	5	Yes	No
35. Coaxes to get bite accepted	1	2	3	4	5	Yes	No
36. Uses threats for acceptance	1	2	3	4	5	Yes	No
37. Uses distractions for acceptance	1	2	3	4	5	Yes	No
38. Mixes or coats foods	1	2	3	4	5	Yes	No
39. Always serves preferred foods	1	2	3	4	5	Yes	No
40. Never serves nonpreferred foods	1	2	3	4	5	Yes	No
41. Mom feeds meals	1	2	3	4	5	Yes	No
42. Dad feeds meals	1	2	3	4	5	Yes	No

HANDOUT 7.7

Mealtime Behavior Problems

Mealtime should not only be pleasant family time but also a time when you teach your child the kind of manners and behavior you want him to exhibit when eating. If you allow your child to misbehave during mealtimes at home, the same thing will happen when you go out or have company.

"Company manners" can be taught to your child during regular meals at home. If you *consistently* follow these procedures, mealtime will not be a problem, and "company manners" and "regular manners" will become the same.

1. *Establish reasonable rules for your child.* For example:

   a. You must remain seated.
   b. Food is chewed with your closed mouth and it is swallowed, not spit out.

   The rules will depend on the age of your child. Discuss these rules with your health-care provider.

2. *Be sure to provide a good deal of brief, nonverbal physical contact whenever your child shows appropriate behavior.* Do this often. Prompt the behaviors you want. This is how you teach your child to behave at mealtime.

3. *Teach your child the behaviors you want.* Once he has exhibited the behaviors you want, you can be assured he knows the rules. Any infraction of the rules after that should be considered inappropriate.

4. *Be sure to include your child in the mealtime conversation.* Do not carry on adult conversations for extended periods of time, as this invites your child to misbehave at mealtime.

5. *If your child breaks a rule, remove her from the table* (time-out) and have her practice the correct behavior.

6. *To avoid having a time-out become a game, only use it twice* for any behavior during a meal. The third time a rule is broken, the meal is over.

7. *If your child continues to misbehave, remove him from the table* and take away his plate—regardless of how much he has eaten. This should be done matter-of-factly. There is no need to nag him about what he has done. This will not hurt your child and will not have to be done often.

8. *Do not allow your child to eat or drink anything except water until the next meal.*

9. *Discipline whining* or constantly asking for snacks by placing your child in time-out.

10. *Remind your child of the rules very nicely* right before the next meal, and continue to use the procedures above.

11. *Don't forget to praise all* appropriate behaviors *very* frequently.

12. *Set a specific time limit* during which food can be eaten and after which the plate will be removed. Purchase and use a portable timer to tell you when mealtime is over.

©Edward R. Christophersen, 1992.

Mealtime Problems: Not Eating/Stalling

1. *Mealtimes should be as pleasant as possible.* Make sure you do not nag, threaten, or warn during mealtimes. This is an excellent time to teach your children how you want them to behave in a social situation.

2. *Include your child in the conversation.* Ask him questions about what he did during the day (without interrogating him). Discuss what interests your child.

3. Give your child very small portions, an amount you're sure she will eat. She can always be given more.

4. *Praise him when he is eating,* rather than nagging him to hurry.

5. *Set a reasonable time limit for the meal,* using a portable kitchen timer. When the timer rings, the meal is over and the table should be cleared without any unpleasant comments on your part.

6. *Praise appropriate eating skills frequently:* using utensils properly, sitting quietly, and not playing with food.

7. *Offer desserts and snacks only if your child finished her meal.* If you allow your child to fill up on snacks between meals, she will not be hungry at mealtimes. Limit snacks. Snacks that have nutritional value, for example, carrot sticks, raisins, and fruits, are much better than junk foods like potato chips and will help teach your child good eating habits.

8. *Do not give in* and allow your child to eat between meals if he did not finish his last meal—to do so will only make your teaching take much longer.

©Edward R. Christophersen, 1992.

Chapter 8

Toileting Problems

More than in any other field of medicine, pediatrics must deal with the initial acquisition of skills, in addition to assessment and modification of skills already learned. Every child, with rare exceptions, must learn to toilet independently. Independent toileting includes transferring all liquid and solid waste into an appropriate receptacle without the assistance of an adult. Independent toileting can be categorized into five basic areas:

- Toilet training and related problems
- Toileting refusal
- Encopresis and constipation
- Day wetting
- Enuresis

These areas will be discussed below.

8.1. TOILET TRAINING

No developmental milestone has more potential for problems than toilet training. If the parents perceived no compliance problems prior to toilet training, but were actually avoiding or ignoring compliance, toilet training will make the compliance problems evident.

If there is a single point to be made about toilet training, it is this: Many of the problems parents encounter with toilet training could be avoided by waiting longer before beginning to toilet train their children.

Parents can be cautioned at the 6-month well-child visit that toilet training too early can be very frustrating for them and for their children. Many parents have unrealistic expectations about when a child is ready to be toilet trained (Stephens and Silber, 1977). These unrealistic expectations persist whether they tell their primary-care provider about them or not. That is why it is best to introduce the subject of toilet training before the parents have given any thought to starting it.

The practitioner who convinces parents to wait until their child is an appropriate age to begin toilet training—30 months or more—will probably get far fewer phone calls about toilet training than would otherwise be the case. Anxious parents who want to start toilet training their younger children can be encouraged to work on some of the components of toilet training, such as dressing, undressing, and vocabulary, as well as general behavioral compliance.

In addition to being an appropriate age, the child should be producing consistent, soft, formed stools as a prerequisite for toilet training. Health-care providers should inquire about the size, regularity, and consistency of the child's stools before a parent starts toilet training. Hard, firm stools or infrequent bowel movements should be corrected using dietary changes, medication, or a combination of the two, prior to attempting toilet training.

8.1.1. Physical Considerations

Parents about to begin toilet training their child should be made aware of several physical considerations.

The child must have a comfortable, convenient place to practice toileting; a child-sized potty chair is ideally suited to the young child. When children sit on the potty chair, their feet touch the floor, offering stability as well as a place to put their feet so that they can push for leverage when they are trying to pass a stool. If the child chooses to use the regular toilet, two small steps should be placed on the front sides of the toilet, offering a step to get up on as well as a platform for the child's feet. The platform offers a stable resting place for the child's feet and allows her leverage—the child can put pressure on her feet to help evacuate her bowel.

Without leverage, many children have difficulty expelling stools. That's why children may have a stool in their diaper but not in the toilet: They have substantially better leverage when they are squatting down. The child who squats in a diaper to expel a stool has 100% of his weight on his feet. The child sitting on a toilet without any small steps has 100% of her weight off her feet, providing very little leverage. The child sitting on a toilet with his feet firmly planted on steps has about half his weight on his feet.

8.1.2. Readiness for Toilet Training

Mastery of bowel and bladder control is considered a major milestone in the physical and social development of children. By the age of 36 months, most children have achieved diurnal bowel and bladder control, although occasional accidents occur through 5 years of age.

Central to the task of toilet training children is the concept of readiness. Brazelton (1962) has suggested several physiological and psychological readiness criteria. Physiological readiness criteria include:

- Reflex sphincter control, which can be elicited as early as 9 months.
- Myelinization of pyramidal tracts, which is completed between 12 and 18 months.

Psychological readiness criteria include:

- Established motor milestones of sitting and walking.
- Some verbal understanding.
- Positive relationships with adults whom the child clearly wants to please.
- Identification with and imitation of parents and other significant people in their lives.
- The desire to be autonomous and master primitive impulses.

Brazelton suggests that readiness appears to peak for most children between 18 and 30 months of age.

Azrin and Foxx (1974), in their best-selling book on toilet training, *Toilet Training in Less Than a Day*, have suggested several specific readiness criteria for parents to use, including:

1. *Bladder control.* The child should empty her bladder completely when urinating, stay dry for several hours, and indicate by facial expressions or posturing that she is about to urinate or defecate. When the child consistently empties her bladder completely and stays dry for several hours, bladder control can be considered adequate for training.
2. *Physical readiness.* The child should exhibit sufficient fine- and gross-motor coordination to be able to walk to and from the toilet, be able to dress and undress enough for toileting, and be able to get on and off the toilet without assistance.
3. *Instructional readiness.* This important criterion is often left out of books about toilet training. The child should have enough receptive language to enable him to follow one-stage and two-stage directions, for example, "Show me your nose," or "Put the toy in the wagon." Instructional readiness indicates the child also is reasonably compliant with parental instructions.

Azrin and Foxx (1974) suggested that most children over 20 months can meet these criteria. The present author (Christophersen, 1988) has suggested that parents wait at least 3 months after their children have met the Azrin and Foxx readiness criteria (see Handout 8.1) before actually beginning training. Training with most children, then, will be initiated when the child is between 24 and 30 months of age.

8.2. TOILET-TRAINING METHODS

The two most popular methods for toilet training have been developed by Brazelton and by Azrin and Foxx.

8.2.1. Brazelton's "Indirect" Method

Brazelton (1962) outlined an indirect method of toilet training, often cited in pediatric literature. His approach emphasizes minimal guidance by the parent as the child is allowed to proceed through several phases at her own pace.

During the first phase (around 18 months of age), the child is introduced to the potty chair and invited to sit on it while fully clothed. After a week or two, the child is taken to the potty chair to sit with his diapers off, although no results are expected. Next, the child is taken to the chair once daily to empty soiled diapers, establishing the potty chair as a convenient receptacle for waste. Then, the potty chair is placed in the child's room or play area. The child does not wear diapers and the parent explains that the child may use the potty chair if she wishes.

After cooperation has been achieved through the preceding phases, the child is dressed in training pants and encouraged to use the potty. Of the almost 2,000 charts that Brazelton reviewed retrospectively for parental reports on toilet-training success, 80% of the children were apparently trained by age 3. The average reported age for day training was 28 months; for day and night training, the average age was 33 months.

8.2.2. Azrin and Foxx's "One-Day" Method

Azrin and Foxx (1974) reported a rapid and effective program for toilet training children that has since been popularized in the book *Toilet Training in Less Than a Day*. The major components of this training program are:

- Practice and reinforcement in dressing skills.
- Immediacy of reinforcement for correct toileting.
- Required practice in toilet approach after accidents.
- Learning by imitation.

Although Azrin and Foxx's published results are impressive, our clinical experience with their procedures during the past 18 years has shown that parents who are training their own children, with the advice and counsel of one of our staff, have had slower results than Azrin and Foxx reported. We encourage parents to wait until their child is ready to work on such readiness skills as dressing if they want to, and not to expect to train the child in 1 day.

Realistically, most children, whether they are trained using Brazelton's approach, Azrin and Foxx's approach, or some other approach, can be trained around the time they are 3 years old. In our experience, it really doesn't make much difference which method is used, and, to my knowledge, there is no published research that uses sound scientific methodology to compare various toilet-training protocols. Parents will usually have a preference for one way over another, and, as long as their child is ready to be trained, we encourage using most of the methods that parents propose.

Azrin and Foxx (1974) did describe a procedure they recommended for use with children who had toileting accidents due, apparently, to the child's simply not being motivated to use the toilet. They called this procedure "positive practice," a mild form of punishment that is also educational in nature (see Handout 8.2).

When the child has a toileting accident, the parent is instructed to direct the child to practice what he should have done instead of having an accident: Walk to the bathroom and sit down so that he could urinate in the toilet. Following a urine accident, the child would be instructed to practice walking to the bathroom and sitting down 10 times in a row, five from the place where the child had an accident and five from other places around the house (for example, the front hall, the kitchen, the family room). The rationale for this procedure is that it gives the child many opportunities to rehearse appropriate behavior when he feels the urge to urinate or defecate.

8.3. TOILETING REFUSAL

The verbal skills and verbal comprehension of young children are such that it is virtually impossible to find out why a child refuses to have a bowel movement in the toilet but willingly defecates in his diaper. Often the only logical reasons are comfort or convenience, owing in part to the stability discussed above and in part to the increased leverage offered by the squatting position. Toileting refusal can be due to the child not wanting to eliminate in the toilet.

8.3.1. Toileting Resistance

Schmitt (1991) described procedures for dealing with children who, without a history of constipation, refuse to use the toilet. He states that the most common reason for toileting resistance is that the child was reminded or lectured too much to use the toilet. Handout 8.3 is a reproduction of Schmitt's recommendations for toilet-training resistance.

8.3.2. Toileting Refusal Due to Constipation

Another consideration relating to toileting refusal is the size and consistency of the child's stools (see Handout 8.4). In the majority of cases of toileting refusal, a toileting history will determine whether the child has had problems with hard, large, or difficult-to-pass stools. If necessary, diet and mediation can be used to soften the stools.

For toileting refusal, we often recommend that parents declare a complete moratorium on toilet training for 1 entire month; parents are advised to discontinue any attempts at training, as well as any discussion of training. Just removing the training pressure is enough to facilitate training in some children. If the child has a history of firm or large stools, the recommended changes in diet and medication can be implemented during the moratorium.

The vast majority of children seen for toileting problems are noncompliant in many areas in addition to toileting. During the 1-month moratorium on toilet training, providing that the child is at least 30 months old, parents should be encouraged to work on general compliance, for children who are more compliant are much easier to toilet train.

8.4. CONSTIPATION AND ENCOPRESIS

Approximately 80% of children brought to physicians for encopresis present a history of fecal retention or constipation (Levine, 1975). This constipation can occur involuntarily, because of insufficient roughage or a bland diet, or voluntarily, because of the individual's retention of feces in the colon for abnormal lengths of time.

Several factors are known to have a causative role in constipation:

- Insufficient roughage or bulk in the diet, so that the contents of the colon do not mechanically stimulate a normal pattern of motility.
- Bland diet, such as one too high in dairy products, without enough counteracting bulk, which also reduces colonic motility.
- Insufficient intake of fluids by mouth, allowing normal reabsorption of water from the colon to dehydrate the feces excessively.

Any of these factors, singularly or in combination, can create constipation-like symptoms or actual constipation. If a child recognizes these symptoms, she may associate them with similar symptoms that occurred earlier and were followed by a painful bowel movement. In an attempt to prevent reoccurrence of the painful bowel movement, the child may voluntarily retain the feces to avoid discomfort when, in actuality, retention or withholding will exacerbate the condition.

If constipation continues and worsens in severity, the child may become lethargic and have a decreased appetite. If a constipated child continues consuming a diet compatible with constipation, the entire symptom complex can be exacerbated. Not infrequently, these children experience seepage around the fecal impaction that results from prolonged constipation, producing what has been termed "paradoxical diarrhea." Although the child is actually constipated or impacted, symptomatically the child may present as though he has diarrhea, producing numerous watery, foul-smelling stools each day. Painful defecation, secondary to constipation, frequently precedes chronic fecal impaction and fecal soiling in American children (Partin, Hamill, Fischel, Partin, 1992).

Occasionally these children pass huge fecal amounts, at times enough to cause problems in the household plumbing system. These large stools are followed by a period of inactivity during which there is no fecal soiling until the colon distends again. The constipation returns and is followed by the paradoxical diarrhea. Some parents may even attempt to treat this type of diarrhea with over-the-counter antidiarrheal agents, an approach that, although well intentioned, further exacerbates the condition.

8.4.1. Treatment of Encopresis

To rule out any of the above-described patterns, the primary-care provider needs to take a thorough dietary history and conduct a physical examination that includes an abdominal examination to check for the presence of large amounts of feces and a rectal examination to check for either large amounts of stool or very dry stool in the rectal vault. The physical examination should be performed by someone trained to conduct physical examinations of children with constipation, to reduce the possibility of missing a significant finding. (The primary-care provider may wish to use a Bowel Problem Intake Form, such as the one shown in Handout 8.5.)

If the history and physical examination clearly point to a pattern similar to that described above, the child, at the discretion of the child's primary-care provider, will probably have to be given cathartics—orally, rectally, or both—to deal with the constipation.

Treatment of encopresis secondary to constipation, the most common history, typically involves placing the child on a long-term treatment regimen. The primary-care provider should take the extra effort necessary to describe each treatment component to the parents and provide a summary of the treatment protocol in writing.

The research literature on treating encopresis secondary to constipation shows general agreement on two major phases. Phase one involves cleaning out any excessive stool the child may have. There is substantial discussion in the literature about whether to use oral medications such as stool softeners or laxatives; to institute dietary changes, usually involving the intake of extra fiber; or to use rectal medications such as suppositories and enemas. Regardless of the individual practitioner's preference, there does seem to be good agreement in the literature that the child cannot be adequately treated prior to resolving the constipation.

It is common for the initial cleaning of the bowel to produce a marked reduction in the encopretic episodes, but, without adequate time for the musculature in the large intestine to regain its tone, the initial reduction in soiling can be misleading. The muscle rebuilding program often needs to be maintained for a number of months, sometimes up to 1 or 2 years.

After the initial catharsis, there is little agreement on how to keep the bowel functioning properly. Levine (1982) and his colleagues characterize this phase of the treatment as "bowel retraining."

During this phase, the primary-care provider should supply the child with enough medication to keep the bowel functioning properly while the muscle in the colon regains its tone. In our office, we use a variety of treatments all aimed at keeping the bowel functioning properly, including:

- Decreased intake of dairy products if, as is usually the case, the child is already consuming too many dairy products.
- Increased intake of dietary fiber, preferably some fiber with every meal and snack.
- Increased intake of nondairy fluids.
- Increased vigorous activity.
- Use of facilitating medications, usually rectal glycerin suppositories.

McClung, Boyne, Linsheid, Heitlinger, Murray, Fyda, and Li (1993) examined children who were exposed to a combination of a high-fiber diet, laxatives, and lubricants as part of a treatment program for encopresis. They reported significant improvements in the children's soiling with no demonstrable deleterious effects from the combined therapy.

Handout 8.6 describes our treatment regimen in its entirety and shows the level of detail recommended in written materials for parents.

In Chapter 5 on compliance, reference is made to symptom rating sheets. We have found that using such a sheet for children with encopresis provides us with a great deal of information during follow-up appointments. Handout 8.7 is a blank symptom rating sheet we use with encopresis.

Whenever we recommend that parents administer glycerine suppositories to their children, we provide them with instructions on withdrawing the suppositories from the treatment regimen. Handout 8.8 describes these instructions.

Although the need to include adequate amounts of fiber in the diet is much easier to explain to parents now that the benefits of a high-fiber diet are more well known, there are still many parents who simply do not know much about fiber. We provide the parent of each encopretic child with Handout 8.9, a description of many foods that are high in dietary fiber. The Minneapolis Children's Medical Center has published a comprehensive handbook for parents on encopresis, *Childhood Constipation and Soiling*, that includes an excellent section on dietary management of constipation. For more information, contact the Minneapolis Children's Medical Center, Behavioral Pediatrics Program, 2525 Chicago Avenue South, Minneapolis, MN 55404, or call 612-863-6798.

Several major studies have evaluated treatment programs for encopresis. Levine and Bakow (1976) followed 110 encopretic children for 1 year. Using an initial cleaning out with rectal suppositories and using mineral oil to maintain regular bowel movements, they reported that 78% of the children studied were in the two most successful treatment categories, either marked improvement or some improvement. Wright (1975) used a treatment protocol involving an initial cleaning out followed by daily use of glycerin suppositories. The 100 children in his study averaged 17 bowel accidents per week before the original cleaning out and 2 bowel accidents per week after the cleaning out. By the 10th week, the average child was having less than one accident per week.

8.4.2. Treating Encopretics Who Have Emotional Problems

No discussion of encopresis would be complete without mentioning emotional factors. The vast majority of encopretics typically have the history of constipation that Levine (1982) reported. In these children, the bowel must be treated. Several recent studies have examined whether children who present with encopresis can also be expected to present with emotional problems. Both Friman, Mathews, Finney, Christophersen, and Leibowitz (1988) and Gabel, Chandra, and Shindledecker (1988) provided data that suggest that the encopretic child who presents in the pediatrician's office typically does not have emotional problems.

Some children present with both encopresis and emotional problems. In these cases, although it may be tempting to attribute the encopresis to the emotional problems, it is just as likely that the emotional problems stemmed from the soiling or, alternatively, that the two are actually unrelated.

Both the encopresis and the emotional problems should be treated, perhaps by the same individual, if the health-care professional is well versed in managing children's bowel problems. Otherwise, one professional should treat the bowel dysfunction while another treats the emotional problems.

Because bowel dysfunction is usually much easier to resolve than emotional problems, the bowel should be dealt with either prior to referring the child for psychotherapy or conjointly. A small number of encopretic children present with no bowel dysfunction and with remarkable emotional problems. In these cases, a complete psychological/psychiatric evaluation would be indicated.

8.5. NOCTURNAL ENURESIS

All newborns urinate while sleeping. Somewhere between 3 and 4 years of age, the majority of children cease urinating while sleeping, with a gradual decrease in nocturnal enuresis with age. At age 3, almost half of all children are enuretic. By 15 years of age, 3% are enuretic. A positive history of enuresis among family members of enuretic children frequently has been noted. When both parents have a history of enuresis, 77% of their children are enuretic; when neither parent has a history of enuresis, only 15% of their children are enuretic (Cohen, 1975). Enuresis appears to be a self-limiting condition, with a spontaneous resolution rate of 12 to 15% per year.

A number of factors have been implicated in enuresis, including food allergies, small bladder capacity, developmental delays, deep sleep, and faulty toilet training. However, no specific etiological factor has been identified and proved.

There are as many treatments proposed for nocturnal enuresis as there are postulated causative agents. As in other areas of medicine, however, the burden of proof for demonstrating treatment efficacy remains with those who propose novel or unique causative agents.

Two basic decisions must be made when dealing with children's nocturnal enuresis:

- When to begin making treatment recommendations
- Which treatment modalities to use

Generally, we recommend that parents refrain from any attempts at treating nocturnal enuresis until their child is at least 7 years old and, just as important, that they wait until the child *wants* the enuresis treated. Once the decision to treat enuresis has been made, there are two approaches supported by research literature: medication and behavioral approaches.

8.5.1. Evaluating the Enuretic Child

Regardless of the treatment approach chosen, several general recommendations apply:

1. A thorough history should be taken. Handout 8.10 is a copy of the Enuresis Intake Form used in our office, which allows us to gather a great deal of relevant history in a short amount of time.
2. A thorough physical examination should be given before any treatment, including a urinalysis and urine culture to rule out the possibility of urinary tract infections or other urological problems. This is particularly important with girls, who more often present with urinary tract infections, and any child who wets during the day, urinates frequently, feels a strong urge to urinate, and has an interrupted urination pattern with a staccato or burst-type urine stream.
3. In addition to ruling out organicity, the author routinely recommends that clinicians wait until a child is 7 years old and has expressed concern that nocturnal enuresis is interfering with some of her social activities (that is, the child shows motivation to stop).

4. Verbal or physical punishment, stopping fluids after the evening meal, setting an alarm clock to go off several times during the night, and a variety of other procedures are almost always ineffective. They also convey to the child the parents' disdain for the child's enuresis. Obviously, large quantities of fluids right before bedtime should be avoided, but a small drink before bedtime, particularly when the child is thirsty, is acceptable.
5. Parents should be told that enuresis is rarely caused by emotional problems, regardless of what the parents may have read in the lay press and that, in all but a few cases, the child has no control over the enuresis. There is ample research literature to support this notion, and parents are usually relieved to hear this from a primary-care provider.
6. With very few exceptions, enuresis can be managed on an outpatient basis.

8.5.2. Medical Approaches

Drugs usually stop enuresis completely in 40 to 50% of enuretic children, while another 10 to 20% show considerable improvement. The relapse rate, however, is high; about two-thirds of enuretics resume wetting after the drugs are discontinued (Christophersen and Rapoff, 1992).

Any time medication is considered as a treatment option, the potential benefits of the medication must be weighed against the known side effects. Drug treatment is recommended by the present author only under these circumstances:

- When the child is under undue stress to discontinue the enuresis, perhaps because of his parents' poor coping skills.
- For short periods of time, like an overnight scouting campout.
- As an adjunct to dry-bed training, as described below.

A number of researchers are continuing their work in an attempt to identify effective drug-treatment protocols. The two drugs with the most research activity are Tofranil and desmopressin (DDAVP). Attempts are currently under way to develop procedures for gradually weaning the child off the medication, with the expectation that such a weaning process may reduce the number of children who relapse when the drug is discontinued. Moffat, Harlos, Kirshen, and Burd (1993) reviewed the published literature on the use of DDAVP, concluding that, "on the basis of current knowledge, DDAVP is inferior to conditioning alarms as a primary therapy" (p. 420).

Warady, Alon, and Hellerstein (1991) recommended that, because nocturnal enuresis is essentially a developmental problem, parents should be encouraged to give their children time to outgrow their enuresis. Approximately 15% of all enuretics outgrow their enuresis each year, without any formal treatment (Cohen, 1975).

8.5.3. Urine-Alarm Treatment

For over 40 years, the standard behavioral treatment for enuresis has been the urine-alarm or bell-and-pad procedure originally described by Mowrer and Mowrer in 1938. (Incidentally, this 1938 paper is fascinating to read!)

The urine-alarm procedure involves placing an apparatus on the child's bed that has a mechanism for sensing when urine has been passed. A battery-operated alarm rings when urine passes onto the sensing mechanism (this is an important distinction, since urine will not sound the alarm if it does not come into contact with the sensing mechanism).

Bed-wetting alarms are now sold in most major department stores. The instructions accompanying the mechanism usually instruct the parents, when the alarm rings, to wake the child, turn off the alarm, have the child finish urinating in the toilet, have the child change her own bedding and clean herself up, and have the child return to bed. (In our experience, the sensing mechanism should not be used more than once per night, since parents may become too fatigued to continue with the urine-alarm procedures.)

Studies have shown that the urine-alarm treatment initially eliminates enuresis in about 75% of cases, with treatment lasting anywhere from 5 to 16 weeks (Mowrer and Mowrer, 1938). Relapse rates are generally high, occurring on average with 45% of the children, although reinstatement of the procedures usually results in a substantially higher cure rate than the first time.

Within the last couple of years, the written instructions packaged with the alarms have been improved to the point that, for a motivated, literate family, the urine-alarm treatment is probably the treatment of choice. Although it does not work in all cases, it is considerably less expensive than referral to virtually any subspecialist for a more complete work-up.

The urine alarm has been shown to be superior to no treatment, to psychotherapy, and to imipramine. The disadvantages of using the urine alarm are length of treatment, the inconvenience of having to wake a child in the middle of the night, and malfunctions of the alarm (Christophersen and Rapoff, 1992).

8.5.4. Dry-Bed Training

The most promising treatment, in terms of both effectiveness and speed of managing enuresis, is the "dry-bed training" initially described by Azrin, Sneed, and Foxx (1974).

Dry-bed training combines a number of behavioral procedures (see Handout 8.11). Bollard and Woodroffe (1977) have researched the dry-bed training procedures and documented the efficacy of several changes in Azrin's original protocol that eliminate the need for home visits (the original dry-bed training was conducted in the home by a therapist), so the procedures can be presented in the office, even, in some cases, with groups of children and their parents.

Dry-bed training is a combination of the urine alarm and night awakening. As is described in Handout 8.11, the child is awakened the first time the urine alarm indicates he wet the bed (second and subsequent wettings in one night are to be ignored), and the child is directed to clean up his bed and his wet night clothes and return to bed. The parents are instructed to set their alarm clock so that they can wake their child 5 hours before he is scheduled to be awakened for the day. After six dry night awakenings, the night awakening is moved up 1 hour. The procedure of moving up the night awakening 1 hour for each six consecutive dry awakenings is continued until the night awakening is scheduled for a time close to when the child is put to bed for the night.

8.6. CONCLUDING REMARKS

Promising treatments for nocturnal enuresis, such as dry-bed training, have been developed. The primary-care provider who follows a large number of children can identify one or two practitioners trained to offer the dry-bed training procedures in his or her area. Then, the primary-care provider has the choice between medication and behavioral procedures, the two treatments of choice as of this writing.

When a child presents with both enuresis and significant emotional problems, referral to a mental-health practitioner is, of course, appropriate.

REFERENCES

Azrin NH, Foxx RM: *Toilet Training in Less Than a Day*. New York: Simon and Schuster, 1974.

Azrin NH, Sneed TJ, Foxx RM: Dry-bed training: Rapid elimination of childhood enuresis. *Behav Res Ther* 12:147–156, 1974.

Bollard RJ, Woodroffe P: The effect of parent administered dry-bed training on nocturnal enuresis in children. *Behav Res Ther* 15:159–165, 1977.

Brazelton TB: A child-oriented approach to toilet training, *Pediatrics* 29:121–128, 1962.

Christophersen ER: *Little People: Guidelines for Commonsense Child Rearing*, 3rd ed. Kansas City, MO: Westport Publishers, 1988.

Christophersen ER, Rapoff MR: Toileting problems in children, in Walker CE, Roberts MC (eds.), *The Handbook of Clinical Child Psychology*, 2nd ed. New York: Wiley, 1992, pp. 399–411.

Cohen MW: Enuresis. *Pediatr Clin N Am* 22:545–560, 1975.

Friman PC, Mathews JR, Finney JF, Christophersen ER, Leibowitz JM: Do encopretic children have clinically significant behavior problems? *Pediatrics* 82:407–409, 1988.

Gabel S, Chandra R, Shindledecker R: Behavioral ratings and outcome of medical treatment for encopresis. *J Dev Behav Pediatr* 9:129–133, 1988.

Levine MD: Children with encopresis: A descriptive analysis. *Pediatrics* 56:412–416, 1975.

Levine MD: Encopresis: Its potentiation, evaluation, and alleviation. *Pediatr Clinics N Am* 29:315–331, 1982.

Levine MD, Bakow H: The school child with encopresis: A treatment outcome study. *Pediatrics* 58:845–852, 1976.

McClung HJ, Boyne LJ, Linsheid T, Heitlinger LA, Murray RD, Fyda J, Li B: Is combination therapy for encopresis nutritionally safe? *Pediatrics* 91:591–594, 1993.

Moffatt MEK, Harlos S, Kirshen AJ, Burd L: Desmopressin acetate and nocturnal enuresis: How much do we know? *Pediatrics* 92:420–425, 1993.

Mowrer OH, Mowrer WM: Enuresis: A method for its study and treatment. *Am J Orthopsychiatr* 8:436–459, 1938.

Partin JC, Hamill SK, Fischel JE, Partin JS: Painful defecation and fecal soiling in children. *Pediatrics* 89:1007–1009, 1992.

Schmitt, B: *Your Child's Health*. New York: Bantam Books, 1991.

Stephens JA, Silber DL: Parental expectations in toilet training. *Pediatrics* 48:451–454, 1977.

Warady BA, Alon U, Hellerstein S: Primary nocturnal enuresis: Current concepts about an old problem. *Pediatr Ann* 20:246–255, 1991.

Wright L: Outcome of a standardized program for treating psychogenic encopresis. *Professional Psychol*, November 1975, p. 453.

Sample Handouts

HANDOUT 8.1

Toilet-Training Readiness Checklist

1. Does your child urinate a good deal at one time rather than dribbling through the day? Yes _____ No _____

2. Does your child stay dry for several hours at a time? Yes _____ No _____

3. Does your child have enough finger and hand coordination to pick up objects easily? Yes _____ No _____

4. Does your child walk from room to room easily without help? Yes _____ No _____

5. Can your child carry out the following instructions when asked?
   a. Point to his nose. Yes _____ No _____
   b. Point to her eyes. Yes _____ No _____
   c. Point to his mouth. Yes _____ No _____
   d. Point to her hair. Yes _____ No _____
   e. Sit down on a chair. Yes _____ No _____
   f. Stand up. Yes _____ No _____
   g. Walk to a specific place in another room. Yes _____ No _____
   h. Imitate you in a simple task like playing patty-cake. Yes _____ No _____
   i. Bring you a familiar toy. Yes _____ No _____
   j. Put one familiar object with another, like putting a doll in a wagon. Yes _____ No _____

SCORING

If your answers to questions 1 and 2 are yes, your child has the necessary bladder control to begin toilet training. If your answers to questions 3 and 4 are yes, your child has the physical skills to begin toilet training.

If your child can follow eight of the ten instructions in question 5, your child has the verbal and social skills to begin toilet training.

If your child does not meet all of these criteria, you should delay toilet training until he can meet them.

Source: Azrin NH, Foxx RM: *Toilet Training in Less Than a Day*. New York: Simon and Schuster, 1974, pp. 36–37.

HANDOUT 8.2

Toileting Accidents

After they have been toilet trained, some children occasionally have periods of frequent wetting or soiling. The children should first be examined by a physician to rule out physical conditions, such as urinary tract infections, that may be causing the accidents.

When you find your child with wet or soiled pants, use the following guidelines:

1. *Show verbal disapproval for the wetting or soiling.*
   a. Tell the child why you are displeased, saying something like, "You wet your pants."
   b. Express your disapproval of the accident by saying something like, "You shouldn't wet your pants. You should go in the potty."

2. *Have the child do positive practice of self-toileting.*
   a. Tell your child what you are doing and why by saying something like, "Bobby wet his pants. Bobby has to practice going to the bathroom."
   b. The child walks quickly to the toilet or potty chair.
   c. The child quickly lowers her pants and sits on the potty.
   d. After sitting 1 or 2 seconds (do not allow urination), the child quickly raises his pants.
   e. The child goes to another part of the house and repeats steps b through d for 10 trials. Five of the trials should start where the child had the accident; the other five trials should start from several different places in the house.
   f. If the child refuses to do the positive practice trials or if he has a temper tantrum, put him in time-out. After time-out has ended, begin the positive practice from where you left off.

3. *Make the child responsible for cleaning up.*
   a. If there is wetness on the floor, have the child get a cloth and wipe up the wetness.
   b. With minimum assistance, require the child to remove her soiled pants.
   c. Have the child put her soiled clothes in an appropriate place, like a soiled-clothes hamper.
   d. If the child is dirty, require her to clean herself or take a quick bath.
   e. Have the child put on clean clothes.

4. *After the accident has been corrected, do not continue to talk about it.* Your child should start with a clean slate.

5. *Remember to praise and hug your child when he eliminates in the toilet.* "Catch 'em being good!"

Source: Adapted from Azrin NH, Foxx RM: *Toilet Training in Less Than a Day.* New York: Pocket Books, 1976.

HANDOUT 8.3

Toilet-Training Resistance

Children who refuse to be toilet-trained either wet themselves, soil themselves, or try to hold back their bowel movements (thus becoming constipated). Many of these children also refuse to sit on the toilet or will use the toilet only if a parent brings up the subject and marches them into the bathroom. Any child who is over 2½ years old and not toilet-trained after several months of trying can be assumed to be resistant to the process, rather than untrained. Consider how capable your child is at delaying a BM until he or she is off the toilet or you are on the telephone. More practice runs, such as you used in toilet training, will not help. Your child's control is already impressive. Instead, your child now needs full responsibility and some incentives.

The most common cause of not being toilet-trained is that the child was reminded or lectured too much. Some of the children have been forced to sit on the toilet against their will, occasionally for long periods of time. A few have been spanked or punished in other ways for not cooperating. Many parents make these mistakes, especially if they have a strong-willed child.

Occasional small amounts of wetting and soiling can be normal. If your child has small amounts of wetting that occur while trying to pull down underwear or undo a zipper, this is normal and no special intervention is needed. Occasionally a girl will have some leakage of urine because she stands up too quickly after urinating. She simply needs to sit there an extra 10 seconds. Also, some of the children with small smears of stool in their underwear simply need a careful review of how to wipe themselves "until clean."

Most children less than 5 or 6 years of age with soiling (encopresis) or daytime wetting (without any other symptoms) are simply engaged with you in a power struggle. These children can be helped with the following suggestions. If your child holds back bowel movements and becomes constipated, medicines will also be needed, so first talk with your child's physician. If your child also has bed-wetting, work on the daytime wetting first, because it will be much easier to change.

HELPING THE CHILD WITH DAYTIME WETTING OR SOILING

Transfer all responsibility to your child. Your child will decide to use the toilet only after he realizes that he has nothing left to resist. Have one last talk with him about this subject. Tell your child that his body makes "pee" and "poop" every day and it belongs to him. Explain that his "poop" wants to go in the toilet and his job is to help the "poop" get out. Tell him you're sorry you punished him, forced him to sit on the toilet, or reminded him so much. Tell him from now on you won't try to help him, because he doesn't need any help and he's "in charge." Then stop talking about this subject with your child or with others when your child is present. When your child stops receiving so much attention and conversation for nonperformance (not going), he will eventually decide to perform for attention.

Stop all reminders about using the toilet. Let your child decide when he needs to go to the bathroom. He should not be reminded to go to the bathroom, nor asked if he needs to go. Reminders are a form of pressure, and pressure doesn't work. Your child should not be made to sit on the toilet against his will, because this will foster a negative attitude about the whole process. He knows when his rectum needs to be emptied (the defecation urge), when his bladder is full, and where the bathroom is. If your child doesn't respond when he needs to, the best reminder of wetness is urine dripping down the leg, and the best reminder of soiling is the odor.

Give incentives for using the toilet. If your child stays clean and dry, he or she needs plenty of positive reinforcement. This reinforcement should include praise, smiles, and hugs from everyone in the family. This positive response should occur every time your child passes his bowel movement or urine into the toilet. For the child who soils or wets himself on some days and not others, this recognition should occur whenever he is clean for a complete day. Better yet, on successful days a parent should take 20 minutes to play a special game with the child or take him for a walk.

For turning around a resistant child, special incentives (such as jelly beans, chocolates, or video time) are invaluable—especially under age 5. Take your child to the grocery store to select 2 bags of favorite candies. For using the toilet, err on the side of giving too much (e.g., a handful each time). If you want a breakthrough, make your child "an offer he can't refuse."

Give stars for using the toilet. Get a calendar for your child and post it in a conspicuous location. Place a star on it for every BM or urination into the toilet. This record of progress should be kept until your child has gone 2 weeks without any accidents.

If your child has never sat on the toilet, try to change his attitude. First, give him choices by asking if he wants to use the big toilet or the potty chair. If he chooses the potty chair, be sure to keep it in the room he usually plays in. For wetting, the presence of the chair and the promise of treats will usually bring about a change in behavior. For soiling, your child may need a pleasant reminder once a day when he is clearly holding back. You can say "The poop is trying to get out and go in the toilet. The poop needs your help." A few children temporarily may need treats for simply sitting on the toilet and trying. However, don't accompany your child into the bathroom or stand with him by the potty chair. He needs to get the feeling of success that comes from doing it on his own and then finding you to tell you what he did.

Remind your child to change clothing if he wets or soils himself. Don't ignore soiled or wet clothes. As soon as your child is noted to be soiled or wet by odor or behavior, remind him to clean himself up immediately. The main role you have in this program is to enforce the rule "You can't walk around wet or with a mess in your pants." Don't expect your child to confess to being wet or soiled, nor ask him a question he will probably answer with a lie. If he is wet, he can probably change into dry clothes by himself. This makes it more boring, which is good. Also have your child rinse the wet underwear in the sink and then hang it on the side of the bathtub to dry. If your child is soiled, he will probably need your help with cleanup, but keep him involved. Have your child rinse the soiled underwear in the toilet. This may be "yucky," which is also good. Then store them until washday in a bucket of water with a lid. Your child may also need a 5-minute soak in the bathtub if he is soiled. If he wets or soils himself when you are out in public places, always have him carry a brown bag with extra clothes in it. If your child has an accident, find a public restroom and put him through his paces.

Don't punish or criticize your child for accidents. Respond gently to accidents. Your child should not be criticized or punished. In addition, siblings should not be allowed to tease. Your child should never be put back into diapers unless he needs to be on laxatives or stool softeners. If there is anyone in your family who wants to "crack down" on your youngster, have that person talk to your child's physician, because this kind of pressure will only delay a cure and it could cause secondary emotional problems. Try to keep your family optimistic about this problem. Eventually all children want to be "grown up" and will use the toilet.

Source: Schmitt, B: *Your Child's Health*. New York: Bantam Books, 1991. ©1991 by Barton Schmitt and reprinted by permission.

HANDOUT 8.4

Toileting Refusal

For reasons we can't always explain, some children between 2½ and 4½ years of age refuse to have bowel movements in the toilet but don't have any trouble having bowel movements in their diaper. In such an instance, several separate, but related, aspects should be addressed.

1. *Stool consistency.* It is much easier to retain a firm, hard stool than it is to retain a soft, formed stool. There are a variety of strategies for softening up a child's stool, including stool softeners like mineral oil, fiber (either natural fiber in foods or fiber supplements), and laxatives (either natural laxatives like honey or commercially available laxatives). If the stools are hard, pebble-shaped, or relatively large for a small child, something needs to be done to soften the stools.

2. *Sitting on the toilet.* Small children cannot sit on a regular-sized toilet to have a bowel movement. They should be provided with two footstools, one placed on each side of the toilet toward the front. In this way, they can get up on the toilet more easily, they can balance more easily, and they can push with their feet to make having the bowel movement easier.

3. *Regular bowel habits.* Children seem to do much better when they are on a regular schedule for sleeping and eating. Try to standardize your child's schedule for at least 1 month, keeping bedtimes, getting-up times, and mealtimes fairly standard. Don't hurry mealtimes, either.

4. *Exercise.* Many young children simply do not get enough vigorous exercise. Try to get at least one time period each day, preferably 15 to 20 minutes in duration, when you can take a long walk, go swimming, and so on.

5. *Medication.* In some cases, depending on the child and his bowel history, your doctor may want to use medication to facilitate regular bowel movements. If your doctor thinks medication would help your child, he or she will discuss this with you.

Most children who have problems with toileting refusal can be helped in a relatively short period of time. Your cooperation and your feedback (in the form of phone calls and return appointments) can greatly help in resolving the toileting problems.

©Edward R. Christophersen, 1984.

Bowel Problem Intake Form

What word does your child use for a bowel movement? _____

Has your child ever been "potty trained"? Yes _____ No _____

If yes, bladder trained: Age started _____ Age accomplished _____

If yes, bowel trained: Age started _____ Age accomplished _____

Does your child wet the bed at night? Yes _____ No_____ If yes, how long has bedwetting occurred? _____

If your child was potty trained, what methods were employed to train the child? Describe: _____

If your child was potty trained, when did soiling first occur after training? Age _____

Number of daily soilings _____ Does this occur at the same time each day? Yes _____ No _____ If yes, note the time(s) _____

Note the amount (circle 1): Very Small   Small   Moderate   Large   Very Large

Note the consistency (circle 1): Hard   Soft   Runny   Pebbles

Does your child have a history of constipation? Yes _____ No _____

If yes, for how long? _____ Previous treatment for constipation? _____

Does your child wipe clean after a bowel movement? Yes _____ No _____

How is the soiling discovered? Describe: _____
_____

What action is taken with your child after soiling has been discovered? Describe: _____

What is verbally said to the child? Supply the quotes used:

Father _____

Mother _____

Have you been able to correlate any traumatic experience happening in your child's life with the onset of soiling? Yes _____ No _____

If yes, describe: _____

Food List—Does the child like and eat the following foods? (Circle 1)

Lettuce	Yes	No	Broccoli	Yes	No	Oranges	Yes	No
Spinach	Yes	No	Cauliflower	Yes	No	Grapes	Yes	No
Cabbage	Yes	No	Green Beans	Yes	No	Dried Figs	Yes	No
Peas	Yes	No	Green Peppers	Yes	No	Raisins	Yes	No
Asparagus	Yes	No	Fresh Plums	Yes	No	Prunes	Yes	No
Tomatoes	Yes	No	Fresh Peaches	Yes	No	Honey	Yes	No
Onions	Yes	No	Fresh Apples	Yes	No	Bran	Yes	No
Celery	Yes	No	Pears	Yes	No	Bran Products	Yes	No
Carrots	Yes	No	Grapefruit	Yes	No	Whole-Wheat Bread	Yes	No
Corn	Yes	No	Pineapple	Yes	No			

Questions asked of the child during the clinic visit:

How do you feel when you soil your pants? Good _____ Bad _____

Why? Describe the child's words _____

What do you do when you soil your pants? Describe the child's words _____

_____

What do your mom and dad do when they find out you've soiled?

Describe the child's words _____

Do you want to stop soiling your pants? Yes _____ No _____

Encopretic Treatment: Instructions for Parents

NEED TO BUY

Pediatric Fleet-brand enema (1)
Adult glycerin suppositories (jar of 50)
K-Y Jelly or Lubrafax (optional)
Premoistened towelettes
Milk and molasses (one-to-one mixture)

FIRST NIGHT ROUTINE

1. Begin after dinner and about 2 hours before your child goes to bed.

2. Give one Pediatric Fleet-size enema, with a one-to-one mixture of milk and molasses at room temperature. It should be administered with the child lying on his left side. Squeeze the bottle slowly and constantly until empty. Do not let go of the bottle while squeezing, as this acts as a suction force in the rectum. Squeeze the buttocks together while removing the enema tip. Have the child retain the enema at least 5 minutes (preferably 20 minutes) before expelling it and the fecal matter.

3. Administer a second milk-and-molasses enema 1 hour after the first, whether or not the child had a bowel movement. Again, have the child retain the enema at least 5 minutes.

4. Record the amount and consistency of the results after both enemas on the symptom recording sheet.

DAILY ROUTINE

Follow the procedures for the morning schedule *or* the evening schedule. *Do not* do both or switch between the schedules.

Morning Schedule

1. Awaken the child at least 1 hour before she has to leave the house.

2. Instruct your child to try to defecate when he arises in the morning. Do not have him sit on the toilet for more than 5 minutes. Make this as pleasant as possible. Don't nag. His feet should firmly touch the floor while he is sitting on the toilet. If they don't, place a footstool under his feet.

3. If he cannot defecate at least a quarter-cup after 5 minutes, insert a glycerin rectal suppository. Then encourage your child to eat a high-fiber breakfast and get dressed.

4. After eating breakfast and dressing, instruct her again to go to the bathroom. If she cannot defecate at least a quarter-cup after 5 minutes, insert a second glycerin suppository.

5. If your child goes for 2 days without a bowel movement, please contact your doctor.

6. Instruct your child to sit on the toilet for 5 minutes each afternoon.

Evening Schedule

1. Instruct your child to try to defecate 30 minutes before dinner. Do not have him sit on the toilet for more than 5 minutes. Make this as pleasant as possible. Don't nag. His feet should firmly touch the floor while he is sitting on the toilet. If they don't, place a footstool under his feet.

2. If she cannot defecate at least a quarter-cup after 5 minutes, insert a glycerin suppository. Your child should have a stool within a half-hour after the dinner meal. If she doesn't have a stool of at least a quarter-cup, insert a second suppository approximately 1 hour after the first one was inserted.

3. If your child goes for 2 days without a bowel movement, please contact your doctor.

4. Instruct your child to sit on the toilet for 5 minutes each morning.

WHAT TO DO WHEN PROPER ELIMINATION HAS OCCURRED

Proper elimination means any bowel movement of appropriate size, regardless of whether or not suppositories or enemas were used, that occurred while the child was on the toilet.

1. Check the toilet for stool, and record the amount and consistency on the symptom recording sheet before the child flushes the toilet.

2. Praise your child—this is *very* important.

3. Decide how you will spend your 15 minutes together for her special time reward (child's time). The special time should be used daily (15 minutes of special time for each bowel movement in the toilet) to enhance the reward for proper elimination.

Monitoring

1. Check frequently, and verbally praise your child for not soiling. Be tactful so as not to embarrass him when doing so.

2. **Be aware.** It is important that you catch soiled pants as soon as possible after soiling has occurred.

WHAT TO DO WHEN YOUR CHILD SOILS HIS PANTS

1. After soiling has occurred, instruct your child to:

   a. Rinse and wash out his own underwear and pants.
   b. Bathe quickly (just enough time to clean herself). Use a bathtub with only 1 or 2 inches of water in it to prevent the child from playing in the bathtub.
   c. Put on clean clothes.

2. Use only enough verbal prompts to keep him going—no nagging. Do not mention the soiling episode *during* or *after* any of these procedures.

CLEANLINESS TRAINING

Make sure your child knows how to wipe himself properly by checking to see if any fecal material is still present after the child reportedly has wiped. If your child needs instructions, use the following procedure.

1. Have your child wipe once, then have him look at the tissue. If any fecal matter or coloration is present on the tissue, have him wipe again. Repeat this procedure until the used tissue is clean. Note: Use of a premoistened towelette initially ("Wet Ones" or "Dab-a-Ways") will make this procedure easier. Praise the child and give him feedback after he has finished wiping correctly.

2. Most children require at least several days of cleanliness training. Check her underwear each day for evidence of coloration, and repeat step 1 above until your child has learned to wipe herself properly.

Bowel Symptom Rating Sheet

	Mineral Oil	No. of Suppositories	No. of Enemas	No. of Soilings	No. of Bowel Movements	Size/Consistency	Diet (No. of Servings)	Water (No. of Glasses)	Activity	Time	Comments:
1											
2											
3											
4											
5											
6											
7											
8											
9											
10											
11											
12											
13											
14											
15											
16											
17											
18											
19											
20											
21											

Patient _____

Month _____

	Mineral Oil	No. of Suppositories	No. of Enemas	No. of Soilings	No. of Bowel Movements	Size/Consistency	Diet (No. of Servings)	Water (No. of Glasses)	Activity	Time	
22											
23											
24											
25											
26											
27											
28											
29											
30											
31											

KEY:

Mineral Oil:	Number of tablespoons
Number of Bowel Movements:	In toilet
Size and Consistency:	Approx. no. of cups; H = Hard, S = Soft Formed, D = Diarrhea
Diet:	3 = 3 meals with high-fiber foods; 2 = 2 meals; 1 = 1 meal; 0 = 0 meals
Water:	No. of glasses (6–8 oz.) of water or juices per day
Activity:	3 = very active; 2 = moderately active; 1 = little activity
Time:	Indicates how much time parent spent with child for each BM in toilet (1 BM = 15 minutes; 2 BMs = 30 minutes, etc.)

HANDOUT 8.8

Instructions for Fading Out Suppositories

1. Begin only after 2 weeks without soiling.

2. Stop the use of suppositories for 1 day each week, for example, on a Monday.

3. If your child does not soil for the next 7 days, another day's suppositories are discontinued. Your child does not receive any suppositories, for example, on either Monday or Tuesday morning. The first three potential daily suppositories that are removed should be on alternating days. That way, there aren't 2 successive days without a potential suppository until the fourth suppository has been removed.

4. If another week is completed without any soiling, another day's suppository is discontinued. This totals 3 days when suppositories are not used, for example, Monday, Thursday, and Saturday.

5. If no soiling occurs, drop 1 more suppository for each week that soiling does not occur. Continue until your child is not receiving any suppositories.

6. If soiling occurs, add 1 day's suppository for each soiling episode until the child is receiving suppositories every day or until he again goes a week without soiling.

7. After 1 week with no soiling, go back to step 2 above and begin again.

8. The suppositories are stopped when the child can function for 2 weeks without soiling after all suppositories are discontinued.

High-Fiber Diet Instructions

RECOMMENDATIONS

1. At least one serving of high-fiber food should be eaten at each meal. (See food list below.)

2. Snacks should be restricted to enhance the normal reflex that stimulates a bowel movement that comes after filling an empty stomach.

3. Fresh vegetables and fruits are better than cooked.

4. Six to eight glasses of water or juices should be consumed daily to help keep stools from becoming hard and dry. (See drinks list below.)

5. Honey and prunes have a chemical laxative and should be encouraged.

6. Fats (butter, margarine, and fried foods) aid the intestines in evacuating stool.

7. Protein (meats, poultry, fish, and eggs) should be included in the child's daily diet.

8. Milk and milk products should be restricted until the soiling has improved. No more than one glass of milk or the equivalent per day. (Milk products include cheese, cottage cheese, ice cream, ice milk, sherbet, yogurt, and milkshakes.)

9. If mineral oil has been recommended, mix it with orange juice in a blender, then add soda water or 7-Up. Mineral oil also may be mixed with any juice to make it more palatable or mixed with canned fruit in heavy syrup.

HIGH-FIBER FOODS

Vegetables: 1 serving = ½ cup
   Lettuce, spinach, cabbage, cauliflower, broccoli, asparagus, tomatoes, onions, peas, celery, green pepper, carrots, corn, and green beans

Fruits: 1 serving = ½ cup or 1 whole fruit
   Apples, pears, oranges, grapefruit, grapes, peaches, dried figs, dried apricots, prunes, raisins, pineapple, and plums

Breads: 1 serving = 1 slice bread or ¼–1 cup
   Cereal (see cereal box for equivalent of 1 serving)
   Bran cereal, such as 100 Bran, Honey Bran, Cracklin' Oat Bran, Bran Chex, 40% Bran Flakes, Raisin Bran, Corn Bran, Most, Butternut Light bread, white bread, wheat bread, any whole-grain bread, graham crackers

Drinks: Juices (6 to 8 glasses per day), prune, water, pruneapple apricot, pruneapple (Sunsweet), any fruit juice, Kool-Aid, Hi-C, soda pop

FOOD PREPARATION IDEAS

Julienne salad (tossed with strips of meat, poultry, and hard-boiled egg)
Tossed salads
Carrot, celery, green pepper sticks, raw cauliflower; may be dipped into salad dressing
Celery with chunky peanut butter
Stewed prunes with honey
Bran muffins with prunes or raisins served with honey
Homemade whole-wheat bread with bran
Glass of warm liquid with breakfast. Example: apple juice with a cinnamon stick
Bread with butter and honey
Add soda water or 7-Up to any juice
Substitute whole-wheat flour for white flour when baking cookies
Add ¼ to ½ cup of bran, cracked wheat, or wheat germ to cookies when baking. Add diced, dried fruit, such as prunes.
Cole slaw
Popcorn
To pancake or waffle mix: Add 1 cup 100% bran cereal to ½ cup milk. Let soak 5–10 minutes. Then add to mix.
French toast made with fresh Butternut Light bread

HANDOUT 8.10

Enuresis Intake Form

PARENTS

1. What word does your child use for urinating? _____

2. Has your child ever been potty trained? _____

	Age Started	Age Accomplished
Bladder trained? ____	____	____
Bowel trained? ____	____	____

3. What potty-training method did you use? _____
   _____

4. Was there ever a time when your child did not wet the bed? Yes ____
   No ____

5. If so, when did bed-wetting begin? _____

6. When did you decide it was a problem? _____
   Your spouse? _____
   Your child? _____

7. What about bed-wetting makes it a problem for you? _____
   For your spouse? _____
   For your child? _____

8. Does your child wet the bed every night? _____
   If not, how often? _____

9. Has your child ever gone for any length of time not wetting the bed?
   ____How long? ____ How often? ____

10. What methods have you used in the past to stop the bed-wetting? ____
    _____
    _____

    For how long? _____

11. Are you still using any of these methods? _____

12. What is your child's responsibility when he wets the bed? _____

13. Does your child ever wet her pants during the day? ____ How often? ____
    How much? Small ____ Medium ____ Large ____

14. Does your child ever dribble in his pants during the day? _____

15. Does your child ever complain of burning when she urinates? _____

16. Does your child have to go more frequently than you think is normal? _____

17. Does your child complain that it doesn't feel like he has completely emptied his bladder when finished? _____

18. When your child has to urinate, can she wait a while, or does she have to go right then or have an accident? _____

19. Have you ever noticed any irritation around the end of his penis/her meatus? _____

20. Has your child ever had a work-up for a urinary tract infection or any other urinary problem? _____

    When? _____

    By whom? _____

    Where? _____

    Results? _____

21. Is your child a sound sleeper? _____

22. When your child stays overnight with relatives or a friend, does he wet the bed? _____

23. What do you believe causes bed-wetting? _____

    _____

24. Has your child ever had problems with constipation? Yes _____ No _____

25. Has your child ever soiled? Yes _____ No _____

26. To your knowledge, did anyone in either the biological mother's or father's family wet the bed? If so, who? _____

CHILD

1. Tell me why you're here. _____

   _____

2. Do you want to stop wetting the bed? _____

3. Does wetting the bed cause you any problem? _____

   _____

4. What do Mom and Dad do when you wet the bed? _____

   _____

5. Have you ever gone without wetting the bed? _____

6. When you wet the bed, what do you do about it? _____

   _____

7. What do you like to do with your mom? _____

   _____

   With your dad? _____

HANDOUT 8.11

Dry-Bed Training Procedures

I. Recording: Use calendar progress chart to record dry or wet from previous night.

    A. Parent praises child if dry.

    B. Parent encourages child to keep working if wet.

II. At bedtime

    A. Child feels sheets and comments on their dryness.

    B. Child describes what he will do if he has the urge to urinate.

    C. Child describes current need to urinate and does so.

    D. Parent expresses confidence in child and reviews progress.

    E. Alarm is placed on bed.

    F. Alarm is connected and tested.

    G. Child goes to sleep.

III. Nightly awakening

    A. Awaken child once during night.

        1. Use minimal prompt in awakening, but be sure the child is awake.

        2. Child feels sheets and comments on dryness.

        3. Parent praises child for dry sheets.

        4. Child goes to bathroom, urinates as much as possible, returns to bed.

        5. Child feels sheets again.

        6. Child states what he will do if he feels urge to urinate.

        7. Parent expresses confidence to child.

        8. Keep alarm on bed if it has not sounded before awakening.

        9. If alarm has sounded more than 30 minutes before scheduled awakening, awaken at scheduled time.

       10. If alarm has sounded less than 30 minutes before scheduled awakening, awaken at scheduled time.

    B. Adjust time of nightly awakening.

        1. On first night, awaken child 5 hours before his or her usual time of awakening.

        2. After child has six consecutive dry nights, awaken him or her 1 hour earlier the next night. Continue to move the awakening time 1 hour earlier after each six dry nights until the awakening time is 8 hours before the usual time of awakening.

        3. When dry for 14 nights at 8-hour awakening, discontinue awakening and discontinue alarm.

IV. When alarm sounds

    A. Awaken child and give mild reprimand for wetting.
    B. Child feels sheets and comments on wetness.
    C. Child walks to bathroom and finishes voiding.
    D. Child takes quick bath.
    E. Child changes into dry clothes.
    F. Child removes wet sheets and places them in laundry.
    G. Child remakes bed with dry sheets.
    H. Child feels bed sheets and comments on dryness.
    I. Do not reconnect alarm.
    J. Child returns to sleep.

V. During day

    A. Child and parents describe progress to relevant friend or family member.
    B. Parents repeatedly express confidence in child and praise him or her.
    C. Parent calls therapist at set times to report progress.

Chapter **9**

Attention Deficit Hyperactivity Disorder

While only approximately 3% of the pediatric-age population presents with attention deficit hyperactivity disorder (ADHD), these children can take up a disproportionate amount of the practitioner's time because ADHD is a multifaceted disorder. While we typically think of ADHD children as being impulsive with a short attention span, they may also present with behavior problems, learning disabilities, and social skill deficits. Also, because ADHD tends to run in families, the presence of ADHD in one of the parents can complicate the management of the child.

    While a thorough discussion of ADHD is considerably beyond the scope of this book, the issue of compliance with respect to the management of ADHD is appropriate.

    The most important aspect of managing ADHD is the initial evaluation. Most researchers, physicians, and primary-care practitioners agree that a child should not be placed on medication based only on the parents' verbal report. Similarly, the physician cannot gain enough information from interviewing a child and conducting a physical examination to determine whether he has ADHD, must less determine whether he does or does not need to be placed on medication. Barkley and Murphy (1991) further make the point that, from a medicolegal perspective, children should not be placed on stimulant medication without at least having the parents and day-care personnel or schoolteachers complete behavior rating scales on the child. For these reasons, the evaluation should include at least an interview of the child and his parents, a physical examination, and standardized rating scales completed by the parents and day-care personnel or schoolteachers.

9.1. ASSESSMENT

The assessment of each individual child's level of functioning should be an on-going process for the practitioner. If the practitioner has a thorough family history, she already has some idea of the risk categories for the child. Also, I have always suggested that the primary-care provider request and add school report cards to each child's office file. This allows the provider to archive the child's school progress for later review.

Asking all parents to complete an Eyberg Child Behavior Inventory (ECBI) (discussed at length in Chapter 4 on assessment) at the 2-year visit gives the practitioner a standardized assessment of each child. As a first-stage screening device, the Eyberg results can, in conjunction with the practitioner's own clinical judgment, facilitate identification of areas of higher-than-normal risk, such as behavior problems, attention problems, or anxiety.

This is not to say that children should be diagnosed with ADHD at 2 years of age. Rather, the practitioner needs to convey to the parents an understanding of and a concern for the behavior and development of each child. Asking questions about day-care or preschool performance at 6-month intervals, with brief notes in the child's file, allows the practitioner to look for trends that might be indicative of behavior or development that is outside of the normal range.

There has been some discussion regarding the age at which ADHD can be accurately diagnosed. While more conservative practitioners recommend waiting until a child is 6 or 7 years old to diagnose ADHD, increasingly more attention is being paid to younger children who have symptoms of ADHD. McGee, Partridge, Williams, and Silva (1991) assessed 976 hyperactive children at 3 years of age and continued assessing them every 2 years until they were 15 years old. Compared with both difficult-to-manage and control groups, these children showed poorer speech articulation, lower IQ, and poorer reading ability in primary school. The authors concluded that preschool hyperactivity must be a target for early intervention; unfortunately, they did not specify what kind of intervention would be most appropriate.

9.1.1. Assessing Children Younger Than Age 6

If the initial screen on the ECBI suggests problems, the Conner's Parent Symptom Questionnaire and the Conner's Teacher Rating Scale can be administered fairly quickly and scored in 4 or 5 minutes, or even faster if the practitioner uses the "Quick Score" forms. The Conner's evaluation tools offer both a parent and a teacher form, and both forms, when scored, yield subscales that are not available with the ECBI. Comments from the parents and alternative caregivers can be a useful adjunct to these standardized tests. Observation and examination of the child in the office can provide additional information for the practitioner. While the behavior of ADHD children is quite variable, one finding has been consistently reported: These children behave better in one-on-one settings than they do in larger groups.

9.1.2. Assessing the School-Age Child

The Child Behavior Checklist (CBCL) has forms for both parents and teachers of children over the age of 5. Both forms have subscales for "attention problems" that can be very useful in diagnosing ADHD. Classroom observation, while beyond the scope of what most practitioners can do, is typically part of a full-scale evaluation by the school. The CBCL does have a form for a standardized classroom observation; however, I cannot recall a single case in which the CBCL classroom observation was used by any of our area private or public schools, even when the school completed a comprehensive, multidisciplinary evaluation. Typically, schools report the results of an unstandardized classroom observation.

The length and comprehensiveness of an evaluation for ADHD has been the subject of much discussion. While some practitioners make a diagnosis of ADHD based on a relatively limited assessment, other practitioners prefer a large battery of psychometric and psychoeducational tests before making a preliminary diagnosis. Much of the published literature supports an evaluation that includes rating scales completed by the parents and the teacher, along with examination of the child's school records (report card, incident reports, and so on).

9.1.3. Multidisciplinary School Evaluation

If there is a strong suspicion that a child has ADHD or learning problems or disabilities, usually there is a history of school personnel making comments to the parents, verbally and/or in writing, to the effect that the child is impulsive and immature, has a short attention span, cannot stay seated, talks too much, or is constantly moving. These children will often rush through their work, both schoolwork and homework, and take home more uncompleted work than their peers. If there is a strong suspicion that the child is having significant problems at school, a written request from the parents to the school for a formal, multidisciplinary evaluation is often indicated. Such an evaluation usually consists of an IQ test, a test for learning disabilities, classroom observation, and whatever additional testing the school personnel think is appropriate.

Chapter 11, on public laws for education of the disabled, provides a comprehensive discussion, for the pediatric health-care provider, of federal legislation that guarantees free evaluation and special services, as needed, for children having difficulty in school. Knowledge of these services is essential for any practitioner who is going to be evaluating and recommending testing or services for children with special needs.

9.1.4. Privately Administered Psychoeducational Testing

If a child is having significant difficulties in the classroom that are documented by comments on report cards and in person with the child's parents, the parents have the legal right to request a multidisciplinary evaluation performed by the school at no cost to the parents. Any practitioner who offers to administer a battery of psychoeducational tests should therefore first advise the parents that the same tests probably could be administered, without charge, by the child's school. After being informed of their right to a free, multidisciplinary evaluation from the school, any family that prefers to have the testing conducted by the practitioner can then be tested privately.

9.2. INITIAL MANAGEMENT OF ADHD

ADHD is not a single, one-dimensional condition. Rather, children have ADHD to varying degrees. Some children have ADHD and no additional problems. Other children have ADHD and learning disabilities, social skill deficits, and motor problems. The initial evaluation of the child suspected of having ADHD must, at least initially, establish that the child meets the diagnostic criteria for ADHD.

There are three major treatment options for a child with ADHD: behavior management alone, medication alone, and a combination of behavior management and medication.

Our initial approach to the management of ADHD is to inform the parents of the findings of our initial evaluation and to inform them that there are two approaches that are usually effective with ADHD—behavior management strategies and stimulant medication. We give the parents two handouts to take with them and to read at their leisure. The first, Handout 9.1, on ADHD, is written by Dr. Patricia Purvis of our office. This handout provides a description of ADHD, how it is diagnosed, some of the manifestations of ADHD, and currently available treatment options.

The second handout we use is a copy of Baren's (1989) article on the Ritalin controversy, which addresses some of the myths put forth about Ritalin over the last several years. We have found that many parents appreciate learning more about Ritalin before placing their child on the medication.

9.3. BEHAVIOR MANAGEMENT WITHOUT MEDICATION

There is a significant overlap between the behavior management procedures used with children who present with oppositional behaviors and the procedures used with children who present with ADHD. Therefore, even though a child may need both behavior management and medication, starting the child on behavior management strategies alone can help with some of his noncompliance. Use of behavior management strategies alone is also appropriate when there is some doubt whether the child should be placed on medication. If the parents are able to implement the behavior management procedures and see an improvement in most of the child's inappropriate behaviors, except for distractibility and a short attention span, the provider has a much stronger case for suggesting that the child be placed on a trial of medication.

Some children can function well with a good deal of structure but with no medication. One issue to explore, then, is how much the child is being stimulated by others around her.

9.3.1. Case Study

I saw a child recently who appeared to be quite active but actually paled in comparison to his father. During the office interview, which was conducted in a physical therapy room full of toys and equipment for children working on muscle development, the father, all 250 pounds of him, was sitting and swinging on a physical therapy device. I asked him repeatedly, as you would with an overactive child, to stop swinging so that we could talk. During the course of our conversation (he never really did stop swinging), he stated he had been on Ritalin as a child but didn't need it anymore. In this case, I was willing to work with the parents in an attempt to find a suitable regimen for the child, but I also recommended that the father see his physician to consider being placed on stimulant medication again. If the child's environment is overstimulating him, you have to attempt to reduce the amount of stimulation he's getting, even though another child might not be overstimulated in that same environment.

9.3.2. Structuring the Child's Environment

In terms of behavior management strategies, we usually begin by instructing the parents in the use of time-in and time-out (see Chapter 2 on cognitive development for more details). When a child presents with behavior problems, it is often difficult to determine if it is simply her behavior that is causing problems or if she also has a short attention span. If implementing behavior management strategies produces a noticeable improvement in the child's behavior, as it has many times in our office, the issue of ADHD need not be addressed, at least for the time being.

Because of the poor organizational skills that many ADHD children have, we typically instruct parents to provide a lot of structure for children suspected of having ADHD. For example, if the parent wants the child to clean his room we instruct the parents to go to his room with him, stand in the doorway, and ask him to put his clothes in the clothes basket. When that part is completed, the parents ask him to put his toys in the toy area. Thus, each complex task is broken into component parts, and the parts are handled one at a time. This technique increases the likelihood that the child will be successful and will receive positive attention from his parents instead of the criticism he receives when he is given too complex a task and is unsuccessful at completing it.

In our office, we see over 800 appointments per year for oppositional behavior in 2- to 10-year-old children. Of the younger children, ages 2 to 4, from 30 to 35% will return 1 to 3 years later with more obvious signs of ADHD. In these cases, I feel as though we have postponed the consideration of medication and relied, successfully, on the behavior management strategies as the primary intervention. Because the majority (65 to 70%) never do require a trial on medication, this seems to be a prudent approach.

9.3.2a. Attention Deficit Disorder without Hyperactivity

Of children who present with ADD, the most difficult to diagnose are those who do not exhibit hyperactivity. Characterized by inattentiveness, hyperactivity is not present. Nevertheless, these children still manifest problems with organization and distractibility, and they may be seen as quiet or passive in nature. It has been speculated that ADD without hyperactivity is currently underdiagnosed as these children tend to be overlooked more easily in the classroom. Thus, these children may be at a higher risk for academic failure than those with ADHD (Education Committee of CH.A.D.D., 1988).

The Teacher Form of the Achenbach CBCL is a useful tool in diagnosing the child with ADD without hyperactivity. A fairly characteristic finding for these children is that they will have a significant score on the "inattentive" subscale, but not on the "delinquent" or "aggressive" subscales. This contrasts with the child who has ADHD, who will usually have significant scores on "inattentive," "delinquent," and "aggressive." Also, because the child does not appear to be hyperactive, the parents are often more skeptical about a diagnosis of ADD, primarily because more parents associate ADD with hyperactivity.

Children with ADD without hyperactivity are more likely to respond to low dosages of Ritalin than their counterparts who had ADHD (Barkley, Dupaul, & McMurray, 1991).

9.3.3. Increasing Attention Span without Medication

We also have developed a protocol for parents' use in increasing their child's attention span (Handout 9.2). The protocol for increasing attention span is designed to provide the child with a lot of physical contact and occasional praise for staying focused on a task. Only after a child has learned to stay focused on a task for the length of time necessary to complete it does she experience the feeling of accomplishment many of her peers already experience when they complete something. This repeated feeling of accomplishment, combined with the enjoyment of play activities, is probably what motivates the average child to stay on task as long as he does.

One recent study showed that behavior management training resulted in significant improvements in parents' compliance management skills, in their children's compliance, and in the overall style of parent–child interaction, but failed to improve any of the measures of the children's attention span (Pisterman et al., 1992). The authors concluded that parent training can be effective for behavior problems but that the more biologically driven problems like attention span are less likely to be affected.

Barkley and Murphy (1991) recommended that ADHD children be placed on such structured programs as the token economies discussed in Chapter 15 of this book. Over time, the child in the structured environment can learn to alter her behavior enough to be within acceptable limits. The token economy, when used to teach social skills, can be a valuable tool for the child with ADHD. The strategies for practicing social skills are described in detail in the Home Chip System Manual (Appendix A) and the Home Point System Manual (Appendix B).

One procedure that is incorporated in both of the token economies consists of the child earning tokens for starting tasks and for working on tasks. This reduces the problem of the child never finishing a task, because we don't require that he finish it in order to earn tokens. For example, if the parent instructs a child to pick up the toys from his bedroom floor, the parent would be instructed to give the child chips when he starts walking toward his room, to give chips again when he begins picking up the first toy, and then to give chips again after three or four toys. By providing tokens for much smaller increments, the child is much more likely to earn the tokens and the access to privileges that are gained from earning the tokens.

Similarly, the child might be given tokens for starting his homework, for working on his homework, for checking his homework, and for completing his homework.

9.4. MEDICATION ALONE

Some ADHD children behave very appropriately; they just have short attention spans and are easily distracted. If both the parents and teachers report that the child does not present with behavior problems, behavior management strategies beyond what the parents and teachers are already doing are probably unnecessary. These children should be given a trial on medication. If the child does not have behavior problems, then no changes would typically be indicated in the way the parents or teachers are managing his behavior. When a child is placed on medication, Ritalin has been the drug of choice. This decision is predicated on the fact that Ritalin is at least as safe as Cylert and Dexedrine and can be prescribed in very small doses, has a short half-life, and is well tolerated by most children.

We always address the side effects of medicine with parents. We have found that discussing the Barkley, McMurray, Edelbrock, and Robbins (1990) paper on the side effects of Ritalin, which demonstrated no discernible difference between low doses of Ritalin and a placebo, is reassuring to parents. We do tell them that, in the unlikely event their child should begin to display muscle twitching or tics, they should immediately stop the medication and contact either our office or their child's physician.

9.4.1. Ritalin Dosage

Because there are no widely accepted recommendations for the number of milligrams of medication per kilogram of children's weight, we usually advise that the physician begin each child, including children up to 8 to 10 years of age, on one 2.5-mg (the smallest pill available, broken in half) dose per day, usually with breakfast. Barkley, DuPaul, and McMurray (1991), in a comparison of three doses of Ritalin (5, 10, and 15 mg), reported that the groups "were not found to differ significantly on any measures in their response to methylphenidate" (p. 519).

If there is going to be a therapeutic effect at a given dosage level, it will usually be evidenced within 4 days. Also, if there is a therapeutic effect, parents, day-care providers, and teachers will be able to ascertain how long the medication is effective, which will direct the physician in terms of what time a second dose should be prescribed, if at all. We have a number of children on the 2.5-mg dosage who have shown a satisfactory therapeutic effect.

Whatever side effects may have been experienced appear to be minimized by starting with the 2.5-mg minidose. Once the physician has feedback on the effectiveness of the 2.5-mg dose, there are three additional possibilities.

First, the child may be doing well enough on the single, daily 2.5-mg dose to stay at that dosage without any need for a second daily dose. Second, the 2.5-mg dose may produce a therapeutic effect, in which case the medication does not have to be increased but a decision must be made about the timing of a second daily dose. We have some children whose first dose produces a therapeutic effect for 3 hours, some for 4 hours, and some all the way up to 6 or 7 hours. However long the first dose lasts, the second dose, if indicated, can be prescribed approximately one-half hour prior to the time the therapeutic effect wears off from the first dose. Third, the breakfast dose may need to be increased to 5 mg. If the 5-mg dose produces a therapeutic effect, in some children there is no need for a second daily dose. Others will need a second daily dose, with the duration of the therapeutic effects of the breakfast dose providing information about when to prescribe the second dose. In this fashion, the physician can empirically determine what exact dosages to use and exactly how many doses per day are needed.

One additional consideration has to do with what has been called a Ritalin "rebound." Some children do fine on the medication, but their behavior shows a dramatic deterioration when the medication wears off. These children are good candidates for a third dose at about 4 P.M. If the child is doing all right on 2.5 or 5 mg twice a day, the "rebound" can usually be controlled by a dose of 2.5 mg at about 4 P.M.

Some children need to be medicated every day of the week, every week of the year. The old adage that children need to be medicated only when they are in school is true some of the time. However, each child presents a unique case and must be managed individually. If a child is having problems at home or with his friends that apparently stem from his short attention span or impulsiveness, a medicine trial may well be in order. In many of the milder cases of ADHD, where the child functions fine at home and with friends, there is probably little benefit to be derived from medication outside of school hours.

There are children who need to be medicated only during the school hours. For those parents who express concern about their child taking any kind of medication, dosages only during school hours, only on days when school is in session, reduce the total amount of time the child is on medication to the absolute minimum. These children are taking their medication only one-half of the year for 8 hours each day; as such, they are medicated only one-sixth of the year.

We simply do not know, yet, why some children need medication both at home and at school and some need it in only one of the settings. That's why an empirical trial helps to determine when to dose a child.

9.5. MEDICATION AND BEHAVIOR MANAGEMENT TRAINING

The majority of children with ADHD require both medication and behavior management training (Barkley, 1990). If the greatest problems are with distraction, concentration, and impulsiveness, we recommend establishing therapeutic levels of medication prior to implementing behavior management strategies. Many highly distractible children are not as amenable to behavioral interventions, and, without medication for the child, the parents may become discouraged by the lack of their child's responsiveness to the added behavioral changes. Once the correct dosage has been determined—which normally doesn't take more than 1 or 2 weeks—behavior management strategies can be introduced to the parents and the child.

In children where the medication trial does not produce a therapeutic effect, including trials on several other medications, behavior management procedures are all the more important.

9.6. THE SCHOOL'S ROLE IN THE MANAGEMENT OF ADHD CHILDREN

Many teachers do an excellent job of handling ADHD children in their classroom. Many schools take a very active approach to the management of children with special needs, providing educational forums and support groups for parents. As is pointed out in Chapter 11, since September 1991, the public schools must now provide whatever evaluation and special services might be necessary for children with ADD.

Both the February and April 1991 issues of the *Journal of Learning Disabilities* were devoted to the topic of ADHD as it relates to the schools. Both are excellent reading for the practitioner interested in ADHD.

9.7. SUPPORT GROUPS

Given the complexity of ADHD, the controversies that exist over its management, and the fact that it usually can be controlled but not cured, we have found that many parents benefit from joining the national organization called CH.A.D.D. (Children with Attention Deficit Disorder). Membership in the organization entitles parents to a monthly newsletter (the CHADDer Box) and makes them eligible to attend local monthly support group meetings and the annual national meeting. Many major cities now have chapters of CH.A.D.D.; the national office, located in Florida, can be contacted by calling 305-587-3700.

9.8. CONCLUDING REMARKS

The assessment, diagnosis, and management of ADHD present dramatic challenges to health-care practitioners. Because many of the symptoms of ADHD are present to some extent in all children, and because many different adults can observe the same child and come to varying conclusions about how excessive her behavior is, the provision of clinical services to children suspected of having ADHD is difficult, yet rewarding. Because of the intensity of children who truly have an attention deficit, the successes are very rewarding, to the parents, the child, and the practitioner. However, the intensity of these youngsters also means that treatment failures are more difficult to manage. When the parent of an ADHD child calls to tell you the medication isn't working and the school has asked her to remove the child for the rest of the day, everyone involved feels a sense of failure.

The fact that some ADHD children also present with learning problems and social skill deficits further contributes to the difficulty of managing them. The decisions about medication versus behavior management, and which to implement first, are often easier to discuss at workshops on ADHD than in the office with the child's parents, who are understandably frustrated and want answers. When we have these answers, and our answers benefit their child, the parents are relieved and grateful. When we don't have the answers, the intensity of the parents' feelings is just as great as the intensity of their child's feelings. We hope someday to find out how to prevent ADHD from occurring in the first place, rather than having to make decisions regarding how to manage it.

REFERENCES

Baren M: The case for Ritalin: A fresh look at the controversy. *Contemp Pediatr* 6:17–25, 1989.

Barkley RA: *Attention Deficit Hyperactivity Disorder: A Handbook for Diagnosis and Treatment.* New York: Guilford Press, 1990.

Barkley RA, DuPaul GJ, McMurray MB: Attention deficit disorder with and without hyperactivity: Clinical response to three dose levels of methylphenidate. *Pediatrics* 87:519–531, 1991.

Barkley RA, McMurray MB, Edelbrock CS, Robbins K: Side effects of methylphenidate in children with attention deficit disorder: A systematic, placebo-controlled evaluation. *Pediatrics* 86:184–192, 1990.

Barkley RA, Murphy JV: Treating attention-deficit hyperactivity disorder: Medication and behavior management training. *Pediatr Ann* 20:256–266, 1991.

Education Committee of CH.A.D.D.: *Attention Deficit Disorders: A Guide for Teachers.* Plantation, FL: CH.A.D.D., 1988.

McGee R, Partridge F, Williams S, Silva PA: A twelve-year follow-up study of preschool hyperactive children. *J Am Acad Child Adolesc Psychiatr* 30:224–232, 1991.

Pisterman S, Firestone P, McGrath P, Goodman JT, Webster I, Mallory R, Goffin B: The role of parent training in treatment of preschoolers with ADDH. *Am J Orthopsychiatr* 62:397–408, 1992.

Sample Handouts

Attention Deficit Hyperactivity Disorder

While the information you are about to read may be new to you, researchers have been writing about this topic since 1902. At that time doctors had studied some people who acted impulsively, had problems paying attention, and were easily distracted. One term that was used for this disorder was "Hyperactivity Disorder." Every year, researchers are learning more. The name that is used now is "Attention Deficit Hyperactivity Disorder" (ADHD). This handout will help you get better acquainted with this term.

Approximately 3 percent of the children-age population has this disorder, which can vary from very mild to severe. About six boys to every one girl are treated in clinics for ADHD. There are some behavioral "warning signs" that often cause parents, teachers, and other professionals to think that it might be a good idea to examine a child for ADHD. They must be present for at least 6 months, and may include some or all of the following:

- Fidgets, squirms, or seems restless
- Has difficulty remaining seated
- Easily distracted
- Has difficulty awaiting turns
- Answers questions impulsively
- Has difficulty following instructions
- Has difficulty sustaining attention
- Doesn't complete tasks at home or school
- Has difficulty playing quietly
- Talks excessively
- Often appears to not be listening
- Interrupts or intrudes on others in games or conversations
- Often loses things, like assignments or supplies
- Engages in dangerous activities

While most children do some of the things listed, children with ADHD often do many or all of them and they do them much more often than other children.

More specifically, these youngsters have difficulty with 5 main areas:

1. *Attention.* They seem to shift quickly from task to task.

2. *Impulse control.* They don't stop to think before they act and they don't have the ability to wait for rewards.

3. *Excessive motor movement.* Their bodies move more, especially in places where control is expected such as in the classroom, at parties, or in restaurants.

4. *Diminished ability to follow rules or directions.* Their learning of rule-governed behavior is like a younger child.

5. *Variable performance.* Their behavior may vary from hour to hour, day to day, and even from caretaker to caretaker.

CAUSES AND CORRELATES

While an exact cause of ADHD has not been determined, most experts agree it is biological, usually existing at birth, and has something to do with the chemistry in the brain. Children with ADHD are usually considered as smart as their peers, which means that children from all intelligence levels can have ADHD. The chemistry in their brain makes concentration more difficult and they need to be continually motivated to stay on task.

Heredity is the single factor shown to be a common association of children with ADHD. They are four times more likely to have siblings, relatives, or parents who have the disorder. Other causes have been investigated. While allergies and diet are sometimes suspected of causing increased activity, studies show that only 1 in 20 children respond to a change in diet, and there have been *no* studies that conclusively show that sugar has an effect on behavior. Exposure to alcohol and cigarettes during pregnancy has been found to have some causal effect. No one knows for sure how much of those substances it takes to affect an unborn child, so most experts are saying no level of tobacco, alcohol, or drug consumption during pregnancy is safe.

DEVELOPMENT

Many children with ADHD can be identified by age 3½. Parents may note that their child was a fussy baby who didn't like to cuddle much. They often comment that their child is harder to manage and gets into more dangerous situations than others his age. However, by age 6, when more pressure is put on these youngsters to function in environments with more rules, like school and sports, other professionals may begin to notice a problem.

Children with ADHD continue to have to adjust to the disorder as they grow older. They continue to have difficulty learning to pay attention for longer periods of time. In fact, they often appear to be several years behind others their age in this area. This should be considered when they are asked to do long classroom assignments or a lot of homework. For example, a 10-year-old with

ADHD might have the attention span of a 7-year-old. It would be unrealistic to expect a 7-year-old to sit down and do an hour of homework. Rather it would be helpful to break up that homework into 15 minutes sessions with a break in between.

About one-third of children with ADHD will have difficulty in school because of a learning disability. It is important to work closely with school personnel to monitor your child's progress. Sometimes it is helpful to have the school's special services personnel conduct an evaluation to determine the best way to educate your child.

ADHD is not a disorder that is outgrown. Each developmental stage will present concerns and require monitoring. Expecting to have this disorder "fixed" is not a realistic way to think about it.

SCHOOL BEHAVIOR AND PEER RELATIONSHIPS

The ADHD child's performance will vary at school just as it may vary from day to day at home. A variety of social, organizational, and academic problems may show up as well. Goldstein and Goldstein (1989) describe school problems well:

> One of the most common descriptors of the ADHD child in the classroom, is that of a daydreamer. The research consensus, however, suggests that it is not simply daydreaming, but rather inattentive behavior. The child is not engaged in random, aimless activity, but focusing on other stimuli. Researchers have noted ADHD kids focusing on parts of their bodies, pencils, or clothing, while their non-ADHD peers are attending to classroom activities. Additionally, the ADHD child's impulsivity often results in his beginning tasks before instructions have been presented and before he clearly understands the task. It further interferes with his ability to contribute effectively in the classroom. The classic ADHD child is described as the first to have his hand raised whether he knows the answer or not. These behaviors interfere with the smooth workings of the classroom and further contribute to the child's alienation by peers and even at times the teacher.

ADHD children often have a difficult time making friends and developing friendships. Because of their restlessness and impulsivity, quiet games don't satisfy them. They may often attempt to solve problems aggressively or be very bossy and want to direct everyone's play. Other children may eventually avoid this youngster because of his unpredictable behavior, and they may be afraid of him.

Adults often describe ADHD children as lacking social skills and the ability to make appropriate social decisions. They are described as having fewer friends and they often tease, provoke, interrupt, or fight with other children and adults. At times they may become physically aggressive and/or destructive with their possessions or those of others.

IDENTIFICATION

Information from a number of sources is obtained before a diagnosis of ADHD is made. The most valuable information can be obtained through a thorough family interview.

Parents will be asked to fill out several checklists that provide further information about their child's behavior, how he acts around other people and at home. We may ask you to have your child's classroom teacher fill out several forms regarding school behavior. Sometimes a visit to the school is necessary. Further educational and psychological testing, which should be available from your child's school, is helpful if the child is having academic problems or more severe behavior problems.

An interview with the child can provide insight from his/her point of view. The child can describe the difficulties and frustrations s/he may feel. The child is often relieved to discover that other children have the disorder and someone can understand how he has been feeling.

THERAPY

The most successful method found for improving the condition of an ADHD child is a combination of medication and consistent management of behavior. The younger the child is when therapy is begun the better the prediction for a good outcome. Researchers have also found that assistance should be sought even through adolescence. As new problems arise with each developmental age they should be worked with, not ignored.

Medication. The prescription medication Ritalin is most often recommended and has been shown to be successful with almost 80% of children with ADHD. Parents should not think of the medication as "fixing" their child. It should not be used alone, but along with behavioral and educational changes.

Ritalin is a medication that acts as a stimulant to the attention center of the brain. The attention center of the brain communicates with the rest of the brain to regulate attention, decision making, and concentration. Ritalin helps that attention center perform these activities more efficiently. This medication takes effect within about 30 minutes and is out of the system in 3½ to 4 hours. In most cases children take 2 doses: one in the morning before school, and a second dose at noon. In some cases a third dose is recommended after school to assist the child in completing homework. Dosage is determined individually. Usually a low dose is prescribed at first and adjustments are made according to how well the child responds. Other medications that are sometimes used are Dexedrine and Cylert. Some children experience side effects. Most side effects are transient. Some children may report a mild stomach upset, headache, less of an

256

appetite, or difficulty falling asleep at night. Sometimes parents notice that their child is more sensitive and may "cry at the drop of a hat." Usually these are not noticed at low dosages.

A more serious side effect can occur in children whose family history is positive for tic disorders such as Tourette's syndrome. Ritalin would not be recommended for these children. If it is prescribed and a parent observes the child making a repetitive motor movement that seems to be involuntary (like twitching an eye, jerking a shoulder, or vocalizing), the medication should be discontinued and the child's prescribing physician notified.

Medication must be prescribed by your child's physician and must be refilled on a monthly basis. This ensures that your child is being monitored by a medical professional as well as a psychologist.

A variety of behavioral and educational interventions can be suggested in conjunction with medication. These interventions vary according to the needs of the child and his family. Further information on the methods recommended for your family will be provided. Please feel free to contact our office for further information.

BEHAVIORAL PEDIATRICS CLINIC
AT CHILDREN'S MERCY HOSPITAL

While each child and his/her family's concerns are different, this section will provide you with information regarding what to expect when you make an appointment to see a therapist in the Behavioral Pediatrics Department at the Children's Mercy Hospital or the Johnson County Office.

After your make an appointment, you will be sent several forms to complete and bring with you to the first appointment. An extensive intake form, a Child Behavior Checklist by Achenbach (blue form for parents), and a Home Situations Questionnaire will provide important information for the therapist. During the first appointment, time will be spent interviewing the parents and the child individually. At that time you may be given some forms for your child's teacher to complete and mail back to the clinic (if your child is school age). Those forms include a Child Behavior Checklist by Achenbach (green form for teachers) and a School Situations Questionnaire. It may be determined at this appointment that a visit to the child's classroom for observation is necessary. If this is recommended, the therapist will arrange for the visit with the classroom teacher and charge for that time as for any other appointment.

Parenting is difficult. Parenting a child with ADHD is even more difficult. Some recommendations may be made to manage your child in a different manner than you did before coming to the clinic. Those recommendations may include spending special time with your child, paying attention to him/her in a different way, learning to be a better manager of your child's behavior with rewards, and using a form of Time-out/Time-in that you will be trained to do. Some families are taught to use a management system that is very structured, using chips or points, for a specified period of time, in order to better manage their child's behavior. The system is one that was developed by E. R. Christophersen, Ph.D., Director of this clinic, and is used widely in other clinics in the United States. Often special arrangements are made with the classroom teacher to send brief reports home with the child to let the parents know how his/her behavior is at school. This prevents the loss of time occurring between a problem at school and when the parents or therapist finds out.

Medication may be recommended in conjunction with beginning behavior management, or it may be determined to be necessary later on in therapy. If medication is recommended, your child's physician will be consulted, with your approval, to discuss the possibility of prescribing the medication and to follow your child from a medical point of view. A low dosage of medication will be prescribed to determine the lowest dose necessary to improve your child's ability to attend. Parent reports and further contacts with the classroom teacher will provide that information.

Some children with ADHD often have a difficult time calming themselves down when they get overexcited or angry. Sometimes it is helpful to directly teach them relaxation strategies to practice when they recognize they are getting out of control. This technique is often implemented following an improvement in general behavior management at home. It is also not recommended for children younger than about 6 or 7 years of age.

Initially, approximately 4 to 6 clinic appointments should be expected to establish different ways of managing your child and for you and the therapist to determine if improvement is occurring. Following this initial time, follow-up appointments will be made at 4- to 6-month intervals to "fine tune" your management skills and to determine if your needs are being met. This is a good time to assess the benefit of the medication as well.

Each family has different needs. The information provided herein includes some of the techniques we recommend, but these are not necessarily used with each family. Our clinic has a therapist on-call 24 hours a day to answer any questions you may have during the initial or follow-up periods. If your calls become frequent and/or lengthy, that is an indication that it is time to make an appointment to see your child's therapist. The parents of a child with ADHD have a very hard job. We hope to provide you with some ways to make it a little easier.

©Patricia Purvis, 1990.

Increasing Attention Span

Increasing your child's attention span is a very slow process but well worth your time and effort. The age of your child will determine what type of activities you will use to increase his attention span. For toddler-age children, playing quietly by themselves is a good behavior to use. For older school-age children, reading and small projects can be used. Always begin with behaviors that your child likes and that are enjoyable to him or her—then gradually add more difficult tasks.

1. Determine how long your child is now playing or engaging in any specific behavior (coloring, playing quietly, reading). This may be a very short amount of time (1 to 5 minutes).

2. Pick a time each day to work on this. Your child will need the structure of a specific time each and every day to work on increasing his attention span to make the process easier.

3. Begin by instructing your child to engage in the behavior you have chosen (for example, playing quietly) for an amount of time you feel certain he can do (maybe 5 minutes). Set a timer for that amount of time.

4. Praise your child very briefly (you don't want to distract him/her) as often as possible during this time.

5. If your child engages in the activity for the specified amount of time, praise and reward him. This can be done by spending 5 to 10 minutes playing with him, reading a story, giving snacks, and so on. Tell him how proud you are, and so on.

6. Gradually increase the required time. The amount of time will depend on your child. Try 3 to 4 days at each time to begin with. You may need to stay on one time length for more than 3 to 4 days depending on your child's progress. Don't lengthen the time until your child is doing well at the shorter time interval.

7. If your child has tantrums before or during the time you are working on this behavior, place him in time-out. After a time-out is over, instruct him again to engage in the activity. Praise getting started and trying. Make this as pleasant as possible, but don't give in to the tantrum by allowing your child to stop working for the specified time.

8. Equally important is *modeling* the kind of behavior you expect your child to exhibit. For example, if you would like your child to read more, it's very important that he see you enjoying reading. Don't make the mistake of "waiting until the kids are in bed" to do your reading.

©Edward R. Christophersen, 1984.

Chapter **10**

Management of Habit Disorders

Thumb sucking, hair pulling, and nail biting are representative of a class of behaviors referred to as habit disorders. There are no rigid criteria for determining whether a particular problem should be classified as a habit disorder. For example, while soiling is considered normal until a child reaches 4 years of age, at which time it is considered abnormal, there is no such consensus for thumb sucking. There are many different opinions regarding when thumb sucking should be treated, if at all. There are also many different recommendations for the treatment of thumb sucking. However, there are few published reports that document the efficacy of treatment procedures for habit disorders.

10.1. ENCOURAGING THE DEVELOPMENT OF GOOD HABITS

While the term "habit" often has negative connotations, habits can and do serve a very important purpose in normal, everyday life. Anyone who buckles his seat belt every time he gets into a car has established a habit of seat-belt wearing. Anyone who takes a vitamin pill every morning has established a habit of taking her vitamins. Neither of these examples is negative; rather, both examples are positive.

I have often thought it is much easier to teach a child a good habit than it is to break a bad habit. Thus, the parent who brushes his teeth every day in front of his young toddler has the beginnings of a good habit for his child.

If the parent begins by gently rubbing the toddler's teeth with a wet washcloth, gradually progressing from brief touches of the child's teeth with a toothbrush to actually brushing them briefly, she can progress until the child is having her teeth brushed every night before bedtime without either the parent or the child ever thinking about what she is doing. In time, with practice and with appropriate modeling from the parent, the child will acquire the habit of brushing her teeth.

Similarly, children who are put to bed awake but drowsy, and are allowed to fall asleep on their own, learn their own sleep-onset habits. Children who ride in some kind of automobile restraint from birth to adolescence, in an automobile with parents who always wear their own seat belts, will have a high likelihood of establishing the habit of wearing seat belts—a habit that may well stay with them the rest of their lives.

Primary health-care providers can serve their young patients well by educating parents about the importance of encouraging their children to develop good habits. Parents who exercise regularly, eat balanced meals, and don't smoke are more likely to have children who exercise regularly, eat balanced meals, and don't smoke. Moore, Lombardi, White, Campbell, Oliveria, and Ellison (1991) found that children of active parents were 5.8 times more likely to be active than were children with inactive parents.

To help a child develop good habits, it is best to repeat the habit over and over again, over an extended period of time, using exactly the same sequence each time. Thus, to develop the habit of tooth brushing in their children, parents should brush their own teeth every night before bedtime. They should brush their child's teeth in the same bathroom, in about the same manner every night. In time, the child will develop the habit of brushing his teeth.

10.2. DIFFERENTIAL DIAGNOSIS OF HABITS AND TICS

When children have acquired "bad" habits, the first priority of the health-care provider is to determine whether the child exhibits a simple bad habit or a habit disorder, or whether the habit is a manifestation of an Obsessive-Compulsive Disorder (OCD).

Technically, there are three different diagnostic categories for what may be referred to as habit disorders or tics. These include:

- Habit disorders.
- Tics.
- Obsessive-compulsive disorders.

Each of these disorders is described in more detail below. The differential diagnosis of habits and tics is based on the severity of the problem, family history, whether the problem interferes with the child's daily activities, and whether the person can voluntarily produce the habit and voluntarily stop the habit for a period of at least a couple of hours.

10.3. STEREOTYPY/HABIT DISORDER

According to the *Diagnostic and Statistical Manual of Mental Disorders*, habit disorders:

1. Are intentional, repetitive, nonfunctional behaviors such as hand shaking or hand waving, body rocking, head banging, mouthing of objects, nail biting, and picking at the nose or skin.
2. Either cause physical injury to the child or markedly interfere with normal activities, for example, injury to the head from head banging or inability to fall asleep because of constant rocking.
3. Do not meet the criteria for either a Pervasive Developmental Disorder or a Tic Disorder. Generally, such childhood habits as thumb sucking and nail biting come under the heading of habit disorders

The most organized and comprehensive research in the area of behavioral treatment of habit disorders has been published by Azrin and Nunn (1977). Under the heading of habit disorders, Azrin and Nunn include nail biting, stuttering, hair pulling, and nervous tics such as shoulder jerks, head jerks, elbow jerks, trembling of the hand, eye blinking, twitching or squinting of the eyes, and jerking of the mouth and cheek. Habit disorders can be distinguished from organically caused movement disorders because habit disorders can be produced voluntarily, can be temporarily suppressed, and can be modified by distractions or special attention. In addition, muscular atrophy is not present, and nervous tics are not painful. A thorough medical history should always be obtained and, if in doubt, further medical evaluation, by a pediatric neurologist, should be completed prior to management as a habit disorder.

10.3.1. Simple Thumb-Sucking and Nail-Biting Habits

Under the heading of simple habit disorders, I include thumb sucking and nail biting. Azrin and Nunn (1977) report that about 40 million people in the United States bite their nails. There seems to be general agreement in the pediatric literature that thumb sucking and nail biting should not be treated below the age of 4; several authors have recommended waiting until the child is 5 years old. Prior to any attempts to treat thumb sucking or nail biting, advise the parents to ignore these habits if the child is below age 4. Most informal attempts to stop thumb sucking or nail biting will not be successful and may aggravate the relationship between the parents and the child. Therefore, the parents should not constantly take the child's thumb out of her mouth, nag him about thumb sucking, or punish her by taking away privileges or offering rewards that will not be earned and, thus, will be unavailable to the child.

Friman, Barone, and Christophersen (1986) analyzed the effectiveness of a procedure to stop thumb sucking. We began by recommending that the parents use a great deal of time-in (discussed in Chapter 2 on cognitive development), as well as an aversive-tasting solution painted on the child's fingers and thumb. It took an average of 2 minutes to explain treatment to the parents. The procedures resulted in the complete elimination of thumb and finger sucking in all of the children in the study within a matter of weeks. Handout 10.1 was given to parents who participated in the study.

More recently, Friman and Leibowitz (1990) made some minor adaptations to these procedures, including a reward system beyond the simple time-in procedures. They also addressed the issue of procedural acceptability to parents who participated in the study. They reported that parents, pediatricians, and pediatric psychologists, when asked to rate the acceptability of the treatment procedures, found them to be "very acceptable."

10.3.2. Habit Covariance

An interesting phenomenon cited in behavioral literature is called "covariance," referring to behaviors that, while seemingly quite different, vary together; when something affects one of the behaviors, the other also changes.

Friman and Hove (1987) published a report showing that thumb sucking and hair pulling (trichotillomania) covary. They reported that hair-pulling behavior was eliminated concomitantly with successful treatment of thumb sucking in children who chronically demonstrated both behaviors. Decreases in the rates of thumb sucking (which occurred after the parents began using the aversive-taste procedures) were closely followed by similar changes in the rates of hair pulling.

The most important consideration in deciding whether to treat thumb sucking in children who pull their hair is whether the two behaviors always occur together. In their 1987 research, Friman and Hove reported that the children were always sucking their thumb while pulling their hair, but did suck their thumbs without pulling their hair. When this is true, treatment of thumb sucking is certainly a viable option. Because thumb sucking almost always occurs more often than hair pulling, it is usually easier to treat. If both thumb sucking and hair pulling cease, fine. If just thumb sucking stops, hair pulling can always be treated separately.

We have successfully used the aversive-taste treatment of thumb sucking in a number of children who both sucked their thumbs and pulled their hair. The Friman and Hove (1987) article provided experimental evidence that the procedures were effective.

10.3.3. Importance of Self-Quieting Skills

In my opinion, most children's habit disorders are related to self-quieting skills. Most thumb sucking gets started by children who suck their thumbs as a means of self-quieting. Parents usually find this quite acceptable in young children yet become concerned when the child reaches 3 or 4 years of age and is still sucking his thumb. Encouraging the development of a variety of self-quieting skills may be an effective way of reducing the child's need for thumb sucking in the first place—before the thumb-sucking habit becomes well established.

Friman and Schmitt (1989) recommend that if a child is over 6 years of age, has a malocclusion, and has failed the recommended combined-treatment procedures above, she should be referred to a dentist who can provide an intraoral appliance that virtually prevents thumb sucking.

10.3.4. Masturbation by the Toddler

Another habit common for children and upsetting to parents is masturbation by toddlers. The vast majority of the time, masturbation is not a sign of child abuse or emotional problems. Rather, it is usually a completely innocuous behavior (Spitz and Wolf, 1949). In fact, McCray (1978) described a procedure for reducing masturbation in 4- to 8-year-olds that involved instructing the parents to provide the child with a great deal of physical contact throughout the day. He reported a dramatic reduction in masturbation on initiation of increased nonsexual tactile contact by the parents. This kind of contact has been discussed at length in Chapter 2, in the section on time-in. There are no data available on the effectiveness of McCray's procedures with toddlers.

Our handout for managing masturbation in toddlers (Handout 10.2) includes McCray's (1978) recommendations and instructs the parents on what to do when they find their child masturbating.

We do not recommend any treatment for the child who holds his genitals at bedtime or for children who engage in rhythmic rocking. This is one of the most common ways that children self-quiet in preparation for sleep onset.

10.4. HABIT AND TIC DISORDERS

For most habit disorders other than thumb sucking and nail biting, there aren't any simple solutions like using an aversive-tasting solution.

Azrin and Nunn (1977) provide a comprehensive approach to dealing with habit disorders that they call "habit control" or "habit reversal." They reportedly treated over 300 patients, with an average reduction of the habit of 99.5% at 6 months. Their standard treatment (which is outlined below) was conducted during a single counseling session that lasted about 2 hours. For the more difficult habits of tics and stuttering, they reported treatment sessions of 2 to 2½ hours in length. For less difficult habits of nail biting and hair pulling, they reported treatment sessions lasting 1½ to 2 hours; a second session was not provided unless the client experienced difficulties after many days or weeks had lapsed. Patients were instructed to call the researchers on the phone each day for a few minutes to review their progress. These calls were made progressively less often as the habits became progressively less of a problem.

Several major components to habit-reversal procedures include:

- *Motivation*—helping the patient realize the full inconvenience caused by the habit.
- *Awareness*—helping the patient become aware of the specific details of the habit.
- *Competing reaction*—instructing the patient to learn to use muscles that directly compete with the muscles used in the habit or tic.
- *Corrective reaction*—instructing the patient to use the competing response intentionally to interrupt the habit or tic.
- *Preventive reaction*—instructing the patient to perform the competing response whenever he is tempted to perform the habit.
- *Associated behavior*—helping the patient learn to recognize behaviors that precede the habit.

- *Habit-prone situations*—helping the patient become aware of the types of situations in which the habit is likely to occur.
- *Relaxation training*—teaching the patient how to use relaxation procedures when she becomes nervous, especially in habit-prone situations.
- *Social support*—teaching parents how to enlist the support of friends to help them become aware of the habit.
- *Practice*—instructing parents to have their child practice the competing response until it becomes automatic.
- *Symbolic rehearsal*—instructing the parents to have their child practice the competing response in many different situations.
- *Display of improvement*—instructing parents to deliberately seek out situations their child would previously have avoided. (Parents should do this only after they have seen definite improvement.)
- *Record keeping*—instructing the parents regarding the importance of keeping daily records of the frequency of the habit so that they can see what progress their child is making.

These procedures, although complex, are not difficult to teach to parents. Handout 10.3 is a summary of the habit-reversal procedures. We have successfully used these habit-reversal procedures for a variety of habit disorders, including head banging and hair pulling (Finney, Rapoff, Hall, Christophersen, 1983). We adapted the habit-reversal protocol, which was developed to treat motivated adults, to procedures that parents could use with their children. In each case, we first ascertained by interview whether the child was motivated to use the habit-reversal procedures.

Interested readers should refer to Azrin and Foxx's (1977) book for a complete description of applying the habit-reversal procedures to a wide variety of habit disorders.

10.5. TICS AND OTHER MOTOR DISORDERS

In 1977, Azrin and Nunn discussed using their habit-reversal procedures for the treatment of motor tics. Azrin recently published a paper on the treatment of Tourette's syndrome using the same habit-reversal procedures (Azrin and Peterson, 1990). Their data are impressive. They reported a 93% mean reduction of tics for all subjects in the last month of treatment. Reductions occurred for vocal tics as well as for each type of motor tic, for children as well as for adults. They report that their procedures are more effective than data published using pharmacological management of Tourette's syndrome. Further, there are no known side effects of the habit-reversal procedures.

10.6. OBSESSIVE-COMPULSIVE DISORDER

Obsessive-Compulsive Disorder (OCD) is much more serious than either habit disorders or motor tics; there are patients who exhibit obsessions or compulsions severe enough to interfere with normal daily functioning, usually social activities and relationships, or to cause marked distress. Current treatment consists of a combination of behavior therapy, often the habit-reversal procedures developed by Azrin and Nunn (1977), and medication. OCD is generally beyond the scope of the primary health-care provider and should be referred to a center where specialized treatment is available.

10.7. CONCLUDING REMARKS

Treatment of simple habit disorders such as thumb sucking and nail biting is usually provided by the primary-care provider rather than being referred to mental-health professionals. Because there has been no standard treatment modality for more serious habit disorders, a variety of providers have used a wide array of treatment modalities to deal with such habit disorders as hair pulling and muscle tics.

The work of Azrin and Nunn (1977) has set new standards for the treatment of habit disorders. Probably because their work has been published in behavioral journals that are not usually subscribed to or read by primary-care providers, their procedures have not been widely used within medical settings. The extension of their habit-reversal procedures to include Tourette's syndrome is even more impressive. As they pointed out in their paper on Tourette's syndrome, while all of the drugs currently available for the treatment of people with Tourette's syndrome have potentially undesirable side effects, the habit-reversal procedures do not. Granted, it takes longer to instruct parents in the use of the habit-reversal procedures than it does to write a prescription, but, if the habit-reversal procedures are more effective, with no side effects, they should at least be considered in the management of habit disorders.

REFERENCES

American Psychiatric Association, Committee on Nomenclature and Statistics. *Diagnostic and Statistical Manual of Mental Disorders*, 3rd ed., revised. Washington, DC: American Psychiatric Association, 1987.

Azrin NH, Nunn RG: *Habit Control in a Day*. New York: Simon and Schuster, 1977.

Azrin NH, Peterson AL: Treatment of Tourette Syndrome by habit reversal: A waiting-list control group comparison. *Behav Ther* 21:305–318, 1990.

Finney JW, Rapoff MA, Hall CL, Christophersen ER: Replication and social validation of habit reversal treatment for tics. *Behav Ther* 14:116–126, 1983.

Friman PC, Barone VJ, Christophersen ER: Aversive taste treatment of finger and thumb sucking. *Pediatrics* 78:174–176, 1986.

Friman PC, Hove G: Apparent covariation between child habit disorders: Effects of successful treatment for thumb sucking on untargeted chronic hair pulling. *J Appl Behav Anal* 20:421–425, 1987.

Friman PC, Leibowitz JM: An effective and acceptable treatment alternative for chronic thumb- and finger-sucking. *J Pediatr Psychol* 15:57–65, 1990.

Friman PC, Schmitt BD: Thumb sucking: Pediatricians' guidelines. *Clin Pediatr* 28:438–440, 1989.

McCray GM: Excessive masturbation of childhood: A symptom of tactile deprivation? *Pediatrics* 62:277–279, 1978.

Moore LL, Lombardi DA, White JF, Campbell JL, Oliveria SA, Ellison RC: Influence of parents' physical activity levels on activity levels of young children. *J Pediatr* 118:215–219, 1991.

Spitz RA, Wolf AM: Autoeroticism. *Psychoanal Study Child* 16:95, 1949.

Sample Handouts

HANDOUT 10.1

Thumb Sucking

The use of aversive-tasting substances for the treatment of thumb sucking in young children can be quite successful if these treatment procedures are carefully followed.

1. Approximately 1 week before starting the treatment, begin increasing the number of times you have brief, nonverbal, physical contact with your child: pats on the head, brief back rubs, or roughing up his hair. Do not talk during these contacts.

2. Purchase a bottle of "StopZit" (or a comparable product) at least a couple of days ahead of time so that you know it is available when you need it. You should be able to find it in most pharmacies.

3. One or 2 days before you begin treatment, discuss the situation with your child (taking no more than 2 to 3 minutes). Mention that she is too old to suck her thumb, that other kids are beginning to tease her, and that both the pediatrician and the dentist are concerned about the effect that the thumb sucking has on her teeth.

4. Begin the procedures on a Friday night. Right before bedtime, paint the thumb and any fingers he sucks. On Saturday morning, paint the thumb and any fingers he sucks immediately after he awakens. Repeat this procedure every time he sucks his thumb and any fingers, continuing for 1 week after he has stopped thumb sucking completely.

5. Never reprimand your child about the thumb sucking. Lectures, explanations, and reasoning are forbidden.

6. If the child refuses to have the "StopZit" applied, place her in time-out until she agrees to the application. While she is in time-out, do not interact with her in any way.

7. Keep up the brief, nonverbal, physical contact throughout the treatment procedures and for a long time after the thumb sucking has stopped. Refrain from verbal reprimands.

8. The treatment of a habit like thumb sucking requires a diligent effort on the parents' part because the child is not engaging in the habit on purpose. There will be times when he is not aware he is sucking his thumb, and he may get upset when you try to apply the "StopZit." It's preferable that you go through the treatment procedures only one time, so follow them religiously for however long it takes for them to be effective. You probably won't have to repeat them.

9. If your child relapses at some future point, repeat exactly the same procedures except for the initial discussion about thumb sucking.

Edward R. Christophersen, *Little People: Guidelines for Commonsense Child Rearing*. Kansas City, MO: Westport Publishers. ©Edward R. Christophersen, 1988.

Managing Masturbation in Toddlers

Most young children explore virtually every part of their bodies, which means they will inevitably discover that it feels good to touch their genitals. This is very common and should not be cause for parental concern.

If this behavior occurs during a bath, while going to the bathroom, or at bedtime, it is perfectly normal. While it is unusual for small children to actually masturbate, they may enjoy rubbing themselves, rocking in a way that places pressure on their genitals, or moving another object, like a blanket, in such a way that they put pressure on their genitals.

If you notice your child is spending a lot of time stimulating herself while with the rest of the family (for example, while watching television, playing board games, or sitting at the dinner table) but not when she is by herself, there are some things you can do to decrease masturbation.

1. Plan activities during the day that you are reasonably sure your child will enjoy. When your child is busy, particularly when her hands are busy, you will find that there is less of a problem with masturbation. Encouraging independent play skills can do a good deal toward reducing the amount of time a child spends masturbating.

2. Provide your child with a great deal of brief, nonverbal, physical contact throughout the day. If your child is in day care, make sure the day-care provider understands and appreciates the importance of providing your child with a great deal of physical contact and comfort.

3. Do not punish your child for masturbation. Do not offer rewards for stopping masturbation.

4. Explain to your child (when he is masturbating in a public area of your house) that if he wants to "do that," he should go either to the bathroom or to the bedroom—it is not something that is done in front of other people. Instructing your child to go to the bathroom removes any secondary gain that he may have been receiving from aggravating his parents. Masturbation should be treated very matter-of-factly.

5. If you notice your child masturbating in the bathtub, while on the toilet, or in bed at bedtime, ignore it completely. In fact, many toddlers discover they can get pleasurable sensations from their bodies while they are placed on the toilet for extended periods of time during toilet training.

6. Although it is perfectly normal for toddlers and preschoolers to want to play "doctor" or to play "house," it is not a good idea to let such play continue for a long period of time. Young children need frequent supervision for a variety of reasons, only one of which is exploring each other's bodies. Safety is another important reason for monitoring children regularly.

7. One medical reason for children rubbing themselves a lot is an infection, either a urinary tract infection or, in girls, a vaginal infection. If you notice your child has redness around the urinary meatus (where he or she urinates from), has a discharge from the meatus, complains about pain when urinating, begins bed-wetting after 6 months of being dry at night, or has a vaginal discharge (girls only), it would be wise to take the child to the pediatrician.

Edward R. Christophersen, *Little People: Guidelines for Commonsense Child Rearing.* Kansas City, MO: Westport Publishers. ©Edward R. Christophersen, 1988.

HANDOUT 10.3

Habit-Reversal Procedures

For reasons that we don't entirely understand, some children develop habits that aren't well accepted socially. To reduce these undesirable habits as much as possible, use the following guidelines:

1. Keep a record each day of your child's habit episodes, starting before treatment begins.

2. List all of the annoyances and inconveniences the habit is causing your child.

3. Identify and list the mannerisms that immediately precede the habit.

4. Describe exactly how and when your child performs the habit.

5. Teach the child to relax when nervous by changing his posture and breathing slowly.

6. Identify the situations, activities, and people that result in the habit occurring more frequently.

7. Teach your child a competing response for his habit, and encourage him to practice it. Examples of competing responses include:

   a. For nail biting and head tics, isometrically contracting the muscles opposing the tic movement.
   b. For body and head tics, isometrically contracting the muscles opposing the tic movement.
   c. For stuttering, breathing smoothly while speaking in short phrases.
   d. For teeth grinding, dropping the jaw and breathing through the mouth.
   e. For eye squinting, relaxing the face muscles and blinking intentionally.
   f. For eye blinking and twitching, blinking intentionally and shifting the gaze.
   g. For nervous throat clearing or coughing, maintaining air flow in breathing.
   h. For lisping, keeping the tongue at the roof of the mouth, closing the jaw.
   i. For cheek and lip biting, closing the mouth and jaw.
   j. For hand or foot tapping, maintaining steady hand or foot pressure.

8. Teach your child to mentally rehearse and act out how he will deal with the habit in different situations.

9. Ask your child's friends to comment on his progress and to remind him of habit episodes.

10. Seek out situations your child has avoided because of the habit.

11. Each day have your child practice the competing response and rehearse how he will use it.

Adapted from Azrin NH, Nunn RG: *Habit Control in a Day*. New York: Simon and Schuster, 1977.

PART III

EDUCATIONAL INTERVENTION STRATEGIES

Pediatricians are often called upon to assist in the evaluation and/or management of a child with special educational needs. Chapter 11 has important information for the practitioner who must make recommendations to parents and teachers of children with special needs. The legal protections available for these children are also discussed in detail in Chapter 11. For example, a sample of a letter to school personnel, requesting psychoeducational evaluation of special needs children, is included.

Even though the leading cause of death and injury to our nation's children, as well as the leading cause of both physician office visits and hospitalization, is intentional and unintentional injury, many primary health-care providers, and a large percentage of psychologists who provide services to children, do not routinely provide information to parents to reduce the risk of injuries. Chapter 12, "Compliance with Injury-Control Strategies," includes a review and written handouts of several approaches to injury control.

Busy pediatric practitioners simply do not have the time to spend on anticipatory guidance that is required to cover the subject comprehensively. Chapter 13, "Alternatives to Traditional Well-Child Care," describes both group well-child care and continuing education for parents. These alternatives to traditional well-child care can be used to better educate parents while also generating additional revenue for the provider. Many of the details that have been developed by several individuals in their clinical practices are described in this chapter.

Chapter **11**

School Problems

Most parents who receive a note or a phone call from their child's teacher about problems at school will try to accommodate the teacher. If the teacher suggests the child spend more time doing homework or practice more with math, most parents will spend as much time as they can to help. If contacts from the teacher start to occur regularly, or if the teacher expresses a real concern about the child's progress, parents frequently contact their pediatrician for advice.

If school personnel suspect any of a variety of learning problems—mental retardation, problems with hearing and speech, emotional disturbances, behavior disorders, or problems with attention span and distractibility—the pediatrician is even more likely to be called on to help school personnel evaluate the child or to provide medical management of conditions that are affecting the child's performance in school. Although a complete review of this subject is beyond the scope of this book, some of the major issues in cooperating with the schools will be covered. No distinction has been made for different age groups; if one particular age group must be handled differently, it is noted.

11.1. IDENTIFYING PROBLEMS

The primary-care physician who regularly assesses behavior and development in routine well-child care is in the best position to identify problems before they interfere with a child's progress. Routine monitoring of each child's growth and development provides the best possible baseline to track each child. Much as changes in growth and height velocity can be "red flags" for physical problems, routine assessments of a child's behavior can provide red flags for behavioral development.

Many parents either do not notice behavior problems in their children or tend to ignore them, attributing the problems to such extraneous factors as, for example, "He's tired because he didn't get his nap," "He doesn't feel good today," or "She's just getting over a cold." If parents don't notice or appear concerned about their child's behavior, it is the primary-care physician's responsibility to determine whether a potential problem exists and to attempt to convince the parents to intervene early. As I've stated before in this book, prevention and early detection are two of the most important aspects of pediatric practice.

11.2. WHAT CAN BE OBSERVED IN THE OFFICE?

Children who are abusive to their parents in the examination room or who pick up or throw everything in the office that's not bolted down are candidates for more careful screening, as are parents who frequently warn their children without following through. However, just because a child does not exhibit any problems in your office does not mean she is not exhibiting problems at home or in preschool or school. For example, many children who present with Attention Deficit Hyperactivity Disorder in school can be well behaved in the physician's office. For this reason, a standardized screening device should be used. The Eyberg Child Behavior Inventory (Robinson, Eyberg, and Ross, 1980) or the Denver Developmental Screening Test (Frankenburg, 1983) are excellent first-stage screening instruments. Usually the combination of taking a history from the parents, observing the child in the office, and using a screening instrument (particularly if the child's teacher serves as one of the informants) is sufficient to determine whether further evaluation is indicated.

11.3. FURTHER EVALUATION OF THE CHILD

If the initial screening suggests the child may have more problems than would be considered normal, a more comprehensive evaluation of the child is in order. Among the most widely used instruments for evaluating preschool and school-age children are the Conner's Parent Symptom Questionnaire and the Conner's Teacher Rating Scale (Goyette, Conners, and Ulrich, 1978). Both the parent and teacher forms can be used for children ranging in age from 3 to 17 years.

The Child Behavior Checklist also is widely used for evaluating children (Achenbach and Edelbrock, 1983). There are two forms for parents, one for children 2 to 3 years of age, and one for children aged 4 to 16. A teacher form is available for children 6 to 16 years old.

Both the Conner's scales and the Child Behavior Checklist are discussed in more detail in Chapter 4, on assessment.

If you suspect a child has a behavior problem, Attention Deficit Hyperactivity Disorder, or both, getting input from both the parents and the teacher is essential for a complete evaluation. When a child is clearly presenting with problems at school, federal legislation (Public Laws 94-142 and 99-457) provides the child with some very important rights.

11.4. PUBLIC LAWS THAT PROTECT CHILDREN'S RIGHTS

Under Public Law 94-142, a child who has been identified by school personnel as having some type of exceptionality—anything from hearing or visual impairments to behavior problems or Attention Deficit Hyperactivity Disorder—is entitled to a free multidisciplinary evaluation from the school that serves the area in which she lives. That is, any children who are attending either public or private schools and are experiencing difficulties can and usually should be evaluated by their school (Meyen, 1978).

> The Individuals with Disabilities Education Act (IDEA), passed in 1975, and its subsequent amendments (most notably P.L. 99-457) inadvertently have included the pediatrician as a participant in several ways. Requiring a multidisciplinary evaluation that could include a medical, developmental, and/or educational assessment gives the pediatrician an active role (Purvis, 1991, p. 334).

These public laws, which now cover children from birth to age 21, provide for multidisciplinary evaluations—a meeting of all of the professionals involved to discuss the child and to do the following:

- Determine whether any special educational needs exist.
- Develop an Individual Educational Plan (IEP) that details the child's needs, as well as how the school intends to meet those needs.
- Develop objective criteria for determining whether the needs have, in fact, been met.
- Determine a time frame for formal reevaluation to verify that the child is benefiting from added intervention by the school.

11.5. REQUESTING A FORMAL EVALUATION BY THE SCHOOL

Schools often initiate the evaluation of a child who presents with significant problems, but there are situations where a school does not. In these cases, the parents should be encouraged to request, in writing, a formal evaluation. Handout 11.1 describes the process to be used when a child is suspected of having special education needs; also included is a sample letter (Handout 11.2) that could be written by the parents to request services for their child.

When the school receives such a letter, and the school personnel have, in fact, observed that the child may have special educational needs, the school is obligated to provide an evaluation. If the evaluation identifies special needs, the school is further obligated to offer the special services necessary to address those needs. In the unlikely event that a parent requests an evaluation but the school personnel have not noted anything remarkable about the child, there would be no obligation to provide a formal evaluation of the child.

For a more detailed discussion of the pediatrician's role in educating children with special needs, see Purvis (1991).

11.6. MULTIDISCIPLINARY EVALUATIONS

The multidisciplinary team usually consists of the teacher, the principal, a representative from the school's special services section, the school psychologist, and other specialists as needed (speech/language or occupational or physical therapists). The team usually meets to determine what evaluations are necessary; this, in turn, determines which professionals are included in the evaluation. While there is no requirement that the child's physician or psychologist attend the team staffing, there are many situations where their presence would be very helpful.

On completion of the evaluation, the team is required to meet with the parents to discuss the team's findings and to arrive at a plan to meet the individual child's educational needs.

11.7. PRIVATE EVALUATIONS

In my experience, it is not uncommon for parents to try to expedite the evaluation of their child by arranging to have the testing performed by a practitioner outside of the school system. There are two disadvantages to following this practice. First, the parents will be charged a fee for services that would have been free had they been performed by the school. Second, while the school is obligated to follow all of the recommendations made by the interdisciplinary team, they are not obligated to follow any recommendation made a private evaluator.

If some testing should be done that cannot be done by the multidisciplinary team (for example, a medical examination), enlisting the services of a practitioner outside of the school system would, of course, be indicated.

11.8. THE INDIVIDUAL EDUCATIONAL PLAN (IEP)

The educational program for any child with special needs must be individualized to meet the specific needs of each child. This may be the most critical provision for school principals and teaching staff because the IEP serves as a record that each student's needs and abilities have been considered and addressed individually.

11.8.1. Least Restrictive Environment (LRE)

If the school evaluation determines that a child has special educational needs, the school is obligated to provide the child with the least restrictive environment (LRE) that will meet the child's special needs. The LRE refers to the fact that the child must be mainstreamed—kept in a normal classroom—if possible. The most restrictive environment would be in a school for children with special educational needs.

In between these two extremes, from least restrictive to most restrictive, are the:

- Regular teacher receiving consultation services from a special education teacher.
- Child attending a special education classroom several hours each week.
- Child attending a special education classroom several half-days each week.

11.8.2. Educational Objectives

The multidisciplinary team also must derive both short- and long-range objectives, as well as objective measures for determining whether the child has met those objectives. In this way, it is possible for the school to assess whether the child's special needs are being adequately addressed.

11.9. WHAT ABOUT THE EFFECTS OF A CHILD BEING LABELED?

Many parents will express a concern that, if their child is "labeled" by the school, they will carry that label with them forever. This concern usually stems more from a lack of knowledge about special education than from prior experience. The child with special educational needs is at much greater risk from not receiving those services than from being labeled.

11.10. WHAT ABOUT THE CHILD WITH AN ATTENTION DEFICIT?

As discussed in Chapter 9 on Attention Deficit Hyperactivity Disorder (ADHD), children with ADHD may need a combination of special school services and medication; some also require individual or family therapy. While there are children who can be managed with just special school services or with just medication, ideally this is a determination that should be made by the multidisciplinary team, not by a teacher or by the pediatrician alone.

11.11. INTERACTION BETWEEN THE SCHOOL AND THE HOME

Common sense often dictates that the parents support decisions made by the school, particularly when problems are involved. Some teachers give notes to children to take home to their parents when the children have been in trouble at school; but, alas, the children may "lose" these notes before they get home.

If teachers are going to send notes home notifying parents that their child has had problems at school, we ask that the teacher send these notes on a regular basis, with both good news and bad news. However, before a teacher starts sending notes home to parents, there should be a discussion between the teacher and the parents to determine how these notes will be used. Otherwise, parents may assume they should be punitive with their child when they receive a "bad" note. I have always believed that if a child is disciplined properly at school, he doesn't need to be disciplined again at home.

11.11.1. Home–School Notes for Children under Age 7

When children have significant problems both at home and in school, prior arrangements can be made to reinforce the child's school performance at home. A simple home–school note, developed together by the teacher and the parents, can emphasize behaviors that need to increase in frequency; for example, such a note might include a list of four behaviors:

- Followed directions
- Handed work in on time
- Quiet until called on
- Turned in homework assignments on time

The child can earn a small reward from her parents for each of the behaviors that were checked, instead of being punished for each of the inappropriate behaviors checked.

If the parents and their health-care provider have already decided that the child should be started on a chip token economy, such as the one discussed in Chapter 15 on token economies (and detailed in Appendix A), the home–school note feedback can be formalized. For example, the parent can place the home–school note in the middle of the kitchen table. The child is then asked to place two of his chips in each of four piles, and the parent places two chips from the bank in each of four piles. The parents go through the home–school note one item at a time, and the child either earns or loses all four chips for each behavior, depending on how the note was checked by the teacher.

11.11.2. Home–School Notes for Children over Age 7

If the child is on a home point system, as described in Chapter 15 on token economies and detailed in Appendix B, the parents and the child can discuss, during a family meeting, how many points should be gained or lost for each of the behaviors checked by the teacher. Handout 15.4 is an example of such a note for the child older than age 7.

The rationale for the home–school note is to formalize the rewards that the child earns for appropriate behavior at school—not to punish her for inappropriate behaviors at school. If the child is engaging in too many inappropriate behaviors at school, a determination must be made whether the child is engaging in the inappropriate behaviors because she is oppositional, has attention problems, or simply does not have the desired behaviors in her repertoire.

If the problem is oppositional behavior, the parents can be encouraged to work on behavioral compliance at home, using many of the procedures described in Chapter 2. If the child has a short attention span, a determination must be made as to whether she may benefit from a trial on psychostimulant medication. If the desired behavior simply isn't in the child's repertoire, the parents need to be assisted in teaching the child desirable behaviors at home.

11.12. CONCLUDING REMARKS

School problems typically require the cooperation of school personnel, the parents, and, when indicated, the child's pediatrician or psychologist. A haphazard approach that emphasizes punishing the child for his transgressions not only is unlikely to benefit the child but may engender hostile feelings in the child toward both his parents and his teacher and, in some cases, hostile feelings between the parents and the teacher.

A planned approach that takes into consideration the special needs of the child and the special services available from the school, in conjunction with the skills of the child's physician, can provide the child with exactly what she needs.

The interested reader is referred to Purvis (1991) for a detailed discussion of the pediatrician's role in dealing with children who have special needs.

REFERENCES

Achenbach TM, Edelbrock CS: Behavioral problems and competencies reported to parents of normal and disturbed children aged four through sixteen. *Monogr Soc Res Child Develop* 46(1, Serial No. 188), 1983.

Frankenburg WK: Infant and pre-school developmental screening, in Levine MD, Carey WB, Crocker AC, Gross RT (Eds.), *Developmental-Behavioral Pediatrics*. Philadelphia: W.B. Saunders, 1983, pp. 927–937.

Goyette CH, Conners CK, Ulrich RF: Normative data on Revised Conner's Parent and Teacher Rating Scales. *J Abnorm Child Psychol* 6:221–236, 1978.

Meyen EL: *Exceptional Children and Youth: An Introduction*. Denver: Love Publishing Co., 1978.

Purvis P: The public laws for education of the disabled—the pediatrician's role. *J Develop Behav Pediatr* 12:327–339, 1991.

Robinson EA, Eyberg SM, Ross AW: The standardization of an inventory of child conduct problem behaviors. *J Clin Child Psychol*, Spring:22–29, 1980.

Sample Handouts

HANDOUT 11.1

Educational Referral Procedures

The referral procedure may vary slightly from school district to school district. The following provides a list of steps followed by many.

Step 1. The evaluation process can be initiated by parents or school personnel who identify a child's difficulty with academic progress. If the parents initiate the process, they should send a formal letter of request to the school principal and a copy to the district director of special education. If the teacher begins the process, she often must complete a request that is given to the principal.

Step 2. On a regular basis, all children recommended for evaluation are presented to a school screening team. It is necessary to document that the child's potential for learning is not adequately met in the current class placement. A classroom observation may occur and/or screening instruments may be administered. Adjustments for a specified period of time may be made in the student's curriculum, method of management, and arrangement of the environment in the regular classroom. If these are successful, then further steps are not necessary. If not, the process continues. Handout 11.2 is a sample letter that parents could use as an example when composing their own letter.

Step 3. Children who continue to have difficulty in the classroom are scheduled for a multidisciplinary evaluation. Written approval for this step must be given by the child's parent/guardian. More than one professional must be involved in this evaluation. The specialty areas that may be included are psychology, speech/language, academic learning, social work, occupational or physical therapy, nursing, and medical services in some situations.

Step 4. If the test results indicate the child meets the need requirement established by the district for services, a meeting is held to interpret the results to the parents and outline the program proposal to meet the child's needs. At this meeting an Individual Educational Plan (IEP) is presented that includes the short- and long-term goals proposed for the child, the special services personnel who will be responsible for working with the child, the amount of time per week that this will occur, and the setting in which it will occur. The district must offer a variety of available service settings ranging from assistance in the regular classroom to self-contained small-group classrooms, if necessary. Again, parental input, agreement, and written approval must be received.

Step 5. Periodic review of the child's progress including all personnel involved is to occur. The frequency of these reviews depends on the program and the age of the child. However, the parent/guardian can request a review more frequently. The IEP must be rewritten yearly (minimum). A complete reevaluation must occur every 3 years.

The law specifies which categories of children qualify for services. At birth, those children with discernible developmental anomalies should be identified before leaving the hospital and available services identified. Most pediatricians incorporate developmental screening devices into their well-child visits. Children who appear to be functioning less well than expected in any one of the following areas should be considered for referral for special services. Those areas are cognitive ability, speech/language development, fine/gross motor skills, and behavioral/social/emotional skills. It is well documented that the earlier intervention occurs the better the prognosis. Waiting for a child to "outgrow" an identified problem wastes valuable time, and intervention services are now available to tackle severe delays at birth and less severe delays by age 3.

©Patricia Purvis, 1992. Reprinted by permission.

Sample Letter Requesting Special Services

Mr. and Mrs. Hays
100 Broadway
Bestplace, U.S.A. 10000

October 30, 19___
Mrs. Jane Wright, Principal
School Address
Bestplace, U.S.A. 10000

Dear Mrs. Wright:

We have been concerned with the progress our daughter/son has been making in school. We feel she/he may benefit from some special services support offered through the school district. We would like to request that the process for a special services evaluation be begun on our child's behalf.

Please notify us as soon as this process is begun.

Sincerely,

Anne and James Hays

cc: Mr. Vernon Jacobs, District Director of Special Education
Dr. Linda Bishop, Pediatrician

Chapter 12

Compliance with Injury-Control Strategies

During a well-child visit, the average primary care physician spends very little time on injury-control strategies (or accident prevention as it used to be called), yet more visits to physicians and hospital admissions result from accidents than from any other cause (Rivera and Mueller, 1987). Handout 12.1 shows the dramatic rate at which injuries and deaths occur in the United States.

Perhaps one reason that primary care providers have not spent more time on injury-control strategies is that they have not had a cost-effective way of including these strategies in well-child visits. In this chapter, I will review injury-control strategies, beginning with passive strategies, such as legislation, that require very little actual effort. I will then discuss health education and present active strategies that parents can use in their homes with their children.

12.1. THE ROLE OF LEGISLATION IN CONTROLLING INJURIES

Passive strategies are those strategies where the person being protected doesn't have to do anything in order to be protected. The most familiar example of a passive strategy is the air bag for automobiles. The vehicle driver simply enters the car, starts it, and drives it; the air bag is there to protect him in the event of a frontal collision. The attractiveness of passive strategies is just that—no effort is needed on the part of the person who is protected by the strategy. Most passive strategies are mandated by legislation, sometimes local (for example, the requirement that homes have smoke detectors), and sometimes federal (for example, air bags).

Recent statistics indicate that legislation (which has been passed in all 50 states) requiring child-restraint seats has contributed to a significant reduction in the number of children killed in automobile travel (Insurance Institute for Highway Safety, 1987).

Similarly, legislation mandating installation of window guards on all high-rise residential buildings (Speigel and Lindaman, 1977) has resulted in a 50% decrease in the number of children killed from falling out of windows. Virtually every major city in the United States has passed similar legislation.

Other legislative efforts have been directed at reducing the number of children killed or injured by:

- Ingestion of potentially harmful substances. Child-proof caps on medicine bottles are required, and the number of tablets per bottle is limited.
- Drowning. Automatically locking gates and fences around residential swimming pools are required.
- Suffocation. Magnetic latches on refrigerator doors are required.

Present legislative efforts are directed toward mandating installation of air bags and automatic seat belts in automobiles, smoke detectors in homes, installation of seat belts on school buses, and the use of seat belts in all automobiles.

12.2. HEALTH EDUCATION

While most injury-control initiatives require more than just a brief educational message to parents from their health-care provider, there are a number of strategies that the provider can implement.

One program, The Injury Prevention Program (TIPP) (1989), sponsored by the American Academy of Pediatrics, provides age-appropriate safety handouts for distribution by health-care providers. TIPP has gained widespread acceptance within the pediatric community. Handout 12.2 is a TIPP handout for parents of children 1 to 2 years old.

12.2.1. Prenatal Education

Information about injury control, from the use of infant-restraint devices for automobile travel to smoke detectors, should be provided to expectant parents during prenatal classes and prenatal office visits. Barone, Williams, Hassanein, and Christophersen (unpublished manuscript) reported on the effectiveness of including injury-control material during prenatal classes. They provided parents with handouts on the importance of setting hot-water heater temperatures correctly (see Handout 12.3) and the importance of smoke detectors (see Handout 12.4).

One of the major findings of the research by Barone et al. was that, although couples expecting their first child turned down their hot-water-heater thermostats after hearing a lecture on the dangers of children getting scalded by hot water, parents of toddlers did not turn down their hot-water-heater temperatures. When debriefed after the research study was completed, the parents of toddlers stated that they did not turn down their thermostats because their child had not been injured and they didn't think he was at much risk now that he was older and could protect himself.

Apparently, parents have a false sense of security when they have practiced unsafe procedures in their home but have not experienced any unpleasant effects from doing so. The authors suggest that first-time expectant parents are more receptive to health education messages because they have a different history than the parents of toddlers. The time at which a health education message is delivered is obviously deserving of more study.

12.2.2. Nursery and Hospital Discharge Standing Orders

A relatively simple, yet beneficial, strategy is to include in Standing Orders in the hospital nursery and in Nursery Discharge Orders, the order that nursing personnel discuss the importance of using infant-restraint devices for all automobile travel. We have used Handout 12.5 for parents of newborn infants.

12.2.3. Automobile Travel with Toddlers

Handout 12.6 can be used to encourage parents to obtain and use restraint devices for toddlers. Handout 12.7 is for parents who are about to embark on an automobile trip. Both of these handouts are designed to encourage parents to use restraint devices and include information on how to make automobile travel more enjoyable for both toddlers and their parents.

12.3. BEHAVIORAL APPROACHES

While legislation and health education efforts frequently have been used to encourage individuals to implement changes that will reduce the risk of injury they face each day, a variety of behavioral approaches also have been used in recent studies of injury control.

Numerous researchers have described programs designed to encourage parents always to use restraint devices for their toddlers and preschoolers during automobile travel. Parents and children can be offered rewards for correctly using child-restraint seats and for correct seat belt usage, but to produce any lasting effects, these initiatives must be part of a much bigger effort.

Research studies have contributed to our knowledge of how to encourage individuals to comply with injury-control strategies. In the aggregate, these approaches are complementary and can produce an effect that could not be realized when one approach is used in isolation. Gallagher, Hunter, and Guyer (1985) reported very encouraging results from a Home Injury Prevention Program in which a three-part injury prevention strategy was evaluated:

- Regulatory—identification and abatement of violations of existing housing codes.
- Educational—counseling on potential safety hazards in the home.
- Technological—installation and distribution of inexpensive safety devices at no cost to the family.

12.3.1. Combining Passive and Active Approaches

As numerous researchers already have shown, while passive approaches to injury control are preferred, there are many instances when a passive approach is simply not possible. For example, parents can turn down their water-heater temperature to protect children from scald burns, but there is no way to remove all potential sources of drowning—toilets, bathtubs, and buckets—in a home.

In those instances where a passive approach is not feasible, a combination of active and passive approaches is desirable. In actuality, there is little chance that injury control can be realized without the contributions of both passive and active approaches. Legislation mandating the use of child-resistant caps on medicines and restricting the number of pills contained in a bottle of children's aspirin has resulted in a decrease in the number of children treated for ingestion of aspirin. But for true injury control, parents also must be educated and prepared to child-proof their homes.

The very nature of young children dictates that their parents be constantly vigilant about the child's location and activity. No amount of legislation will negate the parents' responsibility for monitoring their children. A combination of passive and active approaches most likely will result in the highest level of protection for children.

12.4. MULTICOMPONENT PROGRAMS

The author and his colleagues (Christophersen, Sosland-Edelman, and LeClaire, 1985) reported very high rates of compliance with the use of infant-restraint seats in automobiles when a multidimensional program was used. Following the passage of state legislation, a program consisting of a hospital loaner program for child-restraint seats; nurses and physicians who encouraged and educated new parents about the need for restraint-seat use; and a community-wide educational program about the advantages of restraint-seat use was correlated with more than 85% of the parents in the study correctly using restraint seats at the time of hospital discharge and at 3-, 6-, and 12-month follow-up observations.

In an extension of this study, Treiber (1986) reported that similar health education approaches were effective at getting parents to use automobile seat-restraint devices correctly for young children. Treiber showed that parents had the highest compliance rates when they were informed about both the dangers of automobile travel and the advantages inherent in the use of child-restraint devices. Discussions of only the dangers of automobile travel or only the advantages of restraint-seat use produced lower rates than combining the two procedures.

In another study, Thomas and her colleagues (Thomas, Hassanein, and Christophersen, 1985) demonstrated the effectiveness of an alternative health education format, group well-child care, for encouraging parents to lower the hot-water temperatures in their homes.

The practitioner can improve the injury-control efforts in the community by supporting, and in some cases initiating, legislation that mandates passive and active measures; by taking an active educational approach in the office; and by supporting educational efforts put forth by the schools.

The Harborview Injury Control Center's (Seattle, WA) effort on behalf of children's bicycle helmets is a striking example of how much individual providers can do to promote injury control. They have produced videos for television stations and school classrooms and arranged with helmet manufacturers to provide discount coupons for helmets. Their efforts have resulted in a decrease in injuries from bicycle accidents when the riders are wearing helmets.

12.5. CONCLUDING REMARKS

Much can be learned about medical compliance from the work done on injury control. Both injury control and medical compliance have been pursued in the same approximate time frame, from the late 1960s to date. Advances in the two areas, although not necessarily overlapping in the published literature, should be joined together, conceptually, to benefit the general population. The need to persuade individuals to comply with injury-control strategies is similar to the need to persuade individuals to comply with preventive acute and chronic disease regimens. Requiring passive changes by law or administrative rule, instead of or in addition to individual behavior change, although not normally thought to be within the domain of medical compliance, does offer great potential for compliance researchers. The strategies for offering automatic protection that have developed in the area of injury control certainly have applicability for medical compliance. For example, the water sanitation systems that have been instituted across the country offer individuals clean water without each family being responsible for boiling their water. Similarly, the fluoridation of water supplies has resulted in decreases in dental caries, without parents having to take the responsibility for providing their children with the appropriate amounts of fluoride.

Although it is simply not possible for health-care providers to control childhood injuries effectively on their own, their efforts, combined with legislative mandates, educational campaigns in schools and in the media, and behavioral procedures implemented by practitioners, parents, and day-care providers, can help reduce the risk to our nation's youth.

REFERENCES

Barone VJ, Williams G, Hassanin RS, Christophersen ER: A comparison of the effectiveness of group health education messages between expectant parents and parents of toddlers. Unpublished manuscript, 1992.

Christophersen ER, Sosland-Edelman D, LeClaire S: Evaluation of two comprehensive infant car seat loaner programs with 1-year follow-up. *Pediatrics* 76:36–42, 1985.

Gallagher SS, Hunter P, Guyer B: A home injury prevention program for children. *Pediatr Clin N Am* 32(1):95–112, 1985.

Insurance Institute for Highway Safety: *Status Report* (December), Washington, DC, 1987.

National Academy of Sciences: *Injury in America: A Continuing Public Health Problem*. Washington, DC: National Academy Press, 1985.

Rivera FP, Mueller BA: The epidemiology and causes of childhood injuries. *J Soc Issues* 43:13–31, 1987.

Speigel CN, Lindaman FC: Children can't fly: A program to prevent childhood morbidity and mortality from window falls. *Am J Publ Health* 67:1143–1147, 1977.

Thomas KA, Hassanein RS, Christophersen ER: Evaluation of group well-child care for improving burn prevention practices in the home. *Pediatrics* 74:879–922, 1985.

TIPP—The Injury Prevention Program. Elk Grove Village, IL: American Academy of Pediatrics, 1989.

Treiber FA: A comparison of the positive and negative consequences approaches upon car restraint usage. *J Pediatr Psychol* 11:15–24, 1986.

Sample Handouts

HANDOUT 12.1

U.S. Accident Rates

	Number per Hour	Number per Day	Number per Week
Accidents resulting in death	11	253	1,780
Accidents resulting in injuries	1,030	24,700	173,100

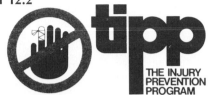

Infant Furniture: Cribs

CHOOSING A CRIB

Special care is required if you are selecting a used crib that may have been manufactured before current crib safety standards were set. To check out an older crib, you will have to take some measurements.

- Cribs should have slats no more than 2-3/8 inches apart. Widely spaced slats pose a strangulation hazard to young infants.
- Check all hardware to make sure all joints and parts fit tightly and snugly. Wood surfaces must be smooth and free of splinters.
- Check for cracked and peeling paint. Be sure that all surfaces are covered with lead-free paint designated for nursery furniture.
- The end panels of the crib should be solid and without decorative "Early American" cutouts. These can trap an infant's head.
- Select only a crib with corner posts that are either flush with the end panels, or else very, very tall (such as a canopy bed). Clothing and ribbons can catch on corner-post extensions, causing strangulation.
- The lowered crib sides should be at least 9 inches above the mattress support to prevent the infant from falling out. Raised crib sides should be at least 26 inches above the mattress support in its lowest position.
- The drop sides should be operated with a locking, hand-operated latch, which is secure from accidental release.
- The mattress should be the same size as the crib so there are no gaps to trap arms, body, or legs. If you can fit two fingers between the mattress and the side of the crib, the crib should not be used.

USING A CRIB

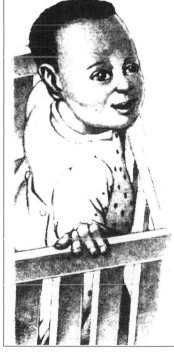

- Carefully read instructions for assembly, use, and maintenance.
- Never leave crib rails down when baby is in the crib.
- No hanging crib toys (mobiles, crib gyms) should be within baby's reach. Any crib toy which is strung across the crib must be removed when your baby first begins to push up on his hands and knees or when he is five months old, whichever occurs first. These toys can cause strangulation.
- Bumper pads should be used around the entire crib until the infant begins to stand. Then they should be removed so that they can't be used as steps.
- Begin to lower the crib mattress before the baby can sit unassisted. Have it at its lowest point before the baby can stand.
- If crib rails are not high enough, safe extenders can be purchased. Children should graduate to a regular bed by the time they are 35 inches tall.
- Never place a crib near hanging window blind or drapery cords. Children can get caught in the cords and strangle.
- Be sure to inspect the crib at grandparent's home, baby-sitter's home, or at day care for safety.

American Academy of Pediatrics

SPONSORED BY SANDOZ PHARMACEUTICAL CORPORATION, PEDIATRIC DIVISION, THE MAKERS OF TRIAMINIC COUGH AND COLD PRODUCTS.
2/90   HE0030

Children and Hot-Water Temperatures

The leading cause of deaths and injuries to children at home is accidents, and scalding from hot water is one of the most dangerous. To show you just how dangerous hot water can be, look at the following chart:

Temperature of Water	Time to Cause a Bad Burn
150° F	2 seconds
140° F	6 seconds
125° F	2 minutes
120° F	10 minutes

You can see from this chart that, if your infant or young child should accidentally, or intentionally, come into contact with hot water, the temperature of the water would make the difference between whether he or she gets burned or not. If your hot-water heater is set at 150° F, and your child should come in contact with the water, he or she would receive a burn bad enough to require medical treatment (known as a full-thickness burn) within *2 seconds*.

The following are some common questions, and their answers, that parents have about hot-water-heater settings.

1. Q: If I turn the hot-water-heater setting down, won't I have trouble getting the dishes in the dishwasher and the clothes in the washing machine clean?

    A: No. The major soap manufacturers design their soap to work best at between 120 and 125° F.

2. Q: Will my baby get more colds if the hot water isn't hot enough?

    A: No. Hot water has nothing to do with getting colds.

3. Q: Will we run out of hot water any sooner if we turn the temperature down?

    A: Yes, you will. But this may be a small price to pay to protect your baby. The recovery time, after using hot water, will be longer when the temperature setting is lower.

4. Q: Will I save any money on utility bills by turning down the temperature setting?

    A: Yes. On the average, for every 10° that you turn the temperature down, you will save 4% on the water-heating portion of your utility bill.

5. Q: I don't know where my hot-water heater is, and I don't know how to tell at what temperature it is set. How can I tell?

A: The first thing to do is to measure the hot-water temperature. The best way to do this is to measure it in the morning, before anyone in your home has used any hot water. Turn on the hot water at the kitchen sink and let it run, straight hot water, for 2 minutes. Then, using either an outdoor thermometer or a candy thermometer, hold the thermometer in the stream of the water until the reading stops going up. If your water-heater setting is at a safe level (between 120 and 125° F) then you don't have to do anything. There is no advantage to setting the thermostat below 120° F. If your hot-water setting is too high, then here are some tips on how to find the thermostat and how to turn it down.

   a. Gas hot-water heaters usually have a thermostat outside the tank at the bottom. Electric water heaters usually have either two panels screwed to the top and bottom of the tank or one panel along the side of the tank. Thermostats are located under these panels.
   b. The thermostat should be set on the "low" setting or within the "energy efficient range." If the temperature at the kitchen sink is still too hot, the setting should be set lower, regardless of what the setting is.
   c. It takes about 24 hours before you can test the temperature again. If you test it in less than 24 hours, you will not get an accurate reading.
   d. Continue to adjust the temperature setting down until you get it down to at least 125° F. If you get it below 120° F, then turn it back up a small amount.

Small children are busy and can get to sinks or bathtubs quickly. They can burn themselves severely before they can get out of the water.

Infants are unable to move away from hot water if it is accidentally left on too hot.

Please, take some time to think about the risk that your child suffers from hot water in your home. Think about whether the convenience of having lots of very hot water is really worth the added risk that you might be taking with your child's health. By the time your youngest child reaches 4 years of age, you can turn your hot-water heater up to a higher temperature, when your child is no longer at significant risk for burn injuries.

Children and Smoke/Heat Detectors

The leading cause of deaths and injuries to children at home is accidents, with fires one of the most dangerous. Most fatal home fires occur at night, while people sleep. If you are asleep or become disoriented from toxic gases produced by a fire, you may not even realize that there is a fire. A smoke/heat detector can sound an alarm and alert you to the danger from a fire in time to escape.

The following are some common questions, and their answers, that parents have about smoke/heat detectors.

1. Q: What are the types of fire alarms or detectors?

   A: There are two types of detectors: (1) the heat detector that sounds an alarm to warn of an abnormally high temperature in the immediate area of the heat detector and (2) the smoke detector that sounds an alarm at the first trace of smoke.

2. Q: What is the power source for smoke/heat detectors?

   A: Some alarms operate on batteries, and some operate on household current, either plugged into a wall outlet or wired directly into the electrical system.

3. Q: What are the advantages and disadvantages of the battery-operated alarm?

   A: The advantages are that they are not affected by a fire that cuts off the electricity to the house and that they can be placed anywhere, even if there are no electrical outlets or wires. The disadvantages are that the batteries need to be changed about once a year, the beep indicating a low battery can be annoying, and false alarms can occur.

4. Q: What are the advantages and disadvantages of the household current-powered detectors?

   A: The advantages include no need to change batteries and no annoying beep indicating a low battery. The disadvantages include the following: Fires that affect the household current will make the alarm not work; detectors must be placed where wiring or outlets are available; and false alarms can occur.

5. Q: Do I have to do anything to maintain smoke/heat detectors?

   A: Yes. You should test the detectors once a month by holding a candle 6 inches away and blowing smoke in the sensing chamber. It should sound in 20 seconds. Some alarms have test buttons, but to be sure the detector works, you must use the smoke-testing method. You need to change batteries when they are low and use the correct kind of battery. You must clean the unit at least once a year by vacuuming the detector. Never paint the alarm.

6. Q: With so many brands of detectors on the market, how do I choose one?

   A: Be sure to buy a detector that has the label of a testing laboratory, e.g., Underwriter's Laboratory (UL), and follow the installation and maintenance recommendations of the manufacturer. Buy the type that best suits your household needs and budget.

7. Q: How many smoke/heat detectors should I buy for my house?

   A: For minimum protection, you should install a smoke detector outside each bedroom area and one on each story of the house. For extra protection, it is recommended that detectors be installed inside bedrooms, dining room, furnace room, utility room, attic, garage, and hallways.

8. Q: Where should the detectors be placed?

   A: Smoke rises, so in order to detect the first traces of smoke, the detector should be mounted on the ceiling (4 inches from any wall) or high on a wall (4 to 12 inches from the ceiling). Heat detectors should be mounted in the center of the ceiling.

9. Q: How much will it cost to install smoke/heat detectors?

   A: Detectors can be purchased for about $7 to $60 each. Packaged fire detection systems may cost $300 and up.

Please take time to think about the risk to your child and family if they are not protected by detectors. The extra time provided by a smoke/heat detector/alarm may allow your family to escape unharmed from a fire. The extra time and money spent on purchasing, installing, and maintaining adequate detectors could save your lives.

Infant Car Seat Handout

Automobile travel can and should be a safe and pleasant time for you and your baby. This is an excellent time for you to talk to your baby and to teach your baby how enjoyable automobile travel can be.

1. If both parents are traveling in the car, one adult and the baby should ride in the back seat. The baby should be in an infant safety seat that is connected to the car with the seat belt so that the baby rides facing backward. If your car has an air bag on the passenger side, the infant seat must be placed in the back seat.

2. If one parent is traveling alone with the baby, the baby should be placed in the front seat next to the parent, in an infant safety seat that is connected to the car with the seat belt so that the baby rides facing backward.

3. Anytime your baby is asleep, don't disturb him; leave him alone. An infant safety seat is a comfortable place for your baby to sleep, and you don't have to worry about his safety.

4. Anytime your baby is awake and behaving nicely—either quiet or jabbering, looking around, and such—make sure you interact with her. This way, your baby will learn to enjoy automobile travel because you are fun to ride with. You can try singing or humming songs and talking about what you are doing or where you are going, for example, "We're going to see Nana and Papa." If your baby has a favorite blanket, place it next to or in the safety seat within her reach.

5. Carry one or two soft, stuffed toys that your baby will learn to associate with quiet travel. It may help to have special quiet riding toys that are played with only in the car. The toys help to decrease boredom, but remember, your baby's attention span is very short. Don't expect him to keep occupied for more than a couple of minutes or less, particularly early in life.

6. Ignore yelling, screaming, and begging. The instant your baby is quiet, begin talking or singing to her again. You should not yell, scream, or nag. Do not take your baby out of her safety seat because she is crying; doing so will only teach her to cry more until you will take her out.

7. Older brothers and sisters also should be expected to behave in the car and to ride with their seat belts fastened correctly. If your baby grows up always riding with his seat belt on, he will not mind having it on at all.

8. By your frequent praise and pleasant conversation, your child will remain interested and busy and will not spend her time crying, because she already will have your attention.

Edward R. Christophersen, *Little People: Guidelines for Commonsense Child Rearing*. Kansas City, MO: Westport Publishers. ©Edward R. Christophersen, 1988.

HANDOUT 12.6

Toddler Car Seat Handout

Automobile trips can and should be a pleasant time for you and your child. This is an excellent time for pleasant conversation and for teaching your child acceptable and appropriate behavior in the car. The car seat is also the safest mode of travel, even for short trips, for your child.

1. Introduce the car seat to your child in a calm, matter-of-fact manner as a learning experience. Allow him to touch it and check it out.

2. Remind the child about the rules of behavior *nicely* before the first ride and between rides.

3. Your first rides with the seat should be short practice rides, perhaps once around the block, to teach your child expected and acceptable behavior. Point out interesting things she can see. Make it a positive experience for both of you.

4. Provide a lot of brief, nonverbal, physical contact throughout the car ride. Praise your child often for appropriate behaviors by saying something like, "Mike, you are sitting quietly in your seat. Mommy is proud of you." This explanation teaches him what you expect and avoids confounding statements like, "Quit that!" Remember to "catch 'em being good." You cannot be too positive with your child.

5. Include the child in pleasant conversation, by saying things like, "That was sure a good lunch. . . . You really like hot dogs, don't you? You were a big help to me in the store. It'll be fun visiting Grandma."

6. This also is a good time to teach your child about her world by saying things like, "Susie, see that *big, red* fire truck? Look at how *fast* it is going. What *do* firemen do? The light on the top is *red.* What else is red?" geared to the age of your child.

7. By your frequent praise, teaching, and pleasant conversation, your child will remain interested and busy and will not spend his time trying to get out of the seat. Rather, he will give you his frequent attention.

8. Ignore yelling, screaming, and begging. The instant your child is quiet, praise her for being quiet. You should not yell, scream, or beg either. Remember to remain calm and matter-of-fact. Keep your child busy in conversation and with observations of her world. Do not give in and let her out of the car seat, which only teaches her that yelling, screaming, and begging will finally get Mom or Dad to let her do what she wants. Show who is the boss.

9. Older siblings also should be expected to behave appropriately. If the young child sees an older sibling climbing or hanging out the window, he will want to become a participant. The older siblings also should be included in the conversation, praise, and teaching.

10. Provide one or two toys that your child associates with quiet play, such as books, stuffed animals, or dolls. It may help to have special quiet riding toys that are played with only in the car. Toys decrease boredom. Remember, the young child's attention span is *very* short. Do not expect her to stay occupied for more than a couple of minutes or less, particularly at the beginning and depending on her age.

11. Immediately after the ride, reward your child with 5 to 10 minutes of your time in an activity he likes, such as reading a story, playing a game, helping prepare lunch, or helping put away the groceries. Do not get into the habit of buying your child favors or presents for good behavior. He enjoys the time spent with you, which is less expensive and more rewarding for both of you. Remember, "catch 'em being good," and praise often.

12. If your child even begins to try to release her seat belt or to climb out of the car seat, immediately tell her "No!" in a firm voice. On your first few trips, which should just be around the block, stop the car if you think it is necessary. Also, state the rule once, clearly, "Do not take off your seat belt."

13. Remember, without the praise and attention for good behavior in the car, your child will learn nothing from the training trips. The combination of praise and attention, with occasional discipline, can and will teach the behavior you want in the car.

Edward R. Christophersen, *Little People: Guidelines for Commonsense Child Rearing*. Kansas City, MO: Westport Publishers. ©Edward R. Christophersen, 1988.

Traveling with Kids

There are a number of practical ways parents can make trips with children more enjoyable for the kids and less stressful for themselves. The most important thing to remember when traveling with children is to try to maintain normalcy as much as possible.

Here are some examples.

1. When taking a trip, wake up the children as close to their normal waking hour as possible and put them to bed at the usual time.

2. Always maintain discipline during an outing or extended trip—kids need and want to have the same structure they are used to having. Parents should not bend their normal rules just because they are away from home.

3. Avoid the temptation of substituting meals with junk food during trips or outings. If the family is taking a long trip in a car, stop regularly for food.

4. Find time while traveling to give your children some exercise. In nearly every age group, children are used to getting some amount of exercise each day. But while traveling, children are sometimes expected to remain seated for hours. If you have time between airplane flights, take long walks in the airport; while traveling by car, stop regularly for walks, foot races, or a swim if possible.

5. When possible, take along little packages of soft toys and nutritious snacks for children. Airlines don't cater to the tastes of children, so snacks can come in handy.

©Edward R. Christophersen, 1992.

Chapter 13

Alternatives to Traditional Well-Child Care

The American Academy of Pediatrics, in its *Standards of Child Health Care* (1977), recommends that a number of topics be covered during routine well-child office visits. In the traditional well-child visit, the practitioner spends from 10 to 15 minutes with each family. During this time, the physician takes a history, performs a physical examination, and answers any questions the parent or caregiver may ask. Of the average 15 minutes spent on a well-child visit, pediatricians have less than 2 minutes to devote to anticipatory guidance (Reisinger and Bires, 1980). Two minutes is simply not enough time to cover what most pediatricians and the Academy think should be

315

covered during a well-child visit. This leaves a substantial amount of material that ideally should be covered but is not.

In 1978, a Task Force on Pediatric Education reported that the most significant body of information that pediatric residents should be exposed to, but are not, is Biosocial or Behavioral Pediatrics—information about child rearing and normal childhood problems.

Wender, Bijur, and Boyce (1992) conducted a study similar to the 1978 Task Force and reported significant differences between the responses on the 1978 report and the responses to their survey in terms of psychosocial or behavioral problems, interviewing and counseling, school health, and community programs. The only area within Behavioral Pediatrics where the recent survey showed insufficient training, compared with the original survey, was in one category that included learning disabilities, Attention Deficit Hyperactivity Disorder (ADHD), and mental retardation. Thus, pediatric residents appear to be receiving better training in Behavioral Pediatrics.

However, given the brevity of the well-child office visit, pediatric health-care practitioners simply do have not have adequate time to cover such issues as behavioral and developmental problems, either in their training programs or in their pediatric practices.

If pediatricians aren't covering enough material during well-child visits, yet agree that the material should be covered, are other options available?

In 1978, Stein was one of the first authors to describe an approach to well-child care that provided the pediatrician with the time necessary to provide more anticipatory guidance by seeing several mothers and their infants at the same time. He referred to this approach as "group well-child care." Osborn (1985) and Osborn and Woolley (1981) also have described providing well-child care to more than one parent at a time. Another option available to provide more comprehensive anticipatory guidance has been called "continuing education for parents." Both of these alternatives to traditional well-child care are discussed below.

13.1. COMBINING GROUP AND INDIVIDUAL WELL-CHILD CARE

Although group well-child care is often presented as an alternative to individual well-child care, it is possible to use such groups as a supplement to a traditional well-child practice. A physician can continue individual well-child care, providing physical examinations and maintaining individual contact with the families, while conducting group well-child classes to provide more time for anticipatory guidance.

13.2. GROUP WELL-CHILD CARE

In both Stein's and Osborn's approaches to group well-child care, five or six mother-child pairs are seen together by the health-care provider for 1 hour. About 45 minutes of this time is spent providing anticipatory guidance on such topics as feeding, sleeping, and infant stimulation, and discussing areas of concern to the parents. The remaining 15 minutes are spent conducting physical examinations. Osborn conducts half of the well-child physicals at the beginning of the group and half at the end. Any immunizations are given at the end to avoid disruption to the group by distressed infants.

We conducted an evaluation of group well-child care through a large, local health maintenance organization and were able to demonstrate the efficacy of the approach in getting parents to implement one major area that is typically considered a part of anticipatory guidance—home injury-control strategies (Thomas, Hassanein, and Christophersen, 1984).

In this study, we demonstrated that parents who were provided with home injury-control strategies were significantly more likely to have safe home injury-control practices than were the parents in the control group classes who did not receive the injury-control training.

13.2.1. Class Topics

Handout 13.1 lists the topics covered in classes for parents of infants and toddlers. As any busy practitioner knows, these are topics that parents frequently ask questions about but that the provider rarely has time to cover adequately. These classes focus on providing parents with information about normal child development and the opportunity to discuss commonly encountered behavioral problems. As such, the classes give practitioners the chance to prevent problems from occurring in the first place, or at least to deal with them as soon as the parents are aware of their existence. The classes for parents of school-age children and adolescents cover such additional topics as cooperation with the schools, homework, overnights, and sporting activities.

13.2.2. Advantages of Group Well-Child Care

According to Osborn (1985), the advantages of group well-child care include:

- More time for parent education.
- Greater parental participation.
- Parental reassurance and support of one another.
- Better opportunities to observe mother-child interactions, because there is more time and there are several mothers interacting with their infants at the same time.

Group well-child care allows more than one mother-child pair to be seen at a time and more time to be spent with each pair. While the mothers are gaining support from one another and benefiting from the others' questions and answers, the provider is reducing the number of times he or she must say the same thing. Many primary health-care providers know only too well the boredom of doing seven well-child visits in one afternoon, trying to maintain their enthusiasm for what they are saying without reducing the amount of material they cover. When six mothers are seen with their infants, all at the same time, you only have to make each point once instead of six different times.

13.2.3. Inviting Parents to Classes

When you see a newborn in the hospital nursery, examine the infant, and talk with the mother, it is an excellent time to mention that you are now offering group well-child care in the office. Instruct the mother, when she phones for her 2-month well-child visit, to schedule a group session if she so desires. Also, instruct your office staff to tell each parent who phones for a 2-month well-child visit that you now offer two options: a 15-minute regular well-child visit or a 1-hour group well-child visit. The individual who sets up appointments must be well informed about the groups in order to answer questions the parents may raise. Initially, there will probably be some resistance to the group well-child visit, simply because parents have never tried group well-child care, but, as more and more mothers take advantage of the groups, more will respond to offers to participate.

13.2.4. Conducting Group Sessions

The actual group is usually started by the group leader (the pediatrician, pediatric nurse, or allied health professional) presenting prepared material. Having material prepared in advance helps to "break the ice" for both the leader and the parents.

Our experience has been that presenting some material on slides prepares the group for the discussion that follows. Once the discussion gets started, the use of slides can help to get the leader back on topic whenever the discussion drifts too far away from what you wanted to cover. Simply pushing the advance button on the slide projector, and projecting a slide on another topic, helps to keep the conversation on the topic.

In conjunction with your group discussion, prepare written materials for distribution at the end of the well-child group. Excellent sources for such materials are the task force reports that appear in the American Academy of Pediatrics newsletter, *AAP News*; these reports are informative and authoritative. We have used two of their reports, one on infant swimming programs and one on infant exercise programs. Because these appear in a professional newsletter, there shouldn't be any problem distributing them to classes as long as there is no fee charged for the task force reports.

13.2.5. Disadvantages of Group Well-Child Care

The major disadvantages of group well-child care are space and scheduling (Osborn, 1985). These problems are not, however, insurmountable.

For example, practitioners can often conduct groups in the office waiting room. If this is done by practitioners in solo practice, it is usually best to schedule groups during the first hour of a morning or afternoon appointment block, for example, at 9:00 A.M. or 1:00 P.M., when other patients are not in the waiting room. However, groups scheduled in such a manner may be disrupted by patients arriving early for the next regularly scheduled individual appointment.

Evening appointments for the groups are well accepted by parents and do not have to be scheduled around other appointments. Obviously, some physicians may not want to conduct groups in the early evening hours. Patients, particularly now that in many families both parents work, like evening appointments because it often means they do not have to take time off work to keep their child's appointment.

While the group-class format allows the provider ample opportunity to cover a great deal of material with a large number of families at a reasonable level of financial recompense, there are obviously questions that parents have that must be handled individually by the physician. These are issues that can often be addressed during regular one-on-one office visits.

13.3. CONTINUING EDUCATION FOR PARENTS

Another format we have been using with parents since 1972 we call "continuing education for parents" (Christophersen, Barrish, Barrish, and Christophersen, 1984). Depending on the age of the children and the purpose of the classes, some classes use only 1 hour from an existing sequence of classes; other classes provide 8 hours of instruction (four 2-hour evening classes). The 1-hour classes, given as part of hospital-based prenatal instruction, include prenatal classes for couples expecting their first child and refresher classes for couples expecting the second or third child. Other classes, which meet for 2 hours each evening for four evenings, for parents of infants, toddlers, and school-age children, are offered for a total of 8 hours.

13.3.1. Prenatal Classes

Approximately 20 years ago, the author began prenatal counseling for expectant couples. The response to these classes has resulted in their continued success in terms of the classes being full each time they are offered, the written evaluations completed by the registrants, and the number of professionals from around the United States who have expressed an interest in offering similar classes.

These classes began from an interest in increasing the use of child-restraint seats during automobile travel but have since been expanded to include a great deal of information on issues that customarily arise during the perinatal period. We are continually developing and evaluating materials and formats for use in these prenatal classes, which currently provide a discussion of:

- The amount and type of sleep that newborns get.
- The amount of fussing that parents can expect.
- How to establish sleep patterns.
- How to help infants develop sleep-onset skills.
- How to test the infant's self-quieting skills.
- How to encourage the development of self-quieting skills.

The classes also provide suggestions for:

- Reducing infant crying.
- Becoming familiar with infant caregiving routines.

- Using baby-sitters.
- Using day care.

For a complete description of the material presented in the prenatal classes, see *The Baby Owner's Manual: What to Expect and How to Survive the First Year*, a book written specifically for prenatal classes (Christophersen, 1988).

13.3.2. Refresher Classes

While much has been written for couples expecting their first baby, much less has been written for parents expecting their second child. Just because little has been written doesn't mean parents are without questions.

Many parents have questions about helping the first child adjust to another child, a newborn infant, in the home. Over the past 15 years, the author has been offering refresher classes to couples expecting their second or third child. These discussions are offered during 1 hour of the 6-hour refresher series (three 2-hour classes at weekly intervals).

During the refresher classes, we recommend that parents:

- Make whatever physical changes they intend to make at least 2 weeks before the new baby is due so that the first child does not associate the new baby with the life-style changes that take place.
- Establish, if necessary, firmer disciplinary limits prior to the birth of the new baby.

The group format is conducive to the practitioner providing much more information than is possible when seeing parents one at a time in prenatal or well-child appointments. And, parents ask far more questions in the groups than they would have time to ask during individual appointments. As a result, the practitioners who conduct such programs with expectant couples (both first- and second-time parents) quickly learn what material parents are interested in and how much time to devote to each topic. As the groups change, the information imparted to the parents changes, as a reflection of the interests of the parents who attend.

The group well-child format gears the information being presented to the parents' interests. At the same time, the groups bring additional revenue into the office; a large number of happy, satisfied patients keeps a practice thriving.

In addition to the prenatal and refresher classes, we have extended the class format to include what we refer to as continuing education for parents. The purpose of these classes is to present material to parents and to allow them a lot of time for group discussion.

Presently, group classes are scheduled to provide 8 hours of lecture and discussion for each age group. The express purpose of the classes is to provide parents with information and the opportunity to discuss issues and concerns that simply cannot be covered within the time constraints of routine well-child care. The original course content was determined by the *Standards of Child Health Care* published by the American Academy of Pediatrics (1977). By cataloging what the Academy indicates should be covered during well-child care, then subtracting what is typically covered, the author arrived at the content for four 2-hour classes.

13.3.3. Mechanics of Conducting Parenting Classes

Most hospitals with obstetrics units have been offering prenatal classes for years. Traditionally, these classes have included information about labor and delivery, pain management, and infant care (bathing, diapering). The addition of more information on parenting was a logical one. Our extension of the class format for parents of infants, toddlers, school-age children, and adolescents was quite easy to do.

13.3.4. Wellness Identification

If classes are offered through the pediatrics office, they are identified with wellness almost automatically. When classes, because of space constraints or personal preference, are offered outside of the pediatrics office, they should be offered through the Education Department of a community hospital. Many hospitals have offered a wide variety of classes as part of a larger wellness campaign. Topics covered have included Sibling Preparation, C-Sections, and Breast Feeding, as well as Heart Programs, Weight Control Programs, and Smoking Cessation Programs.

13.3.5. Program Evaluations

Formal written evaluations should be an integral part of any educational offering. Serving several purposes, they give the hospital the opportunity to solicit feedback on their facility, and can provide feedback on specific aspects of educational offerings after only a short time. Evaluations, in the form of written feedback to the group instructors and the facility sponsoring the groups, can provide valuable suggestions for future educational offerings, including information about the groups' strengths and weaknesses.

13.3.6. Start-Up Time

Most practitioners report it takes up to 2 years for the classes to gain enough popularity to keep the registration full. In the first 6 months of the classes, it is common for enrollment to be as few as four to six couples.

For practitioners who have never taught classes before, starting with four to six couples is probably an advantage because there is less pressure on the faculty and the faculty has more time to learn from the participants in the classes. After several years of classes, it is possible to have an enrollment of 30 couples (which usually results in about 50 individuals in the class).

13.3.7. Class Fees

The fee for classes should be about the same as the cost of one well-child visit, with a maximum enrollment of 30 couples. Thus, if 30 couples enroll at $35 per couple, the four classes will gross $1,050, or about $130 per hour—making the income generated from the classes comparable to what can be generated from routine well-child care.

13.3.8. Advantages of Continuing Education Classes for Parents

Since continuing education groups do not involve physical examinations, the classes can accommodate a large number of parents without the children present. Continuing education classes offer the practitioner and the family several advantages:

- If the provider sees 20 couples together, the same material is presented only once for every 20 families rather than 20 separate times.
- The 20 couples, instead of having only 10 to 15 minutes of contact with their physician, have a full hour of contact.
- The income for 1 hour is derived from 10 or 15 families, instead of four (assuming an office visit typically lasts 15 minutes), increasing the revenue the physician can bill per unit of time.
- Family members benefit from hearing the questions other parents ask and the answers given by both the physician and other parents or caregivers in attendance.
- The greatly increased amount of time allows for coverage of topics that normally would not be able to be covered, such as infant/child care, temperament, nutrition, and home injury control. This makes the sessions more interesting for all attendees—physician and parents alike.
- Practitioners frequently learn a great deal from having a 1-hour discussion with several parents without interruption (Osborn, 1985).
- Couples typically report being very satisfied with such a group format (Osborn, 1985).

These classes can be offered either in the physician's waiting room during evening hours, after the office is closed for the day, or through the Education Department of a local hospital.

Office meetings allow the physician to amortize office expenses over a greater number of hours each week.

Hospital-based meetings usually have hospital staff taking care of registration, fee collection, room arrangements, and so on. In exchange for services rendered, the hospital should receive a portion (for example, 15%) of gross revenue generated from each class. Hospitals also generate goodwill from the classes. For many couples, their first introduction to the hospital was the parenting class. These parents probably stand a much better chance of returning to a hospital if they have had a pleasant experience.

13.3.9. Disadvantages of Continuing Education Classes for Parents

The major disadvantage of the continuing education classes is that the attendance is far better in the evening than during normal office hours.

Also, infrequently, one couple will dominate a class with questions about a child with obvious pathology, for example, Oppositional Defiant Disorder, Attention Deficit Hyperactivity Disorder, or developmental delays. Usually, if a question is clearly outside the realm of the group, the parent can be asked to bring the question up after the class, at which time a referral, if appropriate, can be made to a mental health professional. Over the years, however, it has been interesting to note how many times a parent will ask a question that, superficially, appears to be related to a very narrow range of youngsters but that actually interests many parents.

13.4. MECHANICS OF CONDUCTING CONTINUING EDUCATION FOR PARENTS

The following suggestions, learned from conducting parenting classes for 20 years and from making presentations at professional meetings, make classes more enjoyable for the parents and more successful for the practitioner.

13.4.1. Use Slides

Whenever lecturers use written notes, which is fairly common in classes of 20 hours' duration, attendees are often distracted by the lecturer constantly looking down at the notes. When using slides, the lecturer is literally looking at his notes at the same time the class participants are looking at him. Many parents have said the slides are one of the features of the classes they like most, because it's easier for them to remember material that was covered.

- Whenever possible, use action sides—slides that depict parents or professionals engaging in the activity you are discussing. For example, as we discuss the importance of "time-in" with children, we show a number of slides of parents being affectionate and doing fun things with their children. When we describe the use of time-out with children less than 1 year of age, we show a series of slides of a mother carrying her 11-month-old child facing away from her, placing her in her playpen, then picking her up from her playpen. In this way, parents can see and hear the chronology, particularly if the action slides are also keyed to written handouts.
- Do not use more than six lines of text on a slide. Make the words on the slide as big as is practical. The slides need only contain critical phrases, not the entire text or even complete sentences. Make sure the slides are legible from the back of the room.
- Transparencies are easier to make than slides, and some speakers prefer them. However, it is usually much easier and faster to change slides, and virtually all auditoriums have slide projectors, while only some have transparency projectors.
- Many hospitals have audiovisual departments that can prepare slides for the instructors who are conducting classes for parents. Even if you have to have the slides prepared commercially, the money invested is usually well worth it; they will look better and last longer than homemade slides. Contact the audiovisual department at one of your area hospitals for suggestions about where to have slides prepared, or look in the Yellow Pages under "slides" for a computer graphics designer or presentation specialist near you.
- Polaroid markets high-contrast, black and white slide film that can be used with any 35 mm camera and that can be developed, using a Polaroid slide film

developer, in just 2 minutes. Polaroid also offers slide film that will be blue with white letters for approximately the same cost. At today's prices, the Polaroid slides, with the slide holders, cost about $0.90 each.

13.4.2. Use Written Handouts

Much of the material that is used in parenting classes can be summarized on written handouts. This way, parents can listen because they don't have to take notes, yet they have written supporting materials to take home with them. Obviously, if the written handouts can be keyed to the word slides used in the lecture, the participants will be able to remember the materials more easily.

13.5. CONCLUDING REMARKS

While traditional well-child care has succeeded in aiding in the delivery of health-care services to children, there have been clear limitations in the areas of patient education and anticipatory guidance. Group well-child care and parent education groups offer the pediatric provider greatly increased time to spend with parents for education and discussion. To the interested practitioner, the advantages of seeing parents in a group far outweigh the disadvantages.

REFERENCES

American Academy of Pediatrics: *Standards of Child Health Care*, 3rd ed. Evanston, IL: Author, 1977.

Christophersen ER: *The Baby Owner's Manual: What to Expect and How to Survive the First Year*, 3rd ed. Kansas City, MO: Westport Publishers, 1988.

Christophersen ER, Barrish HH, Barrish IJ, Christophersen MR: Continuing education for parents of infants and toddlers, in Dangel RD, Polster RA (Eds.), *Parent Training: Foundations of Research and Practice*. New York: Guilford Press, 1984.

Osborn LM: Group well-child care. *Pediatr Clin N Am* 12:355–365, 1985.

Osborn LM, Woolley FR: The use of groups in well-child care. *Pediatrics* 67:701–707, 1981.

Reisinger KS, Bires JA: Anticipatory guidance in pediatric practice. *Pediatrics* 66:889–892, 1980.

Stein MT: The providing of well-baby care with parent-infant groups. *Clin Pediatr* 17:825, 1978.

Task Force on Pediatric Education: *The Future of Pediatric Education*. Evanston, IL: American Academy of Pediatrics, 1978.

Thomas KA, Hassanein RS, Christophersen ER: An evaluation of group well-child care for improving parents' home burn prevention practices. *Pediatrics* 74:879–892, 1984.

Wender EH, Bijur PE, Boyce WT: Pediatric residency training: Ten years after the Task Force Report. *Pediatrics* 90:876–890, 1992.

Sample Handout

HANDOUT 13.1

Topics for Group Well-Child Classes

Infant Classes	*Toddler Classes*
Growth/Development	Growth/Development
Temperament	Discipline
Baby/Child Care	Cognitive Development
Parenting	Toilet Training
Stressors	Parent Coping
Illness	Illness
Behavior	Behavior
Baby-Sitters/Day Care	Baby-Sitters/Day Care

PART IV

ADVANCED INTERVENTION TECHNIQUES

Pediatric health-care providers are called on to provide services that are rarely a part of their residency training. Three of these areas—parent coping skills, the use of token economies for motivating and educating children and their parents, and management of pain in the young patient—present unique challenges to the practitioner. Each of these areas is deceptively simple in appearance.

Each area is similar to training parents to manage behavior problems, in the sense that there is a temptation to simply tell parents what they should be doing. Yet, we know from the research literature and from past experience that simply telling someone how to do something is very different from actually teaching him how to do it.

To truly develop coping skills (Chapter 14) takes a good deal of time and practice. As with many other areas of functioning, children often behave in much the same way they have seen their parents behave. Thus, parents with poor coping skills and parents who have problems with their temper are likely, through modeling, to pass these problems on to their children. If parents can learn to deal successfully with their temper, their children will, in time, often come to emulate the same skills.

Token economies (Chapter 15), probably more than any other technique in the behavior literature, are deceptively complicated. Superficially, a token economy involves giving children tokens for appropriate behaviors and taking away tokens for inappropriate behaviors. However, when researchers have analyzed the implementation of token economies either in the natural home or in institutions, they have documented a very complex set of strategies that must come into play in order for the token economy to be a successful intervention technique.

Like many other skills, teaching parents how to implement a token economy is easier the more you do it and harder the less you do it. After practitioners have taught several dozen families how to implement a token economy, they probably have the skills to do so regardless of how many times afterward they implement a token economy. However, a practitioner who has the opportunity to teach these skills only to one or two families a year would be well advised to refer families in need of such assistance to a professional who works more extensively with token economies.

Dealing with painful medical procedures is difficult for the child, his parents, and the practitioner. It is often difficult for health-care providers to realize, or to keep in mind, that the way they handle uncomfortable or painful procedures contributes a great deal to how the child deals with the procedure. A knowledge of the different styles children use to cope with painful procedures determines, in large part, the strategies that will be effective with the child. Chapter 16, "Compliance with Painful Procedures," reviews the strategies children use for dealing with pain, including relaxation and hypnosis, and discusses where the practitioner can get further training in pain-management procedures.

Chapter 14

Coping Skills for Parents

Parents must be proficient in a number of behavioral procedures in order to maintain high levels of compliance in their children. Parents also need reasonable coping skills if they are to carry out the procedures for maintaining compliance. "Coping skills," as used here, refers to the parents' ability to maintain their own composure in the face of noncompliance or oppositional behaviors from their children. One of the foremost authorities on cognitive behavior therapy with adults is Albert Ellis, Ph.D., founder of the Institute for Rational Emotive Therapy in New York. Two of his associate trainers, Drs. Harriet Barrish and Jay Barrish, authors of *Managing Parental Anger* (1988), have adapted Ellis's procedures for use with parents and with older children. What follows is a review of their recommendations for parents. Through our office, we have successfully used these strategies with a number of families from all socioeconomic backgrounds. Many parents find these strategies very helpful.

14.1. IMPORTANCE OF PARENTAL COPING SKILLS IN GAINING COMPLIANCE

Parents must be able to maintain their composure while dealing with inappropriate behaviors from their children or instituting disciplinary procedures. Although in the abstract this sounds relatively easy, in real life it is sometimes very difficult.

During an office visit with the practitioner or while reading a book, it's easy for a parent to talk about how she will handle any variety of inappropriate behaviors her child may engage in. However, when the child has broken a family heirloom or an expensive gift, it may be much more difficult for the parent to remain calm.

When a child engages in a behavior that is detrimental to his medical condition or when he refuses to engage in a behavior likely to benefit him, many parents will immediately become emotional about the situation. For example, after a thorough inpatient endocrine evaluation and successful hospital treatment, a child with a growth hormone deficiency is discharged with a prescription for a synthetic growth hormone. The parents were taught by a nurse in the hospital how to administer the drug (through injection) three evenings a week.

The first time the parents attempt to administer the injection, the child is cooperative but complains afterward that the injection hurts and she never wants to receive such an injection again. The parents are now in a difficult position: They know they must administer the growth hormone injection in order for their child to grow and develop properly, but their child is adamantly opposed to the injection. The parents find it difficult to accept that their child doesn't want to receive the injection.

Although it is easy to understand the child's reluctance to accept the injection, knowing, as is often the case, that the injection is going to leave a sore injection site, it is also easy to understand the parents' frustration. They are holding the solution to their child's problem in their hands but are not able to get the child's cooperation long enough to administer the solution. In a situation such as this one, the parents' ability to cope with the situation will, in large part, determine the success or failure of their intervention attempts. The way the parents address this situation, cognitively, will probably determine whether the child receives the injection.

Many parents, when faced with such a situation, initially attempt to explain to the child why the growth hormone injections are necessary and persist with their attempts at gaining their child's cooperation until they are successful or until they get angry. They may plead with him, offer bribes, become firm with him, or, ultimately, force their child to submit to the injection. In many instances these procedures work.

The way parents handle situations in which they and their child take diametrically opposed positions can make a big difference in how much stress the parents feel and how much resistance they get from their child. While parents actually are in the situation, what they think or say to themselves can produce a dramatic difference.

14.2. HURTFUL SELF-THOUGHTS

In difficult situations, it is common for parents to engage in "hurtful" self-thoughts or self-talk. There are many things parents say to themselves that do not make the situation any easier: "She knows she won't grow properly unless she gets her growth hormone shots," or "I just can't stand it when he fights me like this." In fact, such thoughts frequently make the situation worse.

Hurtful self-thoughts typically are not indicative of any underlying pathology. Rather they are perfectly normal parental reactions to stressful situations where the parents fully understand the importance of getting their child to comply with the physician's treatment recommendations but are unable to do so. Hurtful self-thoughts inevitably make a difficult situation worse.

Parents learn hurtful thoughts much like they learn any other fear-based behavior. Getting a child to engage in a behavior that, although ultimately beneficial to the child, produces immediate discomfort is similar to many other situations adults face, where escaping the situation is, in and of itself, a rewarding experience. The tense parent who gives up trying to coerce her child to comply is likely to feel an immediate sense of relief.

The parents don't feel relief because they gave in. Rather, they feel relief because the tension from the confrontation is relieved. However, over time, the parents may come to resent their child's behavior because they feel the child's behavior "caused" them to give in, or "made" them give in. Then, because the parents feel they are being pushed, they get angry. They blame the child for the anger: "If he had just done what I asked him to do, I wouldn't have had to get angry," or "She knows she has to take her injection; why does she have to be so obnoxious?"

Alternatively, some of the time it "works" for parents to get angry. A child who is refusing to cooperate may give in when facing intense anger from one or both parents. However reinforcing this situation might be to angry parents, it is likely to come up again and again as they are faced with maintaining their child's behavior in a certain way.

14.3. CHALLENGING HURTFUL SELF-THOUGHTS

When parents are in situations where they end up getting angry, they need to learn how to challenge their "hurtful" thoughts. Admittedly, when a child refuses to take medication that is absolutely essential to his growth and development, parents do get stressed. But they don't have to get angry. Rather, they *allow* themselves to get angry. Much of the time, what they are saying to themselves is what leads to them getting angry.

The following examples of hurtful self-thoughts are discussed in the Barrishes' (1988) book:

- My children SHOULD NOT, MUST NOT, CANNOT ACT this way.
- When my children behave this way, they are doing it TO me, and they deserve to be punished.
- My children SHOULD know better.
- It's TERRIBLE and AWFUL when my children behave this way.
- I can't stand it when my children behave this way.
- I HAVE to get angry to make my children act this way.

When parents allow themselves to think these kinds of thoughts, they are much more likely to get angry. It is normal to have these kinds of thoughts; what parents do with them, however, determines whether they deal with them effectively or get angry. If parents give in to these thoughts, if they allow themselves to feel as though their child has no right to behave in a certain way, they are more likely to get angry.

It is important for parents to keep the following axioms in mind:

- Children can and will behave in ways that are detrimental to them.
- Children can and will do things that they will regret later.
- Children can and will do things that are not in their own best interest.

14.3.1. Teaching Parents to Substitute Helpful Thoughts

Parents can be taught how to challenge their hurtful self-thoughts. It is a relatively straightforward procedure, but it is difficult to do during emotional times. Basically, challenging hurtful self-thoughts consists of asking yourself if the hurtful self-thought really is true: Will it happen?

If the parent thinks to himself, "She cannot behave this way," the challenge can be something like, "Yes, she *can* behave this way—she already does." Or, when thinking, "I can't stand it when he behaves this way," the parent can ask herself, "Am I really going to lose my mind?" or "Is it really going to change my life to have her behave the way she is?"

Ultimately, parents need to learn how to substitute "helpful" thoughts, but they may need assistance in doing so. Let's return to the child who needs growth hormone injections. As the child struggles with her parents, the parents begin engaging in hurtful thoughts. The parents need to learn how to control their hurtful thoughts and, whenever possible, to substitute helpful thoughts.

The first step in dealing with intense parental emotions is recognizing and challenging hurtful thoughts as soon as possible, particularly in less intense or less emotionally laden situations. Although it may simply be too difficult for parents to catch themselves during a confrontation with their children, they may be able to find a less stressful situation—a business or traffic situation—in which to practice.

14.3.2. Finding Opportunities to Practice in Everyday Life

Hurtful thoughts are very common when someone is driving too close to the back of your car and you notice yourself getting angry. Typical hurtful thoughts in this situation are, "If I have to stop fast, he's going to run right into the back of my car," or "I ought to slam on my brakes and teach that jerk a real lesson."

Parents need to catch themselves engaging in hurtful thoughts and force themselves to "stop" the hurtful thoughts. This could consist of challenging their hurtful thoughts, in the sense of intellectually questioning them, or merely stopping the hurtful thoughts long enough (usually only 1 or 2 seconds) to think about alternatives. After a 1- or 2-second break, it's much easier to challenge the hurtful thought.

Instead of thinking, "He's got no right to drive that close to the back of my car," an adult can say, "He is driving too close to me. I don't like it, but I can stand it." Then it is possible to explore the options. The immediate option, and the one many people take, is to move out of the other driver's way. Once the "jerk" has passed us, there is very little chance he will drive into the back of our car.

Individuals with bad tempers may have to begin with even more benign situations: for example, where the paper boy left the newspaper. It's one thing to say he has no right to throw it into the middle of your front yard, when he "knows [you] want it on the front steps." It's another thing to acknowledge that the paper is already in the front yard. Through exercising such cognitive coping skills in less emotional situations, the process of identifying exactly when we are engaging in hurtful thoughts begins. The next step consists of disciplining ourselves to substitute more helpful thoughts.

Virtually all of us engage in hurtful thoughts some of the time, so the exercise is rarely a waste of time. Once we gain some experience at identifying when we are engaging in hurtful thoughts, we can begin the process of challenging those hurtful thoughts and acknowledging their very existence.

14.3.3. Applying the Lessons to Medical Situations

The mother of the child who needs growth hormone injections could say to herself, "I really don't like it when Jeff fusses like this, and it does make me uncomfortable, but I know he needs to get his injection and I can stand his fussing." Not only does the parent gain experience in dealing with uncomfortable situations, but the child learns, from seeing his mother deal with the situation, that there are alternatives to fussing every time things don't go his way.

Granted, the responsibility of giving a painful injection to a child is unpleasant, but giving it in spite of her protestations can be rewarding for the parent because he knows he is helping his child. Each time the parent is able to stop long enough to substitute a helpful thought for a hurtful thought, she is one step closer to being able to do it more easily the next time.

14.4. THE ROLE OF THE PRIMARY CARE PHYSICIAN

Let's turn to another child referred to me because he refused to allow his parents to administer growth hormone injections. Although the endocrinologist had made it perfectly clear the child must receive three injections each week, the parents had been able to get only a total of four injections into the child over the course of 1 month. They had resorted to chasing the child around the house, catching him, pulling his pants down, and giving him his injections. By the time this scene was over, the child was nearly hysterical; the parents were furious with him and with themselves. The parents said things to me like, "He has to get his injections or he won't grow normally. We're only doing this for his own good. Why does he have to fight us so?"

Initially, I suggested a moratorium on the injections, mainly because the child wasn't getting them anyway. I checked with his endocrinologist first, who stated the child "must get his injections three times a week." In fact, I think the attitude of the endocrinologist may have inadvertently contributed to the parents' hurtful self-thoughts. He was actually telling the parents, with the best of intentions, that the child "can't refuse his injections." When I pointed out to the physician that the child wasn't currently getting *any* injections, he conceded that, although it would be best if the child were receiving three injections per week, any increase would be an improvement. This admission, in itself, is an example of substituting a helpful thought for a hurtful one.

14.4.1. Modifying Painful Procedures to Gain Compliance

Health-care providers, by the way they approach the parents, may be able to help parents recognize their discomfort and promote helpful self-thoughts; likewise, the health-care provider's approach may cause the parents to ignore the realities of the situation and may unintentionally promote hurtful self-thoughts. The provider needs to acknowledge that it is common for children to complain about painful or uncomfortable procedures and to try anything they can to avoid or escape them. Further, the provider can help the parents by providing them with helpful self-thoughts. For example, the provider might say, "I know from past experience that many children really resist growth hormone injections because they sting. I have found it works best if you try to work out some arrangement with your child so that he gets his injections without having to go through so much unpleasantness. Remember, although he needs to get his injection, he may still refuse it."

With this particular child, after conferring with the endocrinologist and the parents, I asked the child if he thought he could tolerate one-fourth of the dose he was presently being administered. After thinking about it for a while, he said he knew he needed the injections if he was ever going to grow, and he decided it would be much easier to tolerate one-fourth of the dose rather than the entire dose. I also worked with the child on his self-thoughts. We practiced such self-thoughts as, "I know it hurts when I get my injections, but I *can stand it*."

When he received his first injection—one-fourth of the normal dose—he was so surprised by the minimal discomfort that he asked his parents to give him another one-fourth dose in the other buttock. Within 1 week, he was up to the full dose.

14.4.2. Anticipating the Child's Reaction

Chapters 5 and 16 on compliance and pain, respectively, discuss gradually implementing complex medical regimens and assisting children with adopting coping strategies to help them to deal with painful procedures. Rather than insist a child submit to a procedure, risking a negative emotional reaction on both the parents' and the child's part, it is far better to analyze the situation, attempt to anticipate the child's reaction, and deal with it proactively. The provider who is cognizant of the reactions parents and children have to certain medical procedures can help the parents and the child, by the way he approaches the situation, to have helpful self-thoughts about it.

For example, the provider could say, "I know many of the children on this protocol object to it, and you may find yourself getting upset when she does, but this is to be expected. If and when it happens, I recommend you face the situation realistically.

Your child doesn't have to like the procedure; neither do you. Try telling yourself, 'My child may object to this procedure but I can tolerate it when she does. Getting angry only makes the situation worse.' Please give my nurse clinician a call if you have difficulty implementing the protocol. She has extensive experience with it and can probably help you over some of the rough spots."

The Barrishes have developed a self-help worksheet that can make the parents more aware of the way they are approaching a situation and show them that there are alternative ways that may be more productive. Handout 14.1 is an example of the Barrishes' worksheet, completed for a child who has to submit to painful growth hormone injections.

The practitioner would introduce the worksheet by first asking the parents what they were thinking when their son was giving them such a difficult time over the growth hormone injection. By questioning the parents, the practitioner can find out what the parents were thinking or saying to themselves when their child was running from them. Then, he could use examples to point out that the child's behavior didn't *make* them angry—they *allowed* themselves to get angry.

Then the practitioner can point out that the parents had another option. When they caught themselves engaging in hurtful thoughts, they could challenge these thoughts. And, when challenging these thoughts, they could substitute helpful thoughts for the hurtful thoughts. After this discussion, the worksheet can be introduced as an aid to getting the parents to think more about how they are approaching difficult situations. The practitioner and the parents could complete the worksheet together, which, it is hoped, will help the parents to recognize that they have uncomfortable feelings when they have to do something to their child and that they can control these feelings. They can substitute helpful self-thoughts for hurtful self-thoughts. Doing so makes the procedure easier for everyone involved.

The sequence that we want the parents to follow is a three-step process: Stop, think, and act.

14.5. STOPPING HURTFUL SELF-THOUGHTS

Only after we can identify our feelings about a situation can we begin a process the Barrishes (1988) call "STOP, THINK, ACT":

- STOP the hurtful thoughts.
- THINK of at least one or two alternatives that challenge the hurtful thoughts by being less hurtful.
- ACT on one of the alternatives.

Individuals have used several techniques to remind themselves about the 1 or 2 seconds they need to stop and think about a situation in order to substitute helpful thoughts for hurtful thoughts. A rubber band, wrapped around the wrist, can be snapped whenever a parent notices himself thinking hurtful thoughts. Often, just the brief snap of the rubber band is enough to give him a second or two to think.

Another technique is called "thought stopping," which refers to the intentional substitution of a thought that, in comparison with the hurtful thought, carries emotion of a very different kind. The parent might be able to recall, for just an instant, seeing an automobile accident immediately after it happened. As soon as she catches herself thinking hurtful thoughts, she can switch to thinking about the automobile accident. Such a process frequently gives the parent a second or two to pause, making it easier to conclude that the present situation is nowhere near as serious to us as the automobile accident was to the individuals involved.

14.6. PROMOTING HELPFUL SELF-THOUGHTS IN NONMEDICAL SITUATIONS

Many situations that make parents anxious or angry don't involve all of the extenuating circumstances that a growth hormone protocol involves. The example in Handout 14.2, an infant fussing when getting his diaper changed, is familiar to most parents. Parents can get upset with their child for being so stubborn during a diaper change, or they can deal with the situation without getting angry or frustrated.

The child's fussing during a diaper change does not make us angry. It is what we say to ourselves, what we think to ourselves, that allows us to become angry. If we take the whole episode personally and think hurtful thoughts, the situation can get very intense and unpleasant for both parent and child.

Parents need to recognize that their child is operating at an age-appropriate level, not out of malice. By going through the steps the Barrishes (1988) recommend, the parents may identify and recognize how they could have handled the situation differently. When parents begin to learn skills for coping with stressful situations, the blank worksheet in Handout 14.3 helps them analyze situations, to identify what they were thinking that did not help and what they could have thought that may have helped them to handle the specific situation differently.

14.7. RECOGNIZING UNCOMFORTABLE FEELINGS

The blank worksheet provided in Handout 14.3 is intended to be used by parents, often with the assistance of a trained therapist, to identify, recognize, and learn alternative strategies for dealing with difficult or uncomfortable situations.

Unfortunately, there isn't a screening test to identify individuals who frequently engage in hurtful thoughts. Such people may identify themselves as "short-tempered" or say they "get upset easily." Whatever terms are used, some strategy usually has to be implemented to eliminate the hurtful thoughts and substitute helpful thoughts before the individual can implement the desired compliance improvement.

Handout 14.4 is a worksheet filled out for parents of a child who must wear glasses or her vision will deteriorate markedly. In this example, the parents needed to work on their coping skills and had to implement behavior management strategies in order to get their daughter to wear her glasses.

14.8. SUGGESTED SELF-TALK FOR PARENTS

Sometimes we have parents fill out 3-by-5 inch cards that have helpful self-talk on them. We recommend the parents carry their cards around with them and read them as often as necessary, particularly in situations where they need to have more helpful self-talk. Examples of such helpful self-talk are listed in Handout 14.5.

14.9. FEELING GOOD ABOUT YOURSELF

Many parents who are abrupt with children and who have poor coping skills suffer from low self-esteem themselves. The two major options for these parents are entering into therapy and reading self-help books. The best selling of the self-help books is *Feeling Good* by David Burns (1980). His latest book, *The Feeling Good Handbook* (1989), includes a number of homework exercises that can be experimented with independent of any formal therapy. Burns's books provide a lot of suggestions that can be useful to both parents and practitioners. When the practitioner is familiar with Burns's book and the exercises included in it, she can recommend specific exercises for particular parents. Many practitioners also find that a number of the exercises in Burns's book are useful for them in their own personal and professional lives. I have talked with a number of parents and professionals who reported that Dr. Burns's book gave them a healthier perspective on taking responsibility for their own thoughts and actions. In fact, I was originally introduced to Burns's handbook by a child psychiatrist who told me how helpful it had been for her, both personally and in her practice.

14.10. TEACHING CHILDREN TO LIVE WITH THEIR STRONG EMOTIONS

Chapter 2, "Learning, Discipline, and Compliance in Children," discussed how to encourage the development of self-quieting skills in children. It is difficult for adults to develop self-quieting or coping skills if they don't already have them. If parents can help their children develop self-quieting skills early in life, these children may have much better coping skills as adults.

Up to about 10 years of age, it is possible, using procedures such as time-out, to encourage a child's development of self-quieting skills without the child's cooperation and without the child even knowing his parents are working on it. After age 10, most children need to learn coping or relaxation skills in a fashion similar or identical to the way adults learn them. For this reason, it is important to work on children's self-quieting skills while they are still young and can learn them relatively easily. The more trouble children have with dealing with their own tempers, the more important it is to work on their self-quieting skills. There is only one major difference between encouraging self-quieting skills in children and teaching coping skills in adults: Children are learning the skills for the first time, whereas adults have already learned poor self-quieting skills and must retrain themselves. Retraining is virtually always more difficult and more time consuming than learning these skills properly the first time.

14.11. ADVANCED TRAINING

Many excellent training opportunities exist for beginning, intermediate, and advanced training in what has come to be known as either cognitive behavior therapy or rational emotive therapy. Most of these training opportunities are available to physicians, nurses, psychiatrists, and psychologists. Many professional organizations offer workshops and institutes at beginning, intermediate, and advanced levels. Additional information on training dates and locations can be obtained from the following organizations:

- American Psychological Association, 750 First Street NE, Washington DC, 20002. Their annual meeting usually is in late August.
- Association for Advancement of Behavior Therapy, 15 West 36th Street, New York, NY 10018. Their annual meeting usually is in November.
- Center for Cognitive Therapy, University of Pennsylvania, 133 South 36th Street, Philadelphia, PA 19104.
- Institute for Rational Emotive Therapy, 45 East 65th Street, New York, NY 10021.
- Society for Behavioral Pediatrics, 241 Gravers Lane, Philadelphia, PA 19118. Their annual meeting is in mid-spring.
- Society of Behavioral Medicine, 103 South Adams Street, Rockville, MD 20850. Their annual meeting is in mid-spring.

The following professionals offer training workshops for individuals, and they can be contacted directly for more information about training dates and locations:

- Aaron T. Beck, Ph.D., Center for Cognitive Therapy in Philadelphia, Pennsylvania, has pioneered treatment procedures for depression.
- Albert Ellis, Ph.D., Institute for Rational Emotive Therapy, in New York City, developed rational emotive therapy.
- I. Jay Barrish, Ph.D., and Harriet Barrish, Ph.D., Leawood, Kansas, have extensive experience with rational emotive therapy for parents.
- Donald Meichenbaum, Ph.D., Department of Psychology at the University of Waterloo in Ontario, Canada, is considered a pioneer in cognitive behavior therapy.

14.12. CERTIFICATION

At present, there is no board certification available in either cognitive behavior therapy or rational emotive therapy. However, continuing education credit is available at all recognized meetings and workshops.

14.13. CONCLUDING REMARKS

I don't believe it is easy for some parents to deal with their child's misfortune. I believe that some parents exercise more effective coping strategies than others, but I am optimistic that parents with poor coping skills can get assistance, through reading and through contact with professionals, that will help them deal with the intense emotions encountered during the course of raising a child from infancy to adulthood.

Many times, parents have sought help with their child's behavior problems or medical compliance only to find that they don't really benefit from the help. In these cases, the parents may have to learn better and more effective coping skills themselves before they can alter their parenting styles. Only after they are better able to cope with their own emotions will they be in a position to assist their children. The children, in turn, through seeing their parents deal effectively with emotional situations, are more likely to develop effective coping strategies themselves.

REFERENCES

Barrish HH, Barrish IJ: *Managing Parental Anger*. Kansas City, MO: Westport Publishing Group, 1988.

Beck AT: *Cognitive Therapy and the Emotional Disorders*. New York: International Universities Press, 1976.

Burns DD: *The Feeling Good Handbook*. New York: Plume, 1989.

Ellis A, Becker I: *A Guide to Personal Happiness*. Hollywood, CA: Wilshire Book Co., 1982.

Meichenbaum DH: *Cognitive-Behavior Modification*. Cambridge, MA: Ballinger, 1974.

Sample Handouts

HANDOUT 14.1

Self-Help Worksheet for Managing Parental Emotions: Giving a Growth Hormone Injection

1. *What happened/the situation.*

   I tried to give my son his growth hormone injection. He refused to cooperate. He made it very difficult by running away from me. He yelled at me and really hurt my feelings.

2. *What I thought to myself that did not help me handle the situation.*

   You know that I'm just doing this for your own good. I can't stand it when you refuse to cooperate. You're behaving like a little brat!

3. *How I felt.*

   Really angry. I was just trying to help and look at the way he behaved. Look at the thanks I got.

4. *What my behavior looked like.*

   Like I was out of control. Like I was scared.

5. *What I can think to myself to help me handle the situation better.*

   I don't like it when Jeff resists like this, but I certainly don't blame him for not wanting this shot.

6. *How I can feel.*

   Like I'm setting a good example for Jeff. Like I'm in control of my emotions.

7. *What my behavior can look like.*

   Firm and supportive. I can make it easier for him by the way I behave myself.

8. *Discipline strategies/alternative parent behavior options for handling the situation.*

   I can watch a TV show while I give him his shot. I may have to hold him down, but he has to learn that he is going to get his shot regardless of how bad his behavior gets.

Adapted with permission from Barrish HH, Barrish IJ: *Managing Parental Anger*. Kansas City, MO: Westport Publishing Group, 1988.

HANDOUT 14.2

Self-Help Worksheet for Managing Parental Anger: Toddler Example

1. *What happened/the situation.*

   Every time I try to change his diaper, he squirms and makes the task next to impossible.

2. *What I thought to myself that did not help me handle the situation.*

   Don't you know you need changing? I hate this! Cooperate! Why can't you hold still? Change your own diaper!

3. *How I felt.*

   Angry. Intolerant of frustration.

4. *What my behavior looked like.*

   Rough with him. Short, gruff, yelling.

5. *What I can think to myself to help me handle the situation better.*

   It certainly makes changing a diaper more tricky, but it can be done. We'll get through this—we have many times before.

6. *How I can feel.*

   Tolerant but somewhat frustrated and annoyed.

7. *What my behavior can look like.*

   Firm but matter-of-fact.

8. *Discipline strategies/alternative parent behavior options for handling the situation.*

   I can give him something to hold while I change him. I can put him next to a mirror to talk to himself. I can put him on the floor so that he won't roll off the changing table. I can change him and then reward him in some way so that he comes to learn it's fun time.

Adapted with permission from Barrish HH, Barrish IJ: *Managing Parental Anger*. Kansas City, MO: Westport Publishing Group, 1988.

HANDOUT 14.3

Self-Help Worksheet
for Managing Parental Anger

1. *What happened/the situation.*

   _____

   _____

2. *What I thought to myself that did not help me handle the situation.*

   _____

   _____

3. *How I felt.*

   _____

   _____

4. *What my behavior looked like.*

   _____

   _____

5. *What I can think to myself to help me handle the situation better.*

   _____

   _____

6. *How I can feel.*

   _____

   _____

7. *What my behavior can look like.*

   _____

   _____

8. *Discipline strategies/alternative parent behavior options for handling the situation.*

   _____

   _____

Adapted with permission from Barrish HH, Barrish IJ: *Managing Parental Anger*. Kansas City, MO: Westport Publishing Group, 1988.

HANDOUT 14.4

Self-Help Worksheet
for Glasses Wearing

1. *What happened/the situation.*

   My daughter has a condition that requires that she wear her glasses or her vision will deteriorate quickly. So far, she has refused to wear her glasses.

2. *What I thought to myself that did not help me handle the situation.*

   She's so little. I hate to see her so upset. She doesn't understand the importance of wearing her glasses. Maybe, when she gets older, when I can reason with her, it will be easier for her.

3. *How I felt.*

   Caught in a trap. I didn't want to see her upset, but I also didn't want to see her lose her vision.

4. *What my behavior looked like.*

   Like I didn't care. I wasn't concerned enough about her to make her wear her glasses.

5. *What I can think to myself to help me handle the situation better.*

   I don't like it when she fusses, but I'm willing to put up with my own discomfort if I know she will benefit.

6. *How I can feel.*

   Like a parent who is willing to suffer my own discomfort so that my daughter will benefit.

7. *What my behavior can look like.*

   A responsible parent who puts her child's welfare above her own discomfort.

8. *Discipline strategies/alternative parent behavior options for handling the situation.*

   Putting her in time-out for refusing to wear her glasses, and giving her lots of added attention when she does wear them.

Adapted with permission from Barrish HH, Barrish IJ: *Managing Parental Anger*. Kansas City, MO: Westport Publishing Group, 1988.

HANDOUT 14.5

Examples of Helpful Self-Talk

"I don't like it when he behaves that way, but I can stand it."

"Even when she knows the rules, she will break them."

"When he breaks a rule, that's all he has done. Period."

"It's very upsetting when she doesn't follow her doctor's instructions, but I can tolerate it."

"I know that children, like adults, don't always follow the rules."

"I put her in time-out because she needs it, not because I like it."

Chapter 15

Using Token Economies

The United States and most of its economic allies employ a barter system: money. The value of money is determined by consensus of the people working within the barter system, becoming a token of the value it represents.

Parents and professionals can use a similar, though less refined, system of exchange with children. Called a "token economy," it has the same advantages and disadvantages as a monetary system, including a variety of options and opportunities. By earning tokens (poker chips or points) for the behaviors parents want to encourage and losing tokens for the behaviors parents want decreased or eliminated, children are allowed to spend remaining tokens on privileges they desire. Like currency, tokens have many advantages. They:

- Can be more readily carried than the item or activity desired.
- Can be dispensed easily and quickly.
- Have an agreed-on value that can be changed.
- Can be traded for a wide variety of items or activities (rewards or reinforcers) at many different times.
- Can be removed or forfeited, unlike many rewards that, once consumed, cannot be returned.
- Can be added to in large or in small increments.

Child populations served by token economies have ranged from the retarded to the gifted, as well as those with a wide variety of medical problems, including, for example, Attention Deficit Hyperactivity Disorder. Although the research literature is replete with examples of token economies for a wide variety of ages and presenting problems, this discussion applies to the use of token economies in general, with specific examples where necessary to make a point. The use of stickers, stars, happy faces, tickets, and check marks does not constitute a token economy. Rather, stickers or stars provide parents with a means of providing children positive feedback about their behavior. Many families, at one time or another, try something like a "star chart." These types of procedures add a little structure to a family that is already functioning fairly well.

15.1. GENERAL PRINCIPLES OF A TOKEN ECONOMY

Token systems are used to encourage general compliance; in its simplest form, one reward is earned when one task is completed. A child might earn chips, for example, for each activity that is part of getting ready for school on time or helping with household chores. She would lose chips for talking back, interrupting, and other inappropriate behaviors or activities. The privileges she can earn may include such activities as watching television, playing video games, or spending exclusive time with one of her parents.

In many homes, a less-than-formal barter system already is in place. A child might be required to clean his room in order to play a video game for 30 minutes. Or, he may be required to complete several minutes of time-out following an episode of talking back or fighting with a sibling.

A teenager who mows the lawn in exchange for driving the family automobile that evening is making an exchange in her family's token economy. There does not have to be any understanding that the lawn will be mowed again or that the automobile will be available again. In the future, the lawn might be mowed for a variety of different rewards, with use of the car available after any one of a wide variety of tasks is completed. The major disadvantage is that this simple exchange system doesn't have enough variety built into it, and, for some children, it doesn't provide the educational give-and-take experience they need. Although playing video games may be enjoyable one day, it may have little appeal the next day.

The token economy is a simple exchange system that is relatively easy to learn and, in most cases, effective. There must be some agreement, like there is in our monetary economy, about what rewards and punishments are available and what an individual must do to earn them.

In most token economies, the parents and children make written lists, like the examples in this chapter, that detail how many tokens are earned or lost for each of a variety of different behaviors included in the token economy. Once the schedule of rewards and punishments is agreed to, it should be adhered to. Family meetings, as described in the Home Point System Manual (Appendix B), can be used to determine whether the value of tokens needs to be adjusted upward or downward.

In a token economy, a child must, within reason, be allowed to purchase items and activities he has earned. Parents cannot refuse to let a child purchase a previously agreed on item or activity. If a child has earned the right to watch an hour of television, for example, parents can restrict access to certain television shows because they contain offensive scenes, violence, or nudity, but they should not restrict access to all television shows.

Appendixes A and B contain manuals for parents, written to supplement an office discussion and demonstration of a token economy. The Home Chip System (Appendix A) describes how to use poker chips in a token economy for children from approximately 3 to 6 years of age. The Home Point System Manual (Appendix B) describes the use of points in a token economy for children from about 6 years of age to adolescence.

The actual choice of which manual to use depends on the developmental level of the child and her siblings. If a 6-year-old and 4-year-old live in the same home, the chip system would be preferable. If a 6-year-old and a 9-year-old live in the same family, the point system would be preferable. If there is significant doubt whether to use the chip system or the point system, it's probably better to begin with the chip system.

15.2. IMPORTANT CONSIDERATIONS WHEN USING TOKEN ECONOMIES

Tokens become rewarding only when the token exchange takes place almost immediately after the child has engaged in a behavior the parent finds desirable and when the child has the option of exchanging the token for an item or activity he finds enjoyable or rewarding.

The major disadvantage of a home token economy, for some parents, is the level of structure and consistency. Parents must be prepared, within reason, to dispense the rewarding item or activity the child chooses, when the child chooses.

The biggest mistake made in using token economies is the parents' or the professional's assumption that what is reinforcing to one child will be reinforcing to another. Most often, when a caregiver reports that a token economy "didn't work," either the token economy was not providing enough reinforcers to maintain the child's behavior or the people administering the token economy were using it almost exclusively as a vehicle to punish the child.

One of the major advantages of the token economy is its flexibility. The child can exchange a token for any of a variety of items or activities she wants; as her desires change, the rewards can change. As an illustration, adults can usually purchase anything they want to with the money they have. Similarly, children with tokens should be given a good deal of latitude if they have tokens to spend. When severe restrictions are placed on the rewards to which a child has access, the integrity of the token economy is in jeopardy.

Another major advantage of a token economy, beyond its reinforcing value, is its value as a teaching tool for children. Although a child might have only a few opportunities in one day to engage in a particular behavior, the token economy can be used to simulate situations, giving the child many opportunities to practice his skills. Although a child may have little or no interest in practicing French, sharing toys with a sibling, or testing her blood sugar levels, the prospect of earning a lot of tokens exchangeable for some very desirable items can have a markedly strong influence on enhancing positive behaviors.

15.3. WHY USE A TOKEN ECONOMY?

A token economy is a motivational program for children. Indications that a family could benefit from using a token economy include the need to teach children new skills while motivating them to use these new skills. Parents often think that their children need better social skills, coping skills, or negotiating skills, but the only means parents have of teaching their children these skills is to lecture them or to set limits. A token economy, by providing access to a wide variety of items and activities, provides a source of motivation that otherwise may not be possible. While behavioral procedures such as time-out and grounding have been used to encourage children to adapt new behavioral strategies, a token economy can be used to teach children new skills and motivate them to use these skills.

15.4. WHEN TO USE A TOKEN ECONOMY

If a child presents with common behavior problems, standardized behavioral interventions such as those described in Chapter 3, "Behavioral Problems," are probably the first approach to try. Token economies usually are appropriate for children with a mental age of at least 3.

Criteria for considering a token economy are as follows:

- The child is age 3 or older.
- One child presents with multiple behavior problems.
- Several children in the same family present with behavior problems.
- The child lacks age-appropriate social skills, coping skills, or negotiating skills.
- Simpler behavioral treatment has been unsuccessful.

- The child has Attention Deficit Hyperactivity Disorder (ADHD).
- The child presents with medical compliance problems that complicate the child's medical management.

Three basic types of token economies have been developed for use with families: a simple exchange system, a chip system, and a point system.

The simple exchange system provides parents and children with a means of keeping track of household chores, reminding both parent and child what should be done and when it should be completed. Many families without any remarkable behavior problems use the simple exchange system just to add some direction to a complicated lifestyle. The simple exchange system, used in conjunction with the systematic use of time-in and time-out, is suitable for common problems with compliance. If the children have multiple behavior problems, lack good social skills or good coping skills, have problems with medical compliance, have ADHD, or must adhere to a medical regimen for illnesses such as diabetes or arthritis, one of the token economies is more suitable.

Type of Program	Types of Problems
Simple exchange	Scheduling, maintaining consistency
Chip system	Ages 3 to 7, multiple problems, poor social skills, medical compliance, ADHD
Point system	Age 7 and up, multiple problems, poor social skills, medical compliance, ADHD

15.5. SIMPLE EXCHANGE SYSTEM

The simple exchange system involves the parent and the child devising a simple set of rules, often described on a list attached to the refrigerator door with tape or a magnet. The exchange system simply states what behaviors are expected from the child if he wants access to particular items or activities. For example, the child can earn "check marks" for making his bed. Later, these check marks are needed to gain access to activities like playing video games.

The simple exchange system is just that—an exchange system. It is a method of accounting for the rough correlation between what behaviors the child performs and what activities she is allowed. The exchange system is appropriate in those homes where the children are reasonably well behaved but the parents, perhaps because of a hectic schedule or because they are unaccustomed to keeping track of special activities the child has specifically earned, need the simple added structure of the exchange system. The exchange system helps to keep track of children's behavior, whereas the chip and point systems are tools for teaching children new skills.

Dr. Jack Alvord published a booklet that describes a simple exchange system. His *Home Token Economy* (1977) is available by mail order from Research Press in Eugene, Oregon. Handout 15.1 is an example of his exchange system.

In families where children need to be *taught* to behave in substantially different ways, chip and point systems provide the tools for more teaching opportunities, as well as for more effective teaching.

15.6. EXPLAINING THE NEED FOR A TOKEN ECONOMY TO PARENTS

When parents are frustrated with their children's behavior and are yelling at or reprimanding the children excessively (in the parents' opinion), the parents will usually say they are exasperated with their children and they need suggestions regarding what they can do with their children.

If, in the practitioner's opinion, the children actually lack the necessary skills, which is often the case, institution of a token economy is a viable treatment alternative. We explain to families that a child with a broken arm requires an abnormal amount of structure to support the arm while it heals correctly and, although wearing a cast is not a normal state of affairs, the cast is necessary, temporarily, until the bone heals. A token economy is similar in the sense that an abnormal amount of structure is temporarily imposed on the family while children and parents learn more appropriate ways of interacting and coping. Thus, although there is nothing "natural" about using a token economy in the home, the entire family can learn different ways of interacting that are much more natural.

15.6.1. Steps to Follow When Introducing the Token Economy to the Family

After the health-care provider introduces parents to the concept of a token economy, and the parents agree to try it, the parents should be provided with the appropriate manual and scheduled for a return appointment about 1 week later.

The following checklist summarizes the steps to follow:

Step 1. Discuss the need to implement a token economy.
Step 2. Provide parents with the appropriate (chip or token) manual.
Step 3. Schedule a return visit.
Step 4. Assign parents homework:
    a. Make up a list of desirable behaviors.
    b. Estimate the values of tokens.
    c. Purchase chips.
    d. Obtain containers (margarine bowls, Tupperware®, fanny packs).
Step 5. At the return visit:
    a. Go over the list of desirable behaviors.
    b. Go over the estimated value of tokens.
    c. Answer any questions from reading the manual.
    d. Practice giving the child tokens.
    e. Practice with the child taking fines nicely.
    f. Practice purchasing privileges.
    g. Discuss changing token values.

15.7. MEDICAL COMPLIANCE

If a family is having problems with medical compliance, the clinician would have to make an initial determination as to whether to start with general compliance training or with a token economy. The number and types of problems the child is having determine the level of intervention.

If the clinician decides a token economy is necessary, the first step should be teaching the parents to implement a token economy for everyday behaviors and activities, leaving the medically related activities alone until the parent and child are comfortable with the token economy. After the parents and children are acclimated to the token economy, it can be extended to cover behaviors related to medical compliance.

Numerous articles in the pediatric research literature chronicle successes in using token economies with a wide variety of problems with medical compliance. In each case I have read, the clinician has had extensive experience in the implementation of token economies prior to applying this technology to medical compliance. Similarly, the clinician who is relatively naive in the use of a token economy should not start out with medical noncompliance problems. Rather, the clinician should gain initial experience with more common compliance issues in the home.

The most important point for the primary health-care provider to remember about behavioral compliance is that it is easier to promote it in the first place, in young children, than it is to correct it after a long period with problems. Children who have a history of normal levels of compliance are usually much better about accepting the demands of a medical regimen.

The first thing the physician needs to do is to help several sets of parents establish a general pattern of compliance for normal, day-to-day discipline without the use of a token economy. Then, when the physician is accustomed to many of the subtleties of working with behavioral compliance issues, he can begin to apply these principles to problems stemming from prescribed medical regimens. Also, the perspective of having successfully intervened with a number of behavioral compliance problems serves as a good foundation for the physician who is interested in the therapeutic use of procedures that are far more sophisticated and far more difficult to implement, such as token systems.

Although all parents certainly do not have to invest the time and effort into establishing a token economy in the home, they do have to devote a lot of time and effort to teaching their child general behavioral compliance. I've been surprised over the years by the number of parents who have instituted a version of a home token economy without any prior training whatsoever. When asked why they did it, they usually reply that it just made sense to do it. Although some of these "home systems" had to have major adjustments before they were therapeutic for the families, a number of them were helpful, even though their implementation left something to be desired.

Token economies have been successfully used with children following medical regimens for diabetes, arthritis, wearing glasses, growth hormone shots, and a variety of regimens for treating acute diseases such as urinary tract infections, otitis media, and dental hygiene (brushing teeth for children with braces). Instead of the parents constantly trying to verbally encourage the child to complete the components of the medical regimen, tokens are earned or lost for every component of the regimen.

A child on a regimen for arthritis can earn tokens for putting on wrist splints before being asked to do so by his parents, for keeping splints on, for taking medication, for taking a morning bath, and for performing morning and evening exercises (Rapoff, Lindsley, and Christophersen, 1984).

In a study of a token economy used to improve the compliance of a 7-year-old girl with juvenile rheumatoid arthritis, the mean baseline data showed poor compliance with medication (59%), splint wearing (10%), and a prone-lying exercise (0%). Introduction of the token system increased compliance to 95% for medication, 77% for splint wearing, and 71% for prone lying. Through 10 weeks of follow-up, compliance was maintained even though the token economy was withdrawn. Medication, splint wearing, and prone-lying compliance averaged 90%, 91%, and 80%, respectively.

These results were replicated in a second study of a 14-year-old male with juvenile rheumatoid arthritis (Rapoff, Purviance, and Lindsley, 1988). Medication compliance for this boy averaged 44% during baseline, increased to an average of 59% during a simplified regimen condition (when medication was reduced from four to three times a day), and further increased and remained at 100% during the first token economy phase. There was a decreasing trend in compliance during the withdrawal of the token economy (average 77%), an increase during the second token economy phase (average 99%), and an average of 92% during the maintenance phase (where the token economy was withdrawn but could be reinstated if compliance dropped below 80% for 2 consecutive weeks). At the 9-month follow-up visit, when the token economy had been completely withdrawn, compliance averaged 97%. Improvements in clinical outcomes (active joints determined by the rheumatologist and parental ratings of juvenile rheumatoid arthritis symptoms) were noted by the end of the study.

Similarly, a child with insulin-dependent diabetes may earn tokens for performing a finger stick, testing blood properly, calculating diet points, and taking insulin shots calmly. Lowe and Lutzker (1979) demonstrated the effectiveness of using a token economy for getting an insulin-dependent diabetic to perform his daily foot care.

Before a token economy is used to increased medical compliance, a note of caution is necessary: The family must demonstrate some degree of competence using the token economy prior to specifically incorporating a medical regimen. Experience reveals that some families fail to grasp the details of instituting the token economy and may, by improper management, actually make compliance with the medical regimen worse. Requiring that the family demonstrate competence with the token economy prior to incorporating the components of a medical regimen avoids the initial problems associated with emotionally charged behaviors that are usually seen when compliance with a medical regimen is required.

15.7.1. Using the Token Economy to Improve Medical Compliance

After determining that medical compliance is definitely a problem with a given child, the next determination that must be made is whether to start working directly on the medical compliance or to start working on behavioral compliance prior to introducing the token economy for medical compliance.

The following checklist gives the steps to follow:

Step 1. Include behaviors related to medical compliance in the token economy *after* the parents have had success using the token economy with general behavioral compliance.

Step 2. Work with parents to establish behaviors that are to be included in the token economy.

Step 3. Discuss token values with the parents and the child, together.

Step 4. Assign the parents homework:

    a. Use token exchanges frequently for compliance and noncompliance.

    b. Establish the values of tokens such that behaviors related to medical compliance earn more tokens than behaviors related to general compliance.

    c. Have the child practice the appropriate behaviors frequently, with liberal token rewards.

    d. Have the child practice noncompliant behaviors with liberal token fines (with half back for each fine that is accepted nicely).

15.8. IDENTIFYING BEHAVIORS TO INCLUDE IN THE TOKEN ECONOMY

By beginning with the lists of chips (Handout 15.2) or points (Handout 15.3) included in this chapter, the practitioner can add and delete behaviors and privileges that are appropriate or not appropriate for an individual family. For example, if a child practices a musical instrument each day, tokens can be earned for practicing. If a child is active in an after-school activity, she can earn tokens for participation in that activity.

Begin using token values that are easy to remember. For example, begin with two chips for all small jobs around the house, and assign fines of four chips. After a family has used the tokens for about 1 week, they will be very familiar with the values and can usually make changes based on the first week's experience. If a fine of two chips for interrupting hasn't decreased the number of times a child interrupts during the first week, the fine can be increased to four chips during the second week. If four chips the second week doesn't work, increase the fine to six chips. In this way, each level of fines is given 1 week to work or not work. If it works, it stays the same. If it doesn't work, the fine is increased.

Activities through which chips are earned will vary, depending on the individual child. For example, one child may want to earn chips so that she can "purchase" a trip to the playground. Another child who has not been participating in any social activities with other children might be awarded four chips for going to the playground. After a period of weeks during which he goes to the playground many times and learns to enjoy that activity, the number of chips earned can be decreased to two chips. Within another week or two, he could actually be charged two chips for going to the playground.

It is this kind of flexibility that makes the token system so practical for families. Parents can raise and lower the number of tokens earned, lost, or required for an activity, depending on the child's behavior. While it often takes about 2 weeks for the family to acclimate to the tokens, they become almost second nature later.

15.9. INTRODUCING A CHIP SYSTEM TO PARENTS

After taking an extensive family history and securing the parents' agreement that a more structured child-management strategy would be a valuable asset for the family, the health-care professional begins by demonstrating for the child and his parents the giving and returning of chips. The child should be shown how chips are earned and how they are lost.

15.9.1. Purchasing and Banking Chips

Each child needs a container in which to keep her chips. This can be a butter or margarine bowl, a plastic container, or a "fanny pack." The parents need a container for the "bank." The chips, usually poker chips, but any small type of chip is adequate, need to be small enough to carry around and to exchange easily. If more than one child is on the chip economy, each child should have his own chip color.

15.9.2. Practicing Awarding and Taking Away Chips

The professional can begin by offering the child two chips for "listening nicely." As the professional hands two chips to the child, maintaining hold of them, the child is instructed to make eye contact and say, "Thank you." As soon as the child says "Thank you," the practitioner releases the chips and instructs the child to place them in her bowl.

Then, the child might be asked to pick up some toys. As soon as the child begins to pick up the first toy, the practitioner gives the child two chips with a reminder about saying "Thank you" and about placing the chips in the bowl. This procedure is rehearsed several times until the child accepts the chips correctly.

The practitioner can then ask the child to "pretend" she has done something unacceptable by her parents' standards. For example, the practitioner might say, "Allison, please give me two chips for interrupting." The child is instructed to hand the chips to the practitioner, one at a time; count them out as they are handed to the practitioner; and make eye contact with the practitioner during the process. As soon as the child has relinquished the two chips, the practitioner says, "Thank you," and returns one chip to the child for returning the chips nicely. When the child says, "Thank you," the practitioner releases one chip to the child to place in her bowl.

After several rehearsals, the child should be given all the chips that were lost during the practice session. Additional chips are then awarded for practicing nicely. Similarly, the parents can be asked to demonstrate the procedure of giving and taking away chips. The child is then asked what reward she wants to purchase with the accumulated chips (a variety of age-appropriate rewards should be available).

Generally, it is much more important for the child and parents to practice giving and taking away chips correctly than to practice behaviors that result in the child's gaining and losing chips. The rehearsal of the behaviors included in the token economy system can earn a substantial number of tokens for the child. At the completion of this initial rehearsal, earned tokens should be exchanged for some desirable item or activity. The strategy of awarding tokens for beginning an activity, continuing an activity, and completing an activity should be used for all new behaviors introduced.

15.9.3. First Return Visit

At the first return visit, after the parents and child are familiar with the procedures and have performed them for at least a week, such simple jobs as getting up on time, brushing teeth, getting dressed, and combing hair can be combined into one chore called morning hygiene. The child can then earn 10 chips for five combined chores instead of continuing to earn 2 chips for each component of the morning hygiene assignment.

This same strategy can be used to teach a child a variety of complex tasks. For example, the professional might tell the child to pretend he completed his morning chores. The child is then prompted to ask a parent to "check my room." The parent would then check the imaginary room. The parent would give the child two chips for making his imaginary bed while praising the child for doing so.

Thus, if the child has five morning chores (getting up, straightening his bed, brushing his teeth, getting dressed, and picking clothes off the floor) she would have the opportunity to earn 10 chips and to practice accepting chips five separate times. As the child and the parent become more sophisticated at the use of the tokens, the morning chores can be collapsed to just that, "morning chores," with the child earning 10 chips for successfully completing her morning chores.

This illustrates the way the chips are used to teach children social skills. If chips are earned and lost dozens of times each day, the child has dozens of times to practice his social skills. The actual social interaction between the parent and the child is at least as important as the exchange of the tokens.

Similarly, when a child wants to purchase an activity with his chips or has incurred a small chip fine, he is taught to count the chips into the parent's hand one at a time with a neutral attitude and preferably a pleasant one. The parent, in turn, returns half the chip fine because the child "accepted the fine so nicely." These types of interactions, practiced over and over again, teach the child social skills. Over the years, we've found that young children are much more willing to practice social skills when they are on a token system than when they are not. Conversely, as the child learns appropriate social skills, it becomes much easier for the parent to refrain from making negative statements to the child. Parent and child are usually both learning new social interaction skills.

15.10. INTRODUCING THE POINT SYSTEM TO PARENTS

The only significant difference between using chips and using points is the medium of exchange. Where a toddler earns plastic poker chips for each job done correctly, the school-age child earns "points" for each job done correctly (see Handout 15.3).

During the first office visit, the professional engages the child in a discussion about how the point system works, describing how the child gains points for appropriate behavior, loses points for inappropriate behavior, and is required to spend points for privileges.

After such a discussion, the professional asks the child to write her name and the date on the top of the point card. (See Appendix B for a complete discussion of the point system and examples of point cards.)

As soon as the child writes her name, she is instructed, "Give yourself 10 points for filling out the card correctly." Then the professional begins to rehearse a variety of activities in which the child gains and loses points.

Each time the child gains 10 points, he is instructed to give himself 10 points. When the child has written down 10 points and what behavior earned those 10 points, he is instructed to ask the professional to "sign my point card." The professional then initials the card. As soon as the card has been appropriately initialed, the points belong to the child. Several additional examples are rehearsed with the child, each with the child earning points on his point card.

Then the professional introduces the topic of losing points, using examples such as interrupting, stalling, and talking back. The child is asked to "practice" losing points by pretending to interrupt her parents' conversation. The parent says, "Please take off 10 points for interrupting." If the child writes down "talking" under the behavior column and "10" under the point column, the parent says, "Thank you for taking off the points so nicely. I'm going to give you back half the points because you did it so well."

Like the chip system, the child can earns half of every point fine back. If the child stalls while taking off the points, he is fined an additional 10 points for stalling. Then he can earn half of the second fine back but not half of the first one. These point exchanges provide the child with many opportunities to learn appropriate social skills.

15.10.1. Encouraging Children to Use New Skills

If the parent asks the child to do her morning chores, for example, and the child begins walking toward her room, the parent can hold up two chips and tell the child two chips have been earned because the child started the chore right away. The parent can reward the child with two chips because she is working so hard; chips can be given in this manner two or three times.

At the completion of morning chores, the child may have earned 20 chips for a group of chores actually scheduled for only 10 chips. The extra 10 chips are necessary, initially, to reward the child for starting and staying with his chores, in addition to whatever chips are scheduled for completion of the job.

The important point is teaching the child how to get morning chores completed, not punishing her for not doing them. This is true with both the chip system and the point system. The simple act of punishing a child for not doing something is rarely enough to encourage the child to complete a complex set of morning chores.

The token economy using poker chips has been so effective in teaching important social and maintenance skills to children that Russell Barkley (1981), in his book on hyperactive children, recommends that the chip system be considered as a treatment option for all children with Attention Deficit Hyperactivity Disorder. An earlier version of our Home Chip System was included as an appendix in Dr. Barkley's book.

15.11. USING TOKEN ECONOMIES TO MOTIVATE A CHILD TO BE MORE COMPLIANT

Depending on how the parent deals with difficult parent/child situations, token economies can remove some of the emotionalism of parenting. First, parents are very astute when it comes to noting whether their child has engaged in an objectionable behavior. Thus, parents usually remember to fine their children for objectionable behaviors by taking away tokens. Second, children are equally astute at reminding their parents and caregivers when they have earned tokens.

In some families, having the children remind the parents to dispense tokens, in the form of asking them to check the child's job, can help teach the parent that he has been overlooking a lot of good behavior the child has been exhibiting. Few parents, for example, ignore children beginning to fight. With a token economy, rather than criticize the children for fighting, or even spend time ascertaining who was responsible for the fight in the first place, the parents simply request each child to return a previously agreed on number of tokens for fighting and, if the children return the tokens nicely, they receive half of the tokens back.

While a strong admonition can serve to aggravate feelings that resulted in the fight in the first place, the simple and matter-of-fact removal of tokens usually does not make the situation more emotional. Giving back half of the total fine when a child relinquishes the tokens nicely is recommended so that all appropriate token transitions end with the child receiving tokens.

Unlike an admonition, a parent can administer a token fine to a child many, many times in one day with much less chance of getting angry or frustrated. Conversely, when a child has awakened, dressed, made his bed, and arrived at the breakfast table on time, the busy parent is likely, a good deal of the time, to forget to acknowledge that all of these things were accomplished on time. The child on a token economy, however, because she needs tokens to gain access to most of the activities she enjoys, is motivated to remind her mom or dad to "check my jobs." In this way, parents are likely to keep track of the behaviors they do not want their child engaged in, and the child is likely to keep track of the behaviors his parents want him engaged in (the behaviors that earn tokens).

15.12. HOW TOKENS ARE EXCHANGED

The most important consideration is not tokens but rather how parents or professionals dispense them and take them away, and how the child accepts and relinquishes the tokens. If parents remain calm and matter-of-fact, it is much easier for the child to handle earning and losing tokens.

As such, token economies give parents many opportunities for modeling emotions. If the parents handle the tokens in a calm, matter-of-fact manner, they are modeling this behavior for their children. It may require some time for parents to successfully substitute the loss of tokens for more typical emotional outbursts. Children on token economies, however, often report they would rather be yelled at than lose tokens because yelling takes only a minute or two but losing tokens means they must be earned again.

15.13. WHY TOKEN ECONOMIES FAIL

Most failures with token economies are due to two major causes:

• Parents make the token economy too punitive.
• Parents neglect to establish a functional relationship between the number of tokens the child earns and the items and/or activities available to her.

When a token economy is successfully implemented, both children and parents gain experience in handling their reactions in a calm, matter-of-fact manner.

Often, parents, as a crude form of punishment, restrict a child's access to activities the child finds very desirable. The parent's rationale is that the child simply doesn't deserve the activity. After a period of time on a token system, where the child has had an opportunity to demonstrate he "can behave himself," the professional is in a much better position to convince the parent to allow the child more freedom.

For example, parents may say they will not purchase a video game for the child because she can't be trusted. If, after a period of successfully using the token economy, the parent can actually see a marked improvement in the child's behavior, the professional is in a much better position to serve as an advocate for the child and to help to convince the parents to "lighten up." Often, it is only after the child has earned access to really valuable (in the child's mind) activities that the child begins to behave appropriately the majority of the time.

15.14. CHANGING REINFORCERS

Sometimes parents are confused because a child will work for one reward consistently for a month or so, then seemingly doesn't care about that reward anymore. Both adults and children have a natural ebb and flow of reward tastes, sometimes preferring one reward almost exclusively for a time, then, for no discernible reason, switching to another reward. Parents who offer a child only one type of reward may find that, sooner or later, the child tires of that particular reward and subsequently becomes less enthusiastic about working for it. The token economy offers the advantage that the child can, within reason, purchase the items or activities that appeal to him at that particular time; the rewards change as the child's tastes change.

15.15. TAKING THE TIME NECESSARY TO INTRODUCE
A TOKEN ECONOMY

A token economy takes about 1 week to become established in a normal household; it can be expected to last anywhere from a month to a year or more.

Parents may have trouble at first remembering the various behaviors that earn and lose tokens, but it becomes easier each day. After several weeks using a token economy, many parents report that keeping a list of jobs for their children to do is the biggest problem, because the children have learned the value of tokens and now just want to earn as many as they can.

15.16. EXTENDING A TOKEN ECONOMY BEYOND THE HOME

While parents are encouraged to use the token system for most naturally occurring activities within the home, the system can be extended to include behaviors that occur at school. For example, children may earn tokens for doing homework (by the amount of time spent doing homework or by the amount of homework completed) and for papers and grades they bring home from school.

In cases where a child has been having a difficult time at school, we sometimes implement a school note that provides a formal communication link between the school and the home. The child's teachers are asked to complete the home–school note at the end of each class. The child is rewarded for bringing the school note home, regardless of how good or bad the ratings are on the school note. Handout 15.4 provides an example of such a note.

Each day when the child returns from school, he is asked to sit at the kitchen table while one parent and the child review the school note together. For every appropriate behavior indicated by the teacher, the child earns tokens; for every inappropriate behavior that has been checked, the child loses tokens. Following the rule discussed above, every fine is cut in half if the child accepts it appropriately. Ideally, the review of the child's school note and the gaining and losing of tokens based on the school note should take a short time, perhaps no more than 5 minutes.

15.17. WITHDRAWING THE TOKEN ECONOMY

Although many families simply discontinue use of the token system when they feel like it, we have developed procedures for formally withdrawing the system.

With a point system, the parents and the child can come to an agreement regarding how many points the child needs to buy her way off the point system. Children typically set the value of buying their way off of the system far too high—often at a level they can never achieve. The parent's role, in these cases, is to make certain the amount of points required to get off of the point system is reasonable—about the same number of points the child could accumulate in 1 month's time. If the child engages in two major misbehaviors in 1 week, the point system should be reintroduced, with the child starting with no points, as though she was never on the point system in the first place. The child can then start saving her points to purchase her way off of the point system again as soon as she chooses to do so.

With the chip system, parents are encouraged, after at least 2 months on the system, to go a day or two without chips to see how the child behaves. If the child's behavior remains acceptable, he stays off of the chips. If his behavior deteriorates, the chip system should be reintroduced.

15.18. CONCLUDING REMARKS

A token economy is a therapeutic tool that, in the hands of a trained practitioner, and when used appropriately, can be of significant benefit to families who are experiencing behavioral and or medical/behavioral problems with their children. It is not a gimmick, nor is it necessarily an easy procedure to learn to implement. But, when implemented properly by a trained professional, it can produce remarkable results.

REFERENCES

Alvord JR: *Home Token Economy: An Incentive Program for Children and Their Parents*. Eugene, OR: Research Press, 1977.

Barkley RA: *Hyperactive children: A Handbook for Diagnosis and Treatment*. New York: Guilford Press, 1981.

Lowe K, Lutzker JR: Increasing compliance to a medical regimen with a juvenile diabetic. *Behav Ther* 10:57–64, 1979.

Rapoff MA, Lindsley CB, Christophersen ER: Improving compliance with medical regimens: A case study with juvenile rheumatoid arthritis. *Arch Phys Med Rehab* 65:267–269, 1984.

Rapoff MA, Purviance MR, Lindsley CB: Improving medical compliance for juvenile rheumatoid arthritis and its effect on clinical outcome: A single-subject analysis. *Arthritis Care Res* 1:12–16, 1988.

Sample Handouts

Home Token Economy

HANDOUT 15.1

for _____ age _____ for weeks ending _____ & _____

Desirable behavior	Payoff	S	M	T	W	T	F	S	Events	S	M	T	W	T	F	S	Events
1																	
2																	
3																	
4																	
5																	
6																	
7																	
8																	
9																	
10																	

Undesirable behavior	Fine	S	M	T	W	T	F	S		S	M	T	W	T	F	S	
1																	
2																	
3																	
4																	
5																	

Privileges	Cost																
1																	
2																	
3																	
4																	
5																	
6																	
7																	
8																	
9																	
10																	

Parents pay

1 failure to enforce economy																	
2																	
3																	

Token balance

Note: No bankruptcy   No credit   No advances   No millonaires – Please read instruction booklet.

Home Token Economy, Suite 100, 415 East 63rd, Kansas City, Missouri 64110

Chip Values

Behaviors that GAIN chips

Making the bed	+2	Setting the table	+4
Picking up items off the floor	+2	Taking out trash	+4
Brushing teeth	+2	Folding clothes	+4
Picking up toys	+2	Helping Mom or Dad	+2
Dressing self	+2	Beginning homework	+2
Saying please and thank you	+2	Continuing homework	+2
Bathing by self	+2	Finishing homework	+2
Being in bed on time	+2	Beginning jobs immediately	+2
Volunteering to help	+2	Being nice to siblings	+4

Find times to give bonus chips.

Behaviors that LOSE chips

Arguing	−2	Stalling	−2
Talking back	−2	Not having homework sheet	−10
Interrupting	−2	Having a bad school report	−30
Jumping on furniture	−2	Using bad language	−10
Running in the house	−2	Putting coat on floor	−2
Tattling	−2		

Never nag when taking away chips.
Taking off chips nicely always earns back one-half of the fine.

Cost of PRIVILEGES

Watching television	5 per ½ hour
Playing with video games	5 per ½ hour
Extra story	5
Snacks	5 per snack with permission
Toys outside	5
Friends at your home	10
Go to friend's house	30
Friend overnight	100
Overnight at friend's	200

Point Values

Behaviors that EARN points

Brush teeth	10	Carry own dishes to sink	10
Clear table	20	Wash face once a day	10
Close drawers	10	Comb hair before school	10
Dress self without dawdling	10	Dust a room	20
Flush toilet	10	Fold laundry	10
Follow direction first time	10	Get up willingly	10
Use good manners	10	Homework per ½ hour	20
Turn off lights/TV when done	10	Pick up room	10
Put belongings away	10	Put clothes in hamper	10
Volunteer for job	10		

Find times to give bonus points.

Behaviors that LOSE points

Arguing	40	Complaining	20
Leaving clothes on floor	20	Leaving dinner table before	20
Interrupting	40	finished	
Not listening	40	Slamming door	20
Stalling, dawdling	40	Yelling in house	20
Talking back	40		

Never nag when taking away points.
Taking off points nicely always earns back one-half of the fine.

Cost of PRIVILEGES

Basics: 100 points per day
(TV, telephone, play in yard, good snacks, room toys)

Extra Privileges

Bowling	200	Library	30
Park	100	Overnight	200
Picking video	250	Play off property	30
Riding in front seat	200	Skating	100
Snacks	10	Staying up late	30 per ½ hour
Tape player ½ hour	30	TV show	30 per ½ hour

Allowance Money (Once Each Week)

1 point per penny for the first $1.00
5 points per penny for second $1.00
10 points per penny for third $1.00
20 points per penny for each additional $1.00

Daily School Note

Lose 100 points: Note not brought home
Lose 20 points: Argue with note
Gain 20 points: Each acceptable social behavior
Gain 20 points: Work on assignments
Gain 20 points: Hand in assignments

HANDOUT 15.4

Daily School Note for Grade Improvement

_____

_____

_____

Student's Name_____Date_____CLASS _____

Was the student's social behavior acceptable today?	YES							
	NO							
Did the student pay attention and work on class assignments during class?	YES							
	NO							
What grade did the student earn on today's assignment or test handed back?	GRADE							
Has the student failed to hand in any required assignments?	YES, work is not current							
	NO, work is current							
Does the student have a homework assignment that is due tomorrow?	YES							
	NO							
Did the student argue or disagree with the way you marked this note?	YES							
	NO							
	Teacher's Initials (Please use ink)							

Chapter **16**

Compliance with Painful Procedures

Although much has been written about compliance problems, the majority of literature has covered procedures that do not produce direct pain for the patient. When dealing with painful procedures, compliance issues aren't nearly as clearly delineated. For example, while there is the clear implication that outpatients could comply with a medical regimen if they wanted to, many painful procedures conducted with patients demand more than simple compliance. Even a procedure as simple as a venipuncture requires that the patient be able to lie perfectly still while a needle is inserted into a vein. Often, health-care providers must be knowledgeable about a variety of treatment strategies in order to complete their treatments. With a venipuncture, the provider must know what veins are the most accessible and how many venipunctures must ultimately be done so that the initial venipunctures, if there are to be a series of them, are started at the distal point of the vein. A situation such as a patient's presence in an intensive-care unit (ICU) or a burn trauma unit demands more expertise from the health-care provider and typically requires more specific procedures. In ICUs there are more painful procedures, anxiety levels are higher, and there are more aversive procedures for the patient to endure than those normally associated with increasing compliance. Thus, the provider must be prepared to assist the patient in adopting a coping or distraction strategy that is effective for him.

16.1. CHILDREN'S COPING STYLES

Children's adjustment to and subsequent compliance with medical regimens and procedures may be related to their style of coping, that is, use of such individual cognitive strategies as self-instruction, distraction, or information seeking. While coping style has been examined in adults, it has yet to be looked at carefully in children. In a survey administered to 994 school-age children to identify behaviors associated with coping with pain, Ross and Ross (1984) reported that only 21% of children used any type of coping strategy. Of this 21%, the most frequently used strategies were distraction and/or such physical procedures as clenching a fist. A small number used cognitive strategies such as thought stopping and relaxation. While distraction has been reported to be effective anecdotally (Beales, 1983) and empirically in combination with other approaches (Kelley, Jarvie, Middlebrook, McNeer, and Drabman, 1984), it has not been thoroughly evaluated as a single component in reducing noncompliance to medical procedures. Distraction, as a pain-management procedure, refers to the patient, either alone or with the aid of a health-care provider, engaging in a behavior that will take his or her mind off the painful procedure. Although there is no conclusive evidence, McCaul and Malott (1984) suggest that, with adults, distraction may be most effective in mitigating pain behavior if the pain is mild to moderate and of short duration. In children, therefore, it is possible that distraction may best be used when examining a child's ears or giving injections but not during such painful procedures as bone marrow aspiration. In addition, Miller's (1980) finding implies that distraction works best with children known as "blunters," who prefer a minimum of prior or ongoing information. For "monitors," those children who prefer receiving details about upcoming procedures, peer modeling may be the more appropriate strategy.

16.2. MODELING

Modeling refers to the use of an animate or inanimate model, such as a doll, that a child can watch to see what a procedure looks like and to see how the model responds. Modeling has been used in both medical and dental procedures. Melamed and Siegel (1980) reported a series of studies examining the effects of filmed modeling on children's arousal prior to and after hospital operations. Generally, these filmed modeling procedures reduced children's emotional behaviors about their procedures with two possible exceptions:

- Younger children, less than 7 years old, benefit more from the films if they are seen close to the time of surgery.

- Children who have had prior operative procedures showed higher levels of emotion the night before surgery, regardless of whether they were shown a filmed model of the procedure.

Stokes and Kennedy (1980) conducted a series of studies using live models to prepare children for dental procedures. Children who had previously exhibited unacceptable levels of disruptive behavior during dental procedures were used as subjects for the research. The children's behavior was acceptable if:

- They saw the live model receive a reward for cooperating (and no reward for not cooperating).
- They knew they were being observed by another child.

16.3. RELAXATION

Relaxation training has been used to treat a wide variety of medical disorders, including hypertension. Relaxation consists of systematically tensing and relaxing each separate muscle group in the body. Patel (1984) provides a good description of deep muscle relaxation: For the purpose of training in deep muscle relaxation, the patient is asked to lie supine on a couch or a reclining chair, with legs slightly apart and rotated externally at the hip joints so that the heels are pointing inward and the toes are pointing outward. This position reduces the tension in the muscles around the knee joints. The arms are kept by the side, a few inches away from the trunk, and, if possible, the palms are turned upward and the fingers kept slightly flexed. The head, neck, and trunk are kept in a straight line. Although the position of the head is elevated to a comfortable level in the beginning, the patient is encouraged to lie flat; within a few days, most patients are able to do so. The eyes are kept closed. The person is then asked to relax each group of muscles in sequence, starting from the right toes and progressing to include the right heel, ankle, calf, knee, thigh, and hip and then similarly going over the left leg, right arm, left arm, shoulders, neck, jaws, cheeks, forehead, around the eyes, and the scalp. Throughout this process, the patient is asked to become aware of the sensation of relaxation so that he or she would recognize the tension that is inappropriate and be able to relax as soon as it begins to build up in everyday life. Finally, the patient is asked to direct attention to his breathing and to relax the muscles of the chest and abdomen. Relaxation has been shown to be effective in reducing primary hypertension (Patel, 1984), recurrent abdominal pain (Finney, Lemanek, Cataldo, Katz, and Fuqua, 1989), and irritable bowel syndrome (Blanchard, Schwarz, and Neff, 1988). In the study by Finney et al. (1989), children ranging in age from 6½ years to 13¾ years were treated for recurrent abdominal pain with some combination of five treatment components: self-monitoring, relaxation training, limited parental reinforcement for somatic complaints, dietary fiber, and routine activities. At follow-up, after an average of 2.5 office visits, 81% of the participants reported that their pain symptoms were either improved or resolved.

16.4. COMBINATION STRATEGIES

A well-controlled study by Peterson and Shigetomi (1981) found that children who were taught a combination of coping strategies, including relaxation, distraction, and comforting self-talk, in addition to viewing a filmed model, were more cooperative during their hospitalization than those receiving preoperation information or any of the above strategies alone. Children may naturally have different styles of coping (Miller, 1980), which influences the type of preparation most appropriate for each child and further complicates the teaching of coping strategies. More research is needed to determine if children do in fact cope differently and to reliably assess a child's coping style. At present, the practitioner must rely on verbal reports of the parent's and child's past experiences and preferred coping strategies.

16.5. USE OF HYPNOSIS TECHNIQUES

Zeltzer and LeBaron (1982) compared the relative effectiveness of hypnotic and nonhypnotic techniques for children undergoing bone marrow aspirations and lumbar punctures, using both patient report and professional observers. Their procedures follow.

16.5.1. Nonhypnotic Group

Nonhypnotic techniques included a combination of deep breathing, distraction, and practice sessions to help the child control his fear. Distraction involved asking the child to focus on objects in the room rather than on fantasy. During a bone marrow aspiration, for example, a child might be instructed to squeeze her mother's hands, take a few deep breaths, and count the stripes or flowers on her blouse during needle insertion. Patients were helped to notice and discuss various elements of the treatment room. Sometimes this involved jokes or games, such as the therapist counting the child's fingers incorrectly. The manner in which these techniques would be used was determined by knowledge of the patient, family, and situational factors. In general, this nonhypnotic approach involved the use of distraction and encouragement of self-control behaviors; the use of imagery or fantasy was strictly avoided by the therapist.

16.5.2. Hypnosis Group

Patients in this group were helped to become increasingly involved in interesting and pleasant images. The manner in which children were helped to become involved in imagery was designed according to the individual characteristics of the patient, parents, and environment. An exciting or funny story might be told to a child during bone marrow aspirations. Gradually, the story would be made more vivid by filling in with images and surprises and asking the child questions that called on imagination for answers. For example, the child might be asked to "notice the elephant about to squirt water on us" and describe what he "sees." During one procedure, the therapist helped an adolescent girl imagine a visit to a "boyfriend factory," where she described the boyfriend she picked out. She spent the remainder of the procedure "taking her boyfriend on a date." Although patients in this group were also helped to take deep breaths and to have practice sessions, the use of imagery and fantasy were interwoven throughout all aspects of this intervention. While the hypnosis and nonhypnosis groups were similar prior to any intervention, pain during the bone marrow aspiration was significantly reduced by hypnosis alone and to a smaller, but significant, extent by the nonhypnotic techniques. During lumbar punctures, a more painful procedure than bone marrow aspirations according to preintervention data, only hypnosis significantly reduced pain. The authors concluded that hypnosis was shown to be more effective than nonhypnotic techniques for reducing procedural distress in children and adolescents with cancer.

Hypnosis does not and need not involve anything resembling the traditional "trance." Rather, the patient is verbally encouraged to engage in enough visual imagery (with children, in fantasy) that he is no longer concentrating so intently on the painful procedure itself. The patient remains conscious throughout the entire procedure and will usually cry out during particularly painful parts of the procedure, but otherwise appears to experience much lower levels of pain or distress.

16.6. PREVIOUS EXPERIENCE

The probability of compliance may be directly related to a child's previous experience with similar procedures. A greater likelihood exists that a child whose noncompliant behavior has been reinforced by the avoidance of the procedure in the past will be noncompliant under similar circumstances in the future. A child who even temporarily delays an aversive procedure by resisting may be more likely to resist when undergoing future procedures. While children's avoidance behavior has not been specifically evaluated with medical procedures, use of behavior management (usually consisting of reinforcement for compliance and ignoring or time-out for noncompliance) has contributed to increased compliance during various medical procedures.

16.7. PARENTAL FACTORS

Parents can have a direct and immediate impact on their child's compliance during medical procedures. They can serve as a model of appropriate or inappropriate behavior by first simulating the procedure and modeling how they would like their child to behave for the procedure. A number of years ago, my son, my wife, and I had to have gamma globulin shots secondary to exposure to hepatitis. I received my injection first and, although I found it quite painful, I "pretended" that it didn't hurt and thanked the nurse. My wife did exactly the same thing. When my son received his injection, although tears were streaming down his face, he also looked like he had to exert effort to maintain his composure. He also thanked the nurse.

In attempting to determine why some children behave worse with their parents present for a procedure, Gross, Stern, Levin, Dale, and Wojnilower (1983) speculated that negative behavior may be the result of children learning to identify their parents as a potential means of escape from aversive events. During medical procedures, however, the parents' failure to intervene may constitute an extinction contingency. Extinction is the same as ignoring. Typically, when extinction of any behavior is just started, the recipient of the extinction will behave worse initially, exhibiting more of the behavior being extinguished (Drabman and Jarvie, 1977). Parent-training research has demonstrated that clear, concise instructions can be effective in increasing compliance in the home (Roberts, McMahon, Forehand, and Humphreys, 1978). Thus, it may work to simply instruct a normally compliant child to cooperate with a nurse or a doctor.

16.8. INTERACTION WITH HEALTH-CARE PRACTITIONERS

Practitioners who maintain close physical proximity to their patients, give verbal expressions of empathy, and have gentle, but firm, physical contact with their patients are usually perceived as more caring and have fewer problems with compliance (Olness and Gardner, 1988). In contrast, coercion, coaxing, put-downs, and stopping treatment to manage behavior can result in increased fear behaviors. Sometimes there is a circular pattern: The health-care provider's behavior, in response to fearful child behaviors, engenders more fearful behavior and so on, as in the example of a provider who becomes aggravated by avoidance behavior on a child's part and becomes verbally stern with the child, who, in turn, becomes more apprehensive. Prior experience and the nature of that experience can either favorably or unfavorably affect the child's behavior. The more unremarkable the experience a child has with a provider, the more likely that future contacts will be unremarkable.

16.9. ADVANCED TRAINING

There are many excellent organizations that offer training in pain management, including hypnosis. Each year, the Society for Behavioral Pediatrics offers a 3-day training workshop on hypnosis in conjunction with their annual meeting. My experience has been that pediatric health-care providers benefit most from workshops taught by their peers, using pediatric patients and pediatric examples. Organizations include:

- Society for Behavioral Pediatrics, 241 Gravers Lane, Philadelphia, PA 19118. Their annual meeting is in mid-spring.
- Society of Behavioral Medicine, 103 South Adams Street, Rockville, MD 20850. Their annual meeting is in mid-spring.

16.10. CERTIFICATION

Although there are no organizations that offer certification in pain management, there are several societies that offer certification in hypnosis. For more information, contact:

- American Society of Clinical Hypnosis, 2200 Devon Avenue, Suite 291, Des Plaines, IL 60018. Telephone: 708-297-3317.
- Society of Clinical and Experimental Hypnosis, 128A Kings Park Drive, Liverpool, NY 13090. Telephone: 315-652-7299.

16.11. CONCLUDING REMARKS

While there have always been pharmaceutical agents to control patients' pain, only fairly recently have behavioral procedures gained recognition as legitimate intervention strategies both for pain management and for increasing compliance with treatment procedures. As Zeltzer, Barr, McGrath, and Schechter (1992) pointed out, "Pediatric pain is an underdeveloped area ripe for study within the realm of developmental and behavioral pediatrics, as noted by documentation of its undertreatment in children" (p. 816).

REFERENCES

Beales JG: Factors influencing the expectation of pain among patients in a children's burn unit. *Burns Thermal Injury* 9:187–192, 1983.

Blanchard EB, Schwarz SP, Neff DF: Two-year follow-up of behavioral treatment of irritable bowel syndrome. *Behavior Therapy* 19:67–73, 1988.

Drabman RS, Jarvie G: Counseling parents of children with behavior problems: The use of extinction and time-out techniques. *Pediatrics* 59(1):78–85, 1977.

Finney JW, Lemanek KL, Cataldo MF, Katz HP, Fuqua RW: Pediatric psychology in primary health care: Brief targeted therapy for recurrent abdominal pain. *Behav Ther* 20(2):283–291, 1989.

Gross AM, Stern RM, Levin RB, Dale J, Wojnilower DA: The effect of mother-child separation on the behavior of children experiencing a diagnostic medical procedure. *J Consult Clin Psychol* 51(5):783–785, 1983.

Kelley ML, Jarvie GJ, Middlebrook JL, McNeer MF, Drabman RS: Decreasing burned children's pain behavior: Impacting the trauma of hydrotherapy. *J Appl Behav Anal* 17:147–158, 1984.

McCaul KD, Malott JM: Distraction and coping with pain. *Psychol Bull* 95(3):516–533, 1984.

Melamed BG, Siegel LJ: Psychological preparation for hospitalization, in Melamed BG, Siegel LJ (Eds.), *Behavioral Medicine: Practical Applications in Health Care*. New York: Springer, 1980.

Miller SM: When is a little information a dangerous thing? Coping with stressful events by monitoring vs. blunting, in Levine S, Ursin H (Eds.), *Coping and Health*. New York: Plenum Press, 1980.

Olness K, Gardner GG: *Hypnosis and Hypnotherapy with Children*. Philadelphia: Grune and Stratton, 1988.

Patel C: A relaxation-centered behavioral package for reducing hypertension, in Matarazzo JD, Weiss SM, Herd JA, Miller NE, Weiss SM (Eds.), *Behavioral health: A handbook of health enhancement and disease prevention*. New York: Wiley & Sons, 1984.

Peterson L, Shigetomi C: One-year follow-up of elective surgery child patients receiving preoperative preparation. *J Pediatr Psychol* 7(1):43–48, 1981.

Roberts MW, McMahon RJ, Forehand R, Humphreys L: The effect of parental instruction-giving on child compliance. *Behav Ther* 9(5):793–798, 1978.

Ross DM, Ross SA: Childhood pain: The school-aged child's viewpoint. *Pain* 20:179–191, 1984.

Stokes TF, Kennedy SH: Reducing child uncooperative behavior during dental treatment through modeling and reinforcement. *J Appl Behav Anal* 13:41–49, 1980.

Zeltzer LK, Barr RG, McGrath PA, Schechter NL: Pediatric pain: Interacting behavioral and physical factors. *Pediatrics* 90:816–821, 1992.

Zeltzer LK, LeBaron S: Hypnosis and nonhypnotic techniques for reduction of pain and anxiety during painful procedures in children and adolescents with cancer. *J Pediatr* 101(6):1032–1035, 1982.

PART V

OFFICE MANAGEMENT STRATEGIES

Historically, medical schools have not concentrated much of their effort on office management strategies. Issues such as appointment keeping and collection of fees have often been out of the mainstream, such that medical students and residents learn some effective strategies if they spend time with certain staff members, and they learn almost nothing about these strategies if they do not spend time with those staff members.

At Children's Mercy Hospital in Kansas City, Missouri, the Behavioral Pediatrics Section has consistently had one of the highest collection rates. At our satellite office, our collection rate has averaged above 95%, which, by most clinicians' estimates, is very good. This hasn't been due to luck, to good fortune, or to the population we serve. Fee collection is an integral part of the clinical service that we offer. Strategies that we have researched and incorporated into our clinic are discussed in Chapter 17.

Usually, referral—that is, which patients should be referred, when they should be referred, and how they should be referred—is a topic that is learned in residency training. However, because common behavior problems have not been given extensive coverage in residency training programs, pediatric health-care providers often do not have as much experience deciding when and to whom these problems should be referred. There usually aren't grand rounds or seminars devoted to this topic.

Policies and procedures that contribute to getting referrals and to making referrals are also discussed in Chapter 18.

Chapter **17**

Office Management

Although the connection between Behavioral Pediatrics and office management may not be immediately obvious, there are a number of behavioral considerations that can affect how your office functions. For example, the best treatment procedures available can't provide any benefit to a child who doesn't keep his scheduled appointment. And, the provider who has trouble collecting the fees for his services may well become distracted from treatment, feeling that his time might better be concentrated on collections. A number of issues, many of which can be feasibly addressed by the practitioner, maximize patient compliance with treatment recommendations. These include practice management issues as well as the provider's approach to patient care.

Patients prefer seeing the same provider for each scheduled appointment; they don't like to wait an excessive amount of time to see their provider; and they are responsive to mailed and phoned reminders prior to scheduled appointments (Friman, Finney, Rapoff, and Christophersen, 1985). Each of these issues will be discussed below.

17.1. PROVIDER CONTINUITY

Patients who see the same health-care practitioner at each scheduled office visit are more likely to comply with treatment recommendations and to keep follow-up appointments (Rapoff and Christophersen, 1982). Although patients understand that their own provider can't be on call every day and night, they do prefer to see their provider during most scheduled office visits.

17.2. TIME SPENT WAITING

The time a patient spends waiting should be kept to a minimum. Patients can generally accommodate a delay in seeing their health-care practitioner if the office staff is polite and periodically informs them when they can expect to see the practitioner. Offering the patient an opportunity to make a phone call is usually perceived as a sign that the health-care practitioner is concerned about having patients wait. Perhaps the major reason providers will schedule several patients at the same time is because of the history of patients not keeping scheduled appointments. When the appointment-keeping strategies discussed below are implemented, the number of patients who do not keep their appointments is reduced, which, in turn, reduces the need to double- and triple-book appointments.

17.3. TREATMENT REMINDERS

Various studies have shown that compliance with medical regimens can be improved by environmental modifications that cue parental compliance (Mathews and Christophersen, 1989). When we treat a typical toddler for such oppositional behaviors as tantrums, defiant behavior, arguing, and annoying their parents, we explain to the parents what our treatment recommendations are and, after answering their questions, provide them with written summaries of our treatment recommendations, such as those discussed in most of the chapters in this book. At the end of our first office visit for treatment of common behavior problems, we give the parents a 3-by-5 inch card to remind them of our recommendations. Handout 17.1 is a copy of one of those cards. We suggest that they attach the reminder to their refrigerator door with a magnet.

17.3.1. Written Handouts

Throughout much of this book there are written handouts that have been included so that the practitioner can photocopy them for distribution to parents of their patients. These handouts can either be used exactly as they now read or they can be revised and edited prior to distribution to parents. If they are used in their present form, the attribution statement at the bottom of each handout should be included. If they are edited, the attribution statement should be changed to reflect that the handout is "adapted from" the original handout.

Another option that has recently become available to the practitioner is the Pediatric Advisor. The Pediatric Advisor is a computer software program that includes several hundred written handouts that cover most of the conditions encountered by the primary health-care provider, including, by way of example, allergic rhinitis, diarrhea, fever, and vomiting. The Advisor also includes handouts on many of the behavior problems addressed in this book. The Advisor is user-friendly, which means that almost anyone with the slightest familiarity with computers can use it. The handouts contained in the Advisor can be used in their original form or edited, or completely new handouts can be added. The software is written so that the handouts can be printed on any office letterhead.

For more information on the Pediatric Advisor, contact Clinical Reference Systems, Ltd., 7100 E. Belleview Avenue, Suite 305, Greenwood Village, CO 80111-1636. Their telephone number is 800-237-8401.

17.4. TAILORING REGIMENS TO PARENTAL LIFESTYLES

Tailoring a regimen to the individual's routine also has been shown to improve compliance (Rapoff and Christophersen, 1982). For example, parents are more likely to remember to administer medication if it coincides with eating meals, leaving for work, or brushing their teeth. In these instances, a reminder note on the refrigerator, near the car keys, or by the toothpaste can serve as a cue for administering medication in a regular pattern.

17.5. APPOINTMENT-KEEPING STRATEGIES

There are several well-documented strategies for encouraging patients to keep their scheduled appointments. These strategies will be discussed here.

17.5.1. Appointment Reminders

Numerous studies have documented the pervasiveness of patients' failing to keep scheduled appointments with their health-care providers; much of the literature on appointment keeping is epidemiological.

Similar to the studies on compliance, appointment keeping appears to be worse:

1. For the very young and the very old.
2. With patients who are asymptomatic.
3. When the appointment is made by the physician's office instead of by the patient.
4. When the patient must make repeated office visits.

The two best-known and best-documented procedures for improving appointment keeping are written and telephone reminders.

In a study we conducted on appointment keeping (Friman et al., 1985), we demonstrated that patients were more likely to keep their appointments if they received both written and telephone reminders. Similarly, identifying and eliminating structural (for example, parking problems) and financial barriers wherever possible can reduce problems with compliance. This assistance varies from referring the patient to a reliable discount pharmacy to suggesting assistance by a social services agency.

17.5.2. Written Reminders

Written reminders are usually planned to arrive 1 or 2 days before the scheduled appointment. The reminder memo (in an envelope) should include the date, day of the week, and time of the appointment and should be signed by the provider. If the office is difficult to find, or if the physician has more than one office, specific directions should be included with the appointment schedule. Many physicians have printed forms that patients may complete for their next appointment prior to leaving the office, requiring only that office personnel place the form in an envelope and put it in the outgoing mail. The cost involved is minimal: the expense for printing and mailing the reminders. Handout 17.2 is an example of a written reminder used in the study by Friman et al. (1985).

17.5.3. Telephone Reminders

With telephone reminders, a phone call is placed to the patient, usually the day before the appointment, to remind him of the date, time, and location of the appointment (see Handout 17.3). If the patient reports she will be unable to keep the scheduled appointment, there usually is enough time to contact another patient to fill the vacancy.

17.5.4. Increased Convenience

A third strategy, and one less frequently reviewed in the literature, involves making it more convenient for the patient to attend an appointment. In some cases this may involve providing free parking or parking facilities close to the physician's office.

Immediately prior to one of our studies (Friman et al., 1985), patients were required to drive into the parking lot adjacent to a large teaching hospital, park their vehicle, go into the office to obtain a parking pass, return to their vehicle to place the parking pass on the windshield, then return for their appointment. In the study, the parking pass was included in the patient's mailed appointment reminder, alleviating patient inconvenience and possibly engendering a positive psychological attitude about keeping the scheduled visit.

In our study using the three strategies—phoned and mailed reminders, as well as more convenient parking—not only was there an increase in appointment keeping, but 18% more revenue was generated per scheduled appointment time than prior to the study (see Handout 17.4). This revenue gain was more than enough to cover the entire costs of the various appointment-keeping strategies.

17.5.5. Other Appointment-Keeping Strategies

Other strategies include, with varying degrees of success:

- Opening satellite offices that are geographically more convenient for the patient population (a very successful strategy in our experience).
- Providing transportation services for patients, a strategy with varying levels of success depending on the population served, the inconvenience for the patient/ parent, and the cost involved.
- Providing home visits, which are almost always subsidized by some public or private agency and are clearly not feasible on any large scale.

17.6. FEE COLLECTION

Although major teaching hospitals may depend on revenues generated by faculty for clinical services rendered, poor collection rates are a significant problem among these institutions. Very little research has been published on collecting fees for service and its impact on health-care providers. In my opinion, it is perfectly reasonable to expect to collect fees from all patients, except for those for whom you agree in advance to provide pro bono services.

17.6.1. Discussing Fees with Patients

Collection of fees is facilitated by having the person who schedules appointments discuss two items with the patient at the time of the initial appointment.

First, patients should be informed that they will be billed for services rendered and what that fee will be, including a review of any additional fees that may be charged, for example, an additional $20 for immunizations.

Second, patients will be requested to pay for services, at least the co-payment required by their insurance carrier, at the time the service is provided. Arrangements can be made for cash, check, and credit card payments. If provisions are not made for various modes of payment at the time of the visit, collecting at a later date becomes more difficult. When we mail written reminders to each scheduled patient, we include a brochure describing the services available from the office and a reminder that the patient is ultimately responsible for any costs incurred. Mention also is made that the office will assist in the filing of insurance papers but that the responsibility for payment rests with the patients. Handout 17.5 is an excerpt from our brochure, dealing with parents' financial responsibility.

At the time of the appointment, it is not sufficient to simply hand a statement to each parent or patient. The charge for the service should be accompanied by a verbal statement that patients are expected to provide payment for services rendered and should stop at the business office to take care of their bill.

17.6.2. Follow-Up Billing

The sooner patients are billed for the services they receive, the greater the collection rate. If a patient pays part of the fee at the time of the appointment, a bill for the remaining amount should be handed to her with a reminder mailed within 1 week. If patients request additional time in which to pay their bill, discuss how much they are prepared to pay every 2 weeks or each month. Establish routine billings for such patients to remind them of their commitment to make payments on the bill.

The older an unpaid bill is, the less likely the provider is to collect it. Prior to submitting an unpaid bill to a collection service, an office representative should phone the patient to ascertain if any payments will be forthcoming. If the patient indicates he is not in a position to make payments, or if he says a check is "in the mail," he should be informed that any further problems with collections will be handled by a professional collection agency.

17.6.3. Professional Collection Services

The patient should be provided with the name of the agency used by the office. If this financial discussion is handled in a professional and nonthreatening manner, patients are less likely to be annoyed by the collection process. Whether a professional office uses an employee, an attorney, or a collection agency, it is usually cost-effective to send "uncollectible" accounts for collection. It is less effective to give patients time to settle the balance on their account. Receiving only one-half of the amount due through a collection service is better than no reimbursement at all. When patients are impressed that the physician is serious about collections, they are much more likely to pay their bills.

17.7. CONCLUDING REMARKS

In my experience, it is much easier to organize my office in such a way that I maximize patient compliance, rather than deal with the frustration of patients skipping appointments, not following treatment recommendations, and not paying for the services after they have been rendered.

In our study on appointment keeping, conducted in a tertiary-care hospital outpatient pediatrics clinic, we demonstrated the efficacy of reminders for improving the rate of patients who keep their scheduled appointments and also showed that we were able to generate more revenue per unit of time than before we introduced the appointment-keeping strategies.

Similarly, we have demonstrated, by consistently having one of the highest fee collection rates at the hospital, that a proactive approach to fee collection produces acceptable payment levels from patients. Our annual collection rate at our satellite clinic (where we send out written reminders, call patients to confirm appointments the day before, and provide free, nearby parking) is consistently over 95%, which is at least comparable to my colleagues in private practice in the same geographical area.

I have often heard practitioners state they simply cannot offer Behavioral Pediatrics services economically—that Behavioral Pediatrics is a money-losing proposition. Without anticipating problems with patient fee collection, almost any practice would be a money-losing proposition. However, our research suggests that taking a proactive approach to fees can make a substantial difference in fee collections.

REFERENCES

Friman PC, Finney JW, Rapoff MA, Christophersen ER: Improving pediatric appointment keeping with reminders and reduced response requirements. *J Appl Behav Anal* 18(4):315–321, 1985.
Mathews JR, Christophersen ER: Enhancing pediatric compliance in primary care. *Development Behav Disord* 2:193–212, 1989.
Rapoff MA, Christophersen ER: Improving compliance in pediatric practice. *Pediatr Clin N Am* 29:339–357, 1982.

Sample Handouts

HANDOUT 17.1

Treatment Reminders

REMINDERS

I NEED TO KEEP MY MOUTH SHUT
WHEN I DISCIPLINE!

I NEED TO TOUCH MY CHILD MORE!

I NEED TO USE TIME OUT EVERY TIME
MY CHILD MISBEHAVES!

HANDOUT 17.2

Written Appointment Reminder

Dear Parents:

I'm sending you this note to remind you that _____'s appointment with me is scheduled for _____ am/pm on _____ the_____ of _____ . If this time is not convenient for you, please call our office at _____ to cancel and/or reschedule the appointment so that the time will not go unused. I'm also enclosing a Parking Pass that allows you to park in the lot immediately adjacent to the office.

Thank you,

_____
Printed Name

HANDOUT 17.3

Phone Reminder

"This is Dr. _____ 's office calling. May I speak to _____? Hello.
I'm calling to remind you of _____'s appointment with _____ on
_____ the _____ of _____ ."

HANDOUT 17.4

Appointment-Keeping Revenue

Participant	Baseline ($)	Reminders ($)	% Change
PNP1	13.33	18.90	+30
MD2	35.87	39.61	+9
PNP2	15.55	20.04	+23
PNP3	14.19	15.05	+6
MD2	14.42	16.05	+18
$\overline{X}$	17.98	22.08	+18

Note: Changes in Amount Billed per Appointment: $ Billed/No. of Appointments = $ per Appointment.

Excerpt from Office Brochure

FINANCIAL RESPONSIBILITIES

All patients are billed on the basis of the amount of time spent and the services performed. For patients who have insurance, we ask that payment be made by you directly to _____ . The business office will assist you in filing any insurance forms. When you have determined that you are eligible for reimbursement from your insurance company, you should obtain a claims form from them; complete the patient portion of the form, including your signature; and mail the form directly to this office. Receipts for services rendered will be provided. These receipts can be used in submitting your claim. We will cooperate in helping you obtain your benefits from your insurance carrier; however, the responsibility for payment is yours.

If you have any questions about our fees or services, please do not hesitate to contact our office manager.

Chapter **18**

Referrals: When to Treat and When to Refer

Primary-care physicians cannot realistically treat every behavior problem they see and cannot refer every child with common behavior problems to a mental-health professional—the number of referrals would immediately overwhelm the existing mental-health network (Christophersen, 1982).

18.1. COMMON BEHAVIOR PROBLEMS

Several situations suggest referral even though the pediatrician is dealing with common behavior problems:

1. Marital problems
2. Substance abuse
3. Child abuse or neglect
4. Several siblings with behavior problems
5. Depression in either parent

It's been surprising to me, over the years, how many parents will be very straightforward about their family situation. A mother recently told me she had smoked drugs and snorted cocaine during her pregnancy, and she was worried whether this

411

could have had an adverse effect on her child. Having gained this information from my interview, I decided to refer her to a physician who has much more experience dealing with children whose mothers were drug users during pregnancy.

As discussed in Chapter 4, "Recognition and Assessment of Compliance Problems," using detailed intake forms allows you to get a good deal of information about the child and her family in a brief amount of time. There have been many occasions when parents, in completing this form, have indicated they were currently in therapy or on medication for such conditions as depression or bipolar illness. Having this information allows you to decide whether to treat the children in conjunction with the treatment that the mother is getting or to refer the mother to another provider. Either way, having the additional information allows you an option that you would not have had if you didn't have the complete history.

However great the temptation might be to attempt to assist these parents with their child management strategies, the professional who deals regularly with common behavior problems is usually not trained in dealing with significant pathology and may be doing the family a disservice when he or she meets with the parents to discuss child management strategies. Fortunately, there are now physicians who specialize in the treatment of children whose mothers were drug users during pregnancy. Referral to such a practitioner, when possible, is a very reasonable option.

18.2. SIGNIFICANT DISTURBANCE

Pediatricians can exercise the obvious option of referring any child in whom a psychopathological abnormality is either obvious or highly suspected. We occasionally receive calls from families with a child who has been suspended from school because of serious problems at school (for example, pulling a knife on a teacher, or being absent 70 days the first term). We usually screen these families by phone and refer them directly to an appropriate provider without scheduling them for an appointment in our office. In this way, the family is saved the cost of an office visit to see one of us, only to be referred to a mental-health provider who deals with seriously disturbed children.

One article suggested guidelines for determining when referral is indicated (Phillips, Sarles, and Friedman, 1980). The types of behavior the authors identified as clearly needing referral were psychosis (such as infantile autism) and schizophrenia. They stated, "Unfortunately, the majority of problems cannot be identified by the occurrence of a single behavior. . . . Generally, the difference between 'normal' and 'problematic' behavior is not the actual behavior, or behaviors, but, rather, quantity (number of occurrences), distribution (different manifestations), severity (interfering with social or cognitive functioning), and duration (at least four weeks)."

18.3. WHEN ASSESSMENT SUGGESTS REFERRAL

Of the assessment tools discussed in Chapter 4 on assessment, the two Achenbach Child Behavior Checklists (CBCL), one for the parent and one for the teacher, are best suited to identifying children who should be referred for more intensive management.

There are, of course, many other assessment devices available. Of the assessment devices that primary-care physicians can reasonably be expected to administer routinely, the CBCL is, in my opinion, best suited to identifying significant problems.

One of the most difficult behavioral disturbances to deal with in children is "conduct disorder." The CBCL has been constructed in such a way that scores above the 90th percentile on aggressive behavior and delinquent behavior are highly suggestive of a conduct-disordered child (Achenbach and Edelbrock, 1983). Bird, Gould, Rubio-Stipec, Staghezza, and Canino (1991) reported that the combination of the parent CBCL and the teacher CBCL identified 85% of children who were later found to present with conduct or oppositional disorder.

Because conduct-disordered children have, at best, a guarded prognosis (Cantwell, 1989), it is imperative that an accurate diagnosis be made in a timely fashion so that referral to an appropriate practitioner can occur.

18.4. IDENTIFYING APPROPRIATE PRACTITIONERS

I often receive phone calls from pediatricians inquiring whether we see particular kinds of patients in our office. This is usually a tactful way for pediatricians to ascertain whether they should refer patients to us.

Recently, a pediatrician asked me if I saw children who presented with elective mutism (children who refuse to speak in all but a few, usually very familiar, situations). I indicated that I did not but that one of my partners had successfully treated numerous children with elective mutism. I not only routinely refer particular problems to other practitioners whom I know have expertise dealing with them, but I believe we all benefit from doing so. When working up a new child, the first decision that must be made is what course of treatment, if any, the child needs. The second decision is who the best person is to provide that treatment.

Phone inquiry is the easiest way to handle the potentially delicate issue of finding out whether a practitioner has adequate training to deal with a specific type of problem. I think it's appropriate to go so far as to ask specialists to whom you might be referring a patient if they have dealt with the problem before and what kind of clinical outcomes they had. Handled correctly, few practitioners mind such an inquiry. In fact, most of the practitioners to whom we regularly refer patients prefer that we call them prior to referring an unusual case.

In some areas, such as diagnosis and treatment of sexual abuse, our referral patterns are almost constantly changing as new practitioners begin seeing these types of cases and established practitioners decide they will no longer treat this population. Much as the primary health-care provider keeps a mental catalog of individual professionals and the procedures in which they have expertise, a category needs to be included for various behavioral problems and expert practitioners.

18.5. WHAT THE PRIMARY CARE PROVIDER SHOULD TREAT

In my opinion, primary health-care providers should develop the skills for treating minor-to-moderate behavior problems as an adjunct to well-child care, and they should refer children with more severe behavioral disorders elsewhere for assessment and treatment. In this way, primary care providers can deal with "normal" children who have minor problems, and the mental-health system can deal with children who have significant psychopathology.

18.6. THE REFERRAL PROCEDURE

To increase the likelihood that a given patient will follow up on the recommendation to see a certain specialist, several strategies should be considered.

Probably the most effective strategy is to discuss with the parents your intention to refer them to a subspecialist, mention one by name, and offer to call the specialist while the patient is in your office. If the patient agrees, try to get the patient to talk with that provider's office, if only long enough to schedule an appointment. Most physicians follow up the phone call with a brief letter of referral to the new provider.

18.7. THE REFERRED PROVIDER'S RESPONSIBILITY

While most subspecialists in medicine routinely send letters to their referring physicians, it has been my experience that many mental-health professionals do not. We have approached this situation by specifically requesting that the providers to whom we are referring send a note back to us as soon as they have some idea of how the treatment is progressing. If you haven't received a letter back within a reasonable time, a brief phone call often will be the only reminder necessary to get the provider to send you letters in the future.

18.8. CONCLUDING REMARKS

Primary health-care providers frequently refer patients to other professionals for treatment of a specific problem. In so doing, providers have the responsibility to:

- Assess each child thoroughly, to form a judgment regarding what services that child needs.
- Decide which practitioner would benefit the child the most.
- Assist the parents in establishing contact with the subspecialist to whom the provider is referring the parents and their child.
- Make sure they receive feedback from the practitioner to whom they referred the parents and child.

The inclusion of Behavioral Pediatrics in a primary-care practice necessitates that the provider be skilled in assessment, intervention, and referral. Referral patterns, probably as much as any other activity the primary provider engages in, can ensure that children get the services they deserve.

Appropriate referral practices also do a lot to reduce the stress experienced by the primary-care provider. It is far better to refer a child to a practitioner who has experience dealing with the child's presenting problems than to try to treat it yourself and, if you are not appropriately trained, to fail.

REFERENCES

Achenbach TM, Edelbrock C: *Manual for the Child Behavior Checklist and Revised Child Behavior Profile*. Burlington, VT: University of Vermont Department of Psychiatry, 1983.

Bird HR, Gould MS, Rubio-Stipec MA, Staghezza BM, Canino G: Screen for childhood psychopathology in the community using the Child Behavior Checklist. *J Am Acad Child Adolesc Psychiatr* 30:116–123, 1991.

Cantwell DP: Conduct disorder, in Kaplan HI, Sadock BJ (Eds.), *Comprehensive Textbook of Psychiatry* (5th ed.). Baltimore, MD: Williams & Wilkins, 1989, pp. 1821–1828.

Christophersen ER: Incorporating behavioral pediatrics into primary care. *Pediatr Clin N Am* 29(2):261–296, 1982.

Phillips S, Sarles RM, Friedman SB: Consultation and referral: When, why, and how. *Pediatr Ann* 9:36–45, 1980.

POSTSCRIPT

Chapter **19**

Concluding Remarks

This book represents over 20 years of practice in Behavioral Pediatrics, a practice with predominantly middle- to upper-middle-class, mainly two-parent families (although in terms of treating minor-to-moderate behavior problems, we haven't seen that being a single parent is either an asset or a detriment), who are motivated to make a change in their lives and in the lives of their children. The vast majority of the families we see are primary referrals—that is, their primary-care provider has referred them to us as the first recourse for these children. A small percentage, probably less than 10%, have sought help elsewhere prior to scheduling an appointment in our office.

We have a referral base of over 85 pediatricians and family physicians. Over the same 20 years, we have been referred perhaps as few as 10 children from child psychiatrists. When we have discussed these referral patterns with both pediatric health-care providers and child psychiatrists, the feedback has been that we are referred the "simple problems," while the child psychiatrists retain the more complicated cases—as it should be.

In my experience, subspecialty rotations in child psychiatry typically expose medical residents to families far more dysfunctional than those routinely seen by primary-care physicians. I often have had residents say, "I don't see families like this on my other rotations." When I've discussed this with the residents, they usually state that middle- and upper-middle-class families get their care from private-practice pediatricians, not from the teaching hospital. Similarly, many practicing pediatricians have told me they received most of their experience with normal young children after they started their practice.

This does not mean that tertiary-care centers cannot be used as a training ground for Behavioral Pediatrics. The critical issue is whether significant numbers of families are seen who have children with common behavior problems.

Approximately 7% of the total population of 3-year-olds has a behavior problem that can be characterized as ranging from moderate to severe. The most common problems reported included night wetting, poor appetite, soiling, day wetting, and difficulty settling at night (Richman, Stevenson, and Graham, 1975), problems that are typical of the types of compliance problems seen in children. These kinds of problems are seen every day by practicing primary-care physicians; these problems are what Behavioral Pediatrics is all about.

19.1. THE BEHAVIORAL PEDIATRICS CLINIC AT CHILDREN'S MERCY HOSPITAL

In our office at Children's Mercy Hospital in Kansas City, Missouri, we provide a busy service for behavior problems commonly seen in children. We currently have about 2,000 outpatient visits per year. Of these, around 800 are for children who are oppositional—children who have temper tantrums, who don't want to go to bed at night, who don't want to get dressed in the morning, and who don't want to follow simple treatment regimens such as swallowing pills or wearing glasses.

Another 400 appointments are scheduled for children who present with attention problems. The rest of the problems are related to normal toileting habits; adjustment reactions, usually secondary to their parents' separation or divorce; habit disorders; fears and anxiety; and problems secondary to a physical illness or injury.

This base of 2,000 appointments for common behavior problems provides a more-than-adequate teaching population for trainees from pediatrics, family practice, child psychology, and child psychiatry.

In a multisite investigation that examined eight different treatment and training sites, our clinic saw the most families (most of average economic means) and had the fewest number of clinic visits (average of three visits or less), the most minor presenting problems, and the best outcomes (Blechman, Budd, Christophersen, Szykula, Wahler, Embry, Kogan, O'Leary, and Riner, 1981). That is, we intervened early, when problems were minor, with families that wanted help and that followed our recommendations— "competent families," as Dr. Blechman refers to them (Blechman, 1984).

19.2. EVALUATE, THEN REFER?

We treat the vast majority of children seen in our clinic after an initial evaluation. We refer less than 10% to outside sources for treatment. Most of the families that we do refer are referred to child psychiatrists and child psychologists for more extensive therapy because they presented with more serious or more complicated problems than we feel can be treated in a facility that deals with common behavior problems.

The essence of all pediatric care is to intervene early—if you cannot prevent the problem in the first place—with families that you know well because you have been providing their well-child care. Ultimately, the pediatric health-care provider (including the family physician and nurses in both pediatric and family practice offices) is the professional in the best position to deal with common behavior problems.

19.3. PEDIATRIC PSYCHOLOGISTS

Over the past 20 years, more psychologists have begun to treat young children, either directly through the pediatrician's office or on referral from the pediatrician. Generally, because the services offered by pediatric psychologists complement those offered by pediatric health-care providers, the two fields have been synergistic.

19.4. PEDIATRIC PSYCHIATRISTS

The pediatric or child psychiatrist plays a very important role in the treatment of behavior-disordered children. The vast majority of children who present with problems that are thought to have a major organic component (major depression, bipolar disorders, obsessive-compulsive disorders, childhood psychoses) or with severe behavior problems (conduct disorders, childhood autism) are able to receive care from pediatric psychiatrists that is simply beyond the scope of the pediatric health-care provider and of many pediatric psychologists. Over the years, we have had many child psychiatry fellows rotate through our facility during their training. Almost inevitably, they comment that they "never saw children like this." They were saying that, in their tertiary-care centers, child psychiatrists simply were not being referred children with minor behavior problems.

There is also no mention in this book of serious problems that may or may not have a significant organic component, including anorexia nervosa and bulimia, sexual abuse and exploitation of children, alcoholism, or character-disordered adults. These types of problems are, and probably will remain, beyond the scope of the pediatric health-care provider and the pediatric psychologist who deals with common behavior problems.

19.5. ARE WE IGNORING UNDERLYING PATHOLOGY?

Over the years, we periodically have been accused of ignoring or overlooking underlying pathology—that we just treat every child as though he has a simple behavior problem, with no concern for the fact that he comes from a dysfunctional family, a family torn apart by alcoholism, physical abuse, or a wide variety of serious adult psychopathologies.

Our response has been, and will continue to be, that the sophistication of available assessment devices is still crude when it comes to identifying psychopathology in parents.

We have often been able, with our "simple treatment protocols," to determine empirically whether the family needs to be referred for more extensive evaluation and treatment by professionals who deal with more serious problems. This is, in fact, the model that pediatrics and family practice has used for many years. If children present with obvious serious pathology, whether in the form of behavior or medical problems, they are immediately referred to an appropriate practitioner. If a child presents with common, everyday problems, the primary health-care provider typically deals with these problems with no consideration about a referral. It is the child in the middle, the child who may have common behavior problems but who also may have more serious family pathology or more serious organic pathology, who presents the greatest challenge, clinically, to the primary health-care provider.

As Dr. Barbara Korsch (Korsch and Aley, 1973) so eloquently demonstrated in her research on pediatric resident interviewing skills, the skilled interviewer can and often does elicit critical information during a routine office interview. There simply is no substitute for good interviewing skills.

Truly, it is up to individual practitioners to decide, in their best clinical judgment, which children need to be treated and by whom. The art of medicine will probably never be replaced by any technological advance.

19.6. THE ONE TRUE WAY

Is there one true way to evaluate and intervene with any population? Of course not! There are a wide variety of treatment approaches to childhood behavior problems; some of these approaches have not even been mentioned in this book.

This book is not intended to be a scholarly treatise on all of the available approaches to childhood behavior problems. Many good books of this type already are available. Rather, this book presents a comprehensive description of the technology that has been developed for dealing with common behavior problems, including the initial assessment, the forms and tests used in this initial assessment, and the procedures, forms, and materials used in the day-to-day management of common behavior problems.

This is not the one true way. It is one way that has been in use for a number of years, by a number of practitioners, in a number of settings. It has stood that test of time and the rigor of multisite investigation. Still, it is but a piece of technology. In the hands of a skilled practitioner, along with a number of other clinical tools, it can help facilitate the provision of services, by the pediatric health-care provider, to families with children who present with common behavior problems.

19.7. HOW SHOULD THIS BOOK BE USED?

Many primary care physicians, nurses, psychologists, and social workers are called on to evaluate common behavior problems in a primary care situation, or in a practice that receives the majority of its referrals from primary care providers. This book is organized for them.

19.7.1. Assessment Tools

The assessment tools have been selected because they are relatively easy to administer and to score. Office personnel can be trained to administer these tools in a very brief time. Scoring can typically be done within 2 or 3 minutes.

Tested as extensively as they have been, and standardized on normal and deviant populations, they provide the right balance between false negatives (a test score suggesting, incorrectly, that nothing is amiss with a child) and false positives (a test score suggesting, incorrectly, that the child has problems in need of treatment).

Some of these tools can be used directly from this book with no further permission necessary. Some, like the Achenbach Child Behavior Checklist and the Conner's Parent Symptom Questionnaire, should be purchased from the appropriate supplier. The "quick scoring" forms and the computerized scoring forms are available only from the supplier.

Some forms, such as the Eyberg Child Behavior Inventory, are appropriate for administration to almost every child scheduled for, as an example, a 2-year well-child visit. Other forms, such as the Achenbach checklist and the Conner's questionnaire, should be used on an "as needed" basis.

19.7.2. Intake Forms

The intake forms included at the back of some of the chapters are to be used whenever a parent brings up one of these types of problems. The reader is free to reproduce the intake forms, by whatever means available, for use on a day-to-day basis. The forms also may be changed to reflect the individual practitioner's need for more, less, or different history about the child from the family.

The intake forms also can serve as examples for providers who wish to make up a completely different form, based only loosely on the style of the intake forms included in this book.

19.7.3. Written Protocols

The written protocols are meant to supplement a considerable discussion of the problem with parents; they are *not* meant to take the place of a considerable discussion of the problem. Typically, providers discuss their treatment recommendations with the parents and provide the written protocol at the end of the discussion, so that parents "don't have to memorize everything I said today."

Whenever a practitioner makes treatment recommendations, with or without supporting written protocols, follow-up is an important part of the process. Therefore, some form of follow-up, either return office appointments, written symptom ratings scales that are mailed back to the practitioner, or phoned-in summaries of the treatment progress, is virtually mandatory.

19.8. FIELD TESTING

These protocols have been field tested in four different ways.

First, they have been used extensively in our offices at the University of Kansas Medical Center by three of our prior trainees, Drs. Michael Rapoff, Martha Barnard, and Vinnie Barone; in our office at Children's Mercy Hospital (Drs. Linda Ross and Patty Purvis); and by a number of our trainees/colleagues who have been using these and similar written protocols at other sites around the country, including James Barnard and Susan Rainey Barnard (West Palm Beach, Florida), Jack Finney (Virginia Polytechnical Institute), Pat Friman (Father Flanagan's Boys Town), Steve Glasscock (Hopkinsville, Kentucky), Hunter Leake (Ft. Myers, Florida), Nick Long (Arkansas Children's Hospital), Judith Mathews (West Virginia University Medical Center), Jan Myers (Kansas City, Missouri), Shirley O'Brien (Devereux Hospital, Melbourne, Florida), Deborah Sosland-Edelman (Kansas City, Missouri), and George Williams (Lincoln, Nebraska). These individuals have contributed substantially to the development of the technology described in this book. They have written some of the protocols, written some of their own, and trained other professionals in the use of the protocols.

Second, the protocols have been distributed in workshops offered by the present author and some of his colleagues; at meetings of the American Academy of Pediatrics, the American Psychological Association, the Ambulatory Pediatrics Association, the Society for Pediatric Research, the Society for Behavioral Medicine, the Society for Behavioral Pediatrics, and the Association for the Advancement of Behavior Therapy; and at state and local meetings far too many to list here.

Third, over 50 professionals have completed a 1-week Mini-Fellowship in Behavioral Pediatrics, earlier at the University of Kansas Medical Center and more recently at Children's Mercy Hospital, Kansas City, Missouri. The majority have been practicing pediatricians, and some are psychologists. All of the Fellows have been trained in the use of the assessment and treatment procedures for use in their offices.

Fourth, many of the procedures described and recommended in this book have already been published in articles that have appeared in a variety of peer-reviewed journals. Some of this research has been done by past and present members of our office, and some, such as the research on toileting problems and habit disorders, was originally conducted by other individuals who published their work in peer-reviewed journals, where we originally read about it. Appropriate references to these articles appear at the back of each chapter.

Many of these protocols also have been reproduced in prior writings, including two of my books (*Little People* and *Beyond Discipline*); in the chapters that I wrote for the three issues of *Pediatric Clinics of North America* that I edited or coedited; in two monographs that I coauthored (Christophersen and Long, 1987, and Varni and Christophersen, 1990); and in numerous articles.

19.9. ATTRIBUTIONS

The reader is free to reproduce the treatment protocols, by whatever means, for use on a day-to-day basis. The protocols also may be changed to reflect the individual practitioner's need for more, less, or different information for the family. When the protocols are used in their present form, the reader should include an attribution statement, on the front sheet of the form, citing the original authors.

If the reader chooses to change the protocol, but maintains essentially the same material in it, an attribution should be included on the front sheet of the form, stating that the protocol is an adaptation of the original protocol. If the reader chooses to use a completely different written protocol, no attribution statement is necessary.

19.10. FINAL COMMENTS

The time and effort that I have put into Behavioral Pediatrics has been very rewarding. I have received a great deal of joy from the children and parents with whom I have had the pleasure of being associated. And, I've had many wonderful interactions with pediatricians, pediatric nurses, family physicians, and psychologists. I feel as though I have had the *privilege* of practicing Behavioral Pediatrics—the privilege of providing services to parents and children, who report that they benefited from our services and that they appreciated the time and effort I put into helping them with their concerns and questions.

I find great solace in the fact that I have been able to help many families function in a more nurturing fashion. I have been responsible, directly and indirectly, for helping them and I know that I have been able to make their homes a more pleasant place for both parent and child to live and to love.

REFERENCES

Blechman EA: Competent parents, competent children: Behavioral objectives of parent training, in Dangel RF, Polster RA (Eds.), *Parent Training: Foundations of Research and Practice.* New York: Guilford Press, 1984.

Blechman EA, Budd KS, Christophersen ER, Szykula S, Wahler R, Embry LH, Kogan K, O'Leary KD, Riner L: Engagement in behavioral family therapy: A multisite investigation. *Behav Ther* 12:461–472, 1981.

Christophersen ER: Incorporating behavioral pediatrics into primary care. *Pediatr Clin N Am* 29(2):261–296, 1982.

Christophersen ER: Anticipatory guidance on discipline. *Pediatr Clin N Am* 33(4):789–798, 1986.

Christophersen ER: Discipline. *Pediatr Clin N Am* 39:395–411, 1992.

Christophersen ER, Long N: *Pediatric Behavioral Problems* (Monograph 103). Kansas City, MO: American Academy of Family Physicians, 1987.

Korsch BM, Aley EF: Pediatric interviewing techniques, in *Current Problems in Pediatrics.* Chicago: Year Book, 1973.

Richman N, Stevenson JE, Graham PJ: Prevalence of behaviour problems in 3-year-old children: An epidemiological study in a London borough. *Child Psychol Psychiat* 16:277–287, 1975.

Varni J, Christophersen ER: Pediatric behavior problems. *Current Prob Pediatr* 20(11):639–704, 1990.

The Home Chip System Manual for Children Aged 3 to 7

INTRODUCTION

The Home Chip System was developed for children with behavior problems. These procedures have been used with preschool-age children, in families with one to six children, with parents' education ranging from less than high school to postgraduate studies, and with income levels ranging from poverty to upper-income professional. The range of problem behaviors has extended from minor, everyday difficulties, like getting children to bed at night and getting them to keep their rooms neat, to moderate problems like hitting, temper tantrums, hyperactivity, and back talk. Our experience is not sufficient to make any recommendations regarding the use of this program with such severe behavior problems as drug addiction. In the beginning, this program requires dedicated and highly motivated parents willing to put forth the effort necessary to teach their children more appropriate ways of behaving. The program also requires that children be supervised by someone most of the day. We train parents to be teachers. They cannot teach their children if they are not with them. Whether administered by the parents, a nanny, or an alternative caregiver, the program requires that the child(ren) be supervised. We have experience with families from a variety of ethnic and racial backgrounds, including African-American, Hispanic, and Asian-American. The Home Chip System is designed to provide a maximum amount of instruction and feedback to your child through you, the parent. Instruction, feedback, and consequences are the tools you will use to train your child in new desirable behaviors or to eliminate already present undesirable behaviors. The system's effectiveness in changing behaviors will depend on your thoroughness. It will not operate by itself. Its success will depend on the degree to which you actively observe and reward or punish the behaviors you see your child demonstrate.

HOW THE HOME CHIP SYSTEM WORKS

The Home Chip System is based on two simple, yet thoroughly effective, principles:

- Behavior that is immediately followed by a good, rewarding consequence will continue to occur.
- Behavior that is followed by a nonrecurring or punishing consequence will cease to occur or will occur less often.

POKER CHIPS

Like money, chips themselves have no value. Chips must be given meaning or value in order to become effective. It is only through their power to purchase necessary and enjoyable goods or activities that they gain meaning and become useful. They must always be available for you to give and take. However, poker chips serve as rewarding or punishing events only when they immediately follow your child's behavior.

MAKING CHIPS POWERFUL

For chips to be used as an effective consequence for behavior, earning chips (like earning money) must be rewarding for your child; your child must feel like she has indeed gained something. Losing chips (like losing money) must be unpleasant or punishing for your child; your child must feel like he has lost something. Chips will become meaningful for your child as she uses them to buy the "privileges" of having or doing what she desires. Privileges are items or activities usually available in your home or community that your child enjoys and can purchase with his chips.

EARNING PRIVILEGES

Privileges can be anything your child likes to do. Snacks, playing with friends, playing with toys or games, and shopping with Mom all might be considered privileges by some children. The privilege to have snacks, for instance, permits your child to have snacks when they are available and she has paid for them (given you some poker chips). Snacks might be available in the afternoon or before bed. You should decide what constitutes a snack (for example, one scoop of ice cream, two cookies, or one bottle of pop) and the times they are available. For chips to be of value, your child must be required to spend them for his or her privileges. Privileges must be available as often as possible when your child has the chips. Unless the chips are worth something, they will not be effective in changing your child's behavior.

CHIP SYSTEM EXAMPLES

Table A1 shows what a chip system looks like. Both social and maintenance behaviors for your chip system will be taken from a list you fill out. These behaviors, if completed, result in a chip gain; if not completed, they result in a chip loss. For example, if your child brushed his teeth, two chips would be gained. If he failed to brush his teeth, two chips would be lost. It is more important to give chips than it is take chips away. Such behaviors as "being good," "helping," or "playing quietly" only earn chips. These are behaviors you must be aware of and reward consistently, since they are the types of behaviors you would like to see more of every day.

Behaviors that lose chips (see Table A2) are those you would like your child to stop doing. For this system to be effective, you must take the chips away immediately every time one of these behaviors occurs.

The privileges listed on your Home Chip System will be those that your child can "purchase" if he has the requisite number of chips (see Table A3). However, the list may change. You will need to be aware of what your child is doing for fun and add those activities to the list as necessary (see Table A4). Most of the activities children naturally do in their spare time are things they enjoy. Thus, they can be viewed as privileges and added to the list of privileges.

Your child is capable of doing many small jobs around the house. It is important that your child share the responsibilities of the house. This is also an excellent time for you to interact with and to teach your child. A list of jobs, made by you, will help to have jobs available when your child needs chips or wants to help. You can make such a list and attach it to the front of your refrigerator with a piece of tape or a couple of small magnets.

HOW TO GIVE AND TAKE AWAY CHIPS

Both giving and taking away chips should be as pleasant as possible. Here are several things you and your child need to do whenever there is a chip exchange.

TABLE A1.   Behaviors That Gain or Lose Chips

	Number of chips	
	Gained	Lost
Making bed	+2	−2
Picking up bedroom	+2	−2
Brushing teeth	+2	−2
Picking up toys	+2	−2
Picking up clothes	+5	−2
Dressing yourself	+2	−2
Saying "please" and "thank you"	+2	−2

TABLE A2.   Behaviors That Lose Chips

	Number of chips lost
Throwing things	−2
Jumping on furniture	−2
Talking back	−2
Having tantrums	−3
Coming downstairs after bedtime	−2
Interrupting	−4
Running in the house	−2

Rules for Parents

When giving chips remember to:

1. Be near your child and able to touch him (not 20 feet or two rooms away).
2. Look at your child and smile.
3. Use a pleasant voice.
4. Make sure your child is facing you and looking at you.
5. Praise your child by saying something like, "Hey, that's great. You're really doing a nice job. That's really helping me."
6. Reward your child with chips and say, "Here are two chips for being so good."
7. Describe the appropriate behavior for your child so that she knows exactly what behavior she is being praised and rewarded for.
8. Hug your child occasionally—kids love it!
9. Have your child acknowledge you by saying something like, "Thanks, Mom" or "OK."

When taking away chips remember the following:

1. Be near your child and able to touch her.
2. Look at your child and smile.
3. Use a pleasant voice. Your child should not be able to tell by the tone of your voice or your facial expression whether you're going to give or take away chips.
4. Make sure your child is facing you and looking at you.

TABLE A3.   Privileges and Their Value

Privilege	Chip value
Watching television	5 per ½ hour
Playing outside	5
Eating snacks	5 per snack
Going to a friend's	10
Riding bike	5

TABLE A4.   Extra Jobs That Earn Privileges

Setting the table
Sweeping the porch
Picking up trash in the yard
Dusting
Emptying ash trays
Wiping off the table
Folding wash cloths

5. In a calm manner, explain what was inappropriate (see the section on instruction).
6. Be sympathetic: "I know it's hard to lose chips, but that's the rule."
7. Tell the child how much the chip fine costs.
8. Make sure your child gets the chips appropriately (see the next section).
9. Prompting the appropriate responses will sometimes be necessary by saying, for example, "Come on, give me a smile. That's right."
10. If a chip loss is taken well by your child, give him back one-half of the chip fine. "You took off the chips so well, I'm going to give you back half of the chip fine!"
11. If your child is too mad or upset to give you the chips, don't forget the issue. Place your child in time-out (to cool off), and get the chips out of your child's chip container while he is in time-out.

Rules for Children

When getting chips, children should:

1. Be facing their parents, looking at them, and smiling.
2. Acknowledge receiving the chips by saying, "OK," "Thanks," or something else in a pleasant voice.
3. Put the chips in the specified container. (Any chips left lying around are returned to the bank.)

When losing chips, children should:

1. Face their parents, look at them, and smile (not frown).
2. Acknowledge the chip loss with, "OK," "All right," "I'll get the chips," or something else in a pleasant voice. (Children must keep looking at parents and be pleasant.)
3. Give the chips to their parents pleasantly.

PRACTICE GIVING AND TAKING AWAY CHIPS

Once on the Home Chip System, families frequently encounter instances where a child has done something to earn chips but hasn't done it very well. This is an excellent time to teach your child how to do it correctly by having her practice doing it correctly. Practicing can be done with both social and maintenance (jobs) behaviors.

Practicing with Social Behaviors

If your child becomes unpleasant and talks back when he loses points, the following rules will be useful in teaching your child the appropriate response.

Practicing with Back-Talk Example	*Parent Rule*
1. "You came quickly when I called, and I really appreciate that."	Praise a related behavior.
2. "But the rule is that you don't talk back after a chip loss. I'll have to take off two more chips for back talk."	Describe fully the inappropriate or inadequate behavior.
3. "Remember—you're supposed to look at me, be pleasant, and say 'OK, Dad' in a nice tone of voice."	Describe the appropriate behavior.
4. "This way we'll get along better at home, and it will help you take criticism better at school."	Give a reason for the appropriate behavior.
5. "Do you understand what you're supposed to do?"	Request acknowledgment.
6. "Say it pleasantly and give me a big smile— like this" (parent says "OK" and smiles).	Model: Show child how to do it.
7. "Now you try it."	Practice.
8. "That's right; you're looking at me with a pleasant facial expression."	Praise or feedback.
9. "Great—that's how it's done. You practiced very well. You can have a chip back."	Praise and reward.

Practicing with Maintenance Behaviors

When teaching your child how to do a new job correctly or when giving her feedback on a job poorly done, practice is essential. For example, if your child is doing the dishes but, when you check, he is not doing them correctly, the following rules will help you teach your child the correct way.

Practicing with Dishwashing

Dishwashing Example	*Parent Rule*
1. "You're really working steadily, and the table looks really clean. Thanks."	Praise related behavior.

2. "But it looks like you haven't gotten all the food off the plates."	Describe fully the inappropriate or inadequate behavior.
3. "It's important that all the dishes are clean with no food left on the plates."	Describe the appropriate behavior.
4. "Because germs can grow on the dishes, and besides, the next time you use the plate you will want it to be clean."	Give a reason for the appropriate behavior.
5. "Do you understand?"	Request acknowledgment.
6. "When food is stuck, a good way to get it off is to use the scraper instead of the cloth—like this."	Model: Show child how to do it.
7. "Now you try it."	Practice.
8. "Great, you're doing a much better job getting them clean now."	Praise or feedback.
9. "When you get done, come get me and you will get your chips, plus two for practicing so nicely. You're really doing a good job now."	Praise and reward.

When to Practice

The best time to practice is during a pleasant time of the day, preferably when your child hasn't done anything wrong. A great time to do this is when he needs more chips in order to purchase an item or activity that he wants. This teaches your child under pleasant circumstances how to respond to important situations. However, prompting and practicing the correct responses are still important after a rule violation or a poorly done job has occurred. When there has not been a rule violation, you can practice using make-believe violations and make-believe time-out. For example, if your child says that he needs a job to earn some chips, you can tell him that you will give him five chips if he will do a good pretend time-out. If he says, "OK," then direct him to go to time-out. When he has completed his pretend time-out, give him the five chips and tell him what a good job he did. This is a good way for your child to earn chips at the same time that he practices important social behaviors. Another example would be to have your child practice taking off chips. For example:

MOTHER: Jim, let's practice how you're supposed to take a chip loss and you can earn two chips.

JIMMY: OK.

MOTHER: Jim, please take two chips off for throwing the ball in the house. Remember, the rule is that balls must be thrown outside.

JIMMY: Sure, Mom (*with pleasant facial expression and tone of voice*).

MOTHER: That was great! If you can remember to do that the next time you lose chips, I'll give you back half of the chips you lost.

JIMMY: Gee, thanks, Mom.

CHECKING JOBS

Checking jobs, whether daily or extra work, is a vital aspect of the Home Chip System. It not only helps you teach your child the right way to do things, it provides a good opportunity for you to interact with your child in an appropriate way. The rules that apply to practice situations also apply to checking jobs. If the job has been done correctly the first time, you needn't go through all the steps. Instead, make sure you specifically praise the things done well and give chips.

Giving Chips for Jobs Completed Well

The number of chips given for a job should be decided beforehand; that way, you can reward with extra chips a job done especially well and take away chips for a job performed poorly. However, all jobs must be done as specified—a poorly done job is not acceptable and must be done again. For this reason, it is good to define how a job is done, then write the description on the job list so that you can look at it whenever a question comes up. If your child asks you to check the table and all the above things have been done correctly the first time, praise your child and give him the full four chips. However, if the job was not done correctly, go through the practice components and tell your child that if she corrects the faulty job components, she can get back half the chips possible. Be sympathetic but firm. Encourage your child to do it right this time so that he can get the two chips. If, when checked again, the job still is not done correctly, it's probably not because the child doesn't know how. Place the child in time-out (without loss of privileges) to think about it. After the time-out is completed, ask your child, again, to do the things that weren't done right. Be sure to practice each time before asking the child to repeat the job (see the section on the time-out procedure). If, after the time-out, your child cooperates and corrects the job, give chips for correcting the job. If your child will not cooperate, place him in time-out again. Most children will do what is required of them rather than sit in time-out. But, the first couple of times they may choose to go to time-out several times in a row—sort of a test to see if you really intend to follow through. Once in a while, a child will test both you and the rules. Don't give in to such tests, as it may only make it harder to convince your child that you and the rules are here to stay.

MONITORING YOUR CHILD: THE 10-MINUTE RULE

It is important that you be aware of what your child is doing. Periodic checks should be made so that you can reward (give chips and praise) such appropriate behavior as playing quietly or working on a job, and punish (take away chips) inappropriate behavior, like fighting, stalling, or getting into things. You don't have to check every 10 minutes exactly. However, the checks should be done at intervals somewhere between 5 and 20 minutes. This rule should not be used to harass your child. When you go to see what he's doing, you don't need to interrogate him. Instead, look at his behavior and either praise and give chips or take some chips away and give the child feedback. If the child is quietly engaged in a privilege, such as playing with a game in her room with the door closed, you don't need to open the door every 10 minutes to see what she is doing.

PUNISHMENT: WHEN CHIPS DON'T WORK

The use of brief time-outs, when you do not interact with your child in any way until he has calmed himself down, can be used at two different time: when your child refuses to do a job or a chore and when your child is out of chips. Time-out means the temporary revoking of all privileges and social interaction. Traditionally, this has been done by having the child stand in the corner or go to his room. We have changed this somewhat. The time-out place should be a dull, but not ugly, place (no closets or dark places!). The best places are a living-room chair, a kitchen chair, or a front step (if the child is outside). The child should be directed to time-out with no more than three words: for example, "time-out, stalling," or "time-out, talking back." There should be no further words exchanged until your child has calmed himself down. There is no such thing as a time-out within a time-out. Once you have directed your child to a time-out, you should not say another word until he has calmed himself down—regardless of what he does. Time-out should be used when your child has lost as many or more chips than he has gained. This may occur at any time during the day. In other words, when your child has no chips, he must go to time-out. First, practice time-outs when your child is not upset so that it will be easier for him when a time-out actually happens. For example, at a nonemotional time of the day, especially if your child has told you that he needs chips in order to gain access to an activity that he wants, your child can earn chips for practicing time-out.

TIME-OUT PROCEDURE

If your child has either refused to do a job or has run out of chips, you need to direct him to time-out. To institute a time-out, follow these steps:

1. Briefly explain to your child that he has lost all of his chips and that he is in time-out.
2. Do not interact with him until he is calm. If he's really upset, he may get very obnoxious, including yelling, calling you names, or telling you that you can't make him do a time-out if he doesn't want to.
3. When the initial stay in time-out is completed, your child then has the choice either to earn some chips or to stay in time-out. Many children will choose to stay in time-out, hoping that you will give in and let them do what they want to. Don't give in. Just let the time-out last as long as the child wants it. It's far better to have a couple of long time-outs (as long as 30 to 45 minutes) than to have your child think that he doesn't have to follow your rules. Remember, the time-out is not a substitute for doing the work. More than anything else, the time-out provides your child with an opportunity to learn how to calm himself down when he doesn't like the way things are going. Through repeated use of

time-out, children learn how to calm themselves down, without any assistance from one of their parents.

4. Your child must work until she has earned at least five chips and may then go about her business.

Rules for the Child in Time-Out

1. While a child is in time-out, no chips are earned or lost.
2. If undesirable behavior occurs while the child is in time-out, it is best to ignore it.
3. Social interaction is forbidden during time-out. Instruct other family members to observe this rule, and fine the other children each time they interact with anyone in time-out. If the other children are not on the chip system, then at least separate them from the child who is in time-out.
4. Ignore all inappropriate behavior that may follow placement of your child in time-out.
5. As soon as your child is quiet for 2 to 3 *seconds*, tell him that the time-out is over. Do not remind him why he went to time-out. Do not ask him why he went to time-out. If you're going to use time-outs to help a child to learn how to calm himself down, you can't nag him after each time-out.
6. Children of all ages should be started out with these very brief time-outs.
7. As your child learns to calm himself down when he's in time-out, gradually increase the amount of time that passes between when he calms down and when you tell him he's out of time-out.
8. It is critical that your child learn to associate calming down with a time-out.
9. At a later time, after your child can readily calm down in time-out, you can begin using time-out with him when he is angry or frustrated. Each of these situations is a time when a child who has the ability to calm himself down has a decided advantage.

Example of a Time-Out

The following conversation is an example of when time-out should be used:

FATHER: Susie, you were really good about getting home on time, but you forgot to hang up your coat. Remember, the rule is that we all hang up our coats as soon as we get home. Give me two chips and then hang your coat up, please.

SUSIE: I don't want to do it right now.

FATHER: I know it's hard sometimes, but we all have to follow the rules. That's back talk. Remember, you're supposed to say "OK Dad," and then go do it. Give me two more chips for back talk, and we'll try it again.

SUSIE: I'm not going to give you any chips.

FATHER: Right now, you're a little upset, so you'll have to go to time-out and cool off.

As soon as Susie is quiet, father says, "You're really being quiet; that's great. You're out of time-out now."

NINE HELPFUL HINTS FOR PARENTS

1. Nothing good is free. For chips to be powerful and useful as consequences for behavior, it is absolutely necessary that all privileges be purchased with chips.

2. If it bothers you, it's bad. If your child does something that annoys you, it probably annoys other adults too. Explain this to your child, set a chip consequence, fine this behavior, and reward a more appropriate one. Thus, any behavior that bothers you should probably be modified. You should define it, instruct your child in the appropriate behavior, and provide feedback.

3. It is absolutely necessary that you have a baby-sitter you can call on short notice. There will undoubtedly be a time before a family outing when one of your children has no chips to pay for the outing. Because it's not fair to make the rest of the family stay home, you'll need someone to stay with your child or somewhere to take him. If you allow your child to participate in a privilege that he can't purchase, you are only weakening the whole system.

4. Don't be discouraged when a behavior doesn't change overnight. It usually means that you aren't being consistent enough and are letting things go by too often, or the payoff (privilege) isn't big enough. You have to be consistent with both taking away chips and giving chips.

5. Don't get discouraged. Try to keep in mind that your child has, on the average, 70 more years to live. A couple of months of teaching him some critical skills doesn't seem like such a big deal when you put it in this perspective.

6. Preparation is very helpful for teaching your child new skills and for avoiding a show of temper. Prepare your child for the right response before you tell the child what he or she did wrong. Example: "Tommy, I'm going to tell you something that might make you a little angry, but if you keep looking at me, stay pleasant, and take it well, you'll earn an extra five chips." Try it—it works.

7. When chip fines are given, remember that you can express your sympathy with your child's unfortunate situation while at the same time being firm in applying the chip fine. Reassure the child who is receiving a lot of chip fines that when you take away chips it doesn't mean you are mad; it only means she is behaving in a manner unacceptable to you.

8. Don't use nagging, unenforceable threats, warnings, emotional pleading, or anger as methods of changing behavior; data indicate these do not work. Also, parental nagging, tantrums, and anger make life very unpleasant for the whole family. Firm but unemotional, even sympathetic, feedback seems to work best.

9. Chips and praise go together. Chips are not powerful just because they are chips. They must be made to be powerful. *That is the secret to the effectiveness of your chip system.* To make chips powerful, they must be the only way the child can get his or her privileges. When you give chips, also give praise. And, if it is worth a few words of praise, it couldn't hurt to give a few chips.

PHASING OUT THE CHIP SYSTEM

The prime criterion used for deciding when to phase out the chip system should be your child's overall behavior. Your child doesn't need to be "perfect" before the chips are discontinued. Rather, when your child's behavior has been satisfactory to you over a period of time, and he has clearly learned self-quieting skills, it is a good time to begin phasing out the chips. You should check with your health-care practitioner before attempting this phase out!

Trial Days

While you are still using the chips on a daily basis, trial days off the chip system may be initiated. The following steps should be followed for any trial day.

1. Explain to your child that you would like to try a day off the chip system.
2. Stress that if things go well, you'll have another trial day the next day, too.
3. Explain that the child must follow the rules just as if he or she were on the system.
4. Explain what will happen if the rules are not followed—that you will be using time-out for all misbehavior. If time-out is used more than two times for the same behavior, the next day cannot be a trial day. The chips may be started again at any time during any day.
5. Prompting the right response from your child can be very effective in obtaining cooperation, as the following example shows:

MOTHER: Marianne, before I tell you what I saw, I want you to remember that today is a trial day and I'm sure you'll want to take what I say the right way and be pleasant and say 'OK.' Do you understand?

MARIANNE: Yes, I understand.

MOTHER: I was watching you and Michael playing with your toys. You were really nice to share with him, but when you started playing on the swings, I saw you push Michael off one of the swings. That's against the rules, right?

MARIANNE: OK.

MOTHER: Usually you lose chips for that, but since we're not doing that today, let's say that you'll have to wait 15 minutes before playing on the swings again.

MARIANNE: OK, Mom.

It is important for parents to remember that not all trial days will be successful and that it may take some time before the chips can be completely phased out. Chips can always be used again, whether it has been 1 day off the system or 4 weeks. After your child once knows how you want him to behave, it is up to you to follow through when a rule is broken. When your child is on the chip system, breaking a rule should result in a chip loss. When she is off the system, breaking a rule should result in time-out. If you do not follow these procedures, your child will not follow the rules. Praise for desirable behavior is also a must, whether on or off the system. If being good doesn't have a reward (attention, praise, or extra privileges), the desired behavior will not occur as often. When phasing out the chip system, all the procedures for practicing, checking jobs, and time-out should still be followed consistently but with praise rather than chips.

Making photocopies of this manual violates copyright law. If you would like to have more copies of the manual, please order them.

For parents:

Home Chip System (Ages 3–7) $7.00
Home Point System (Ages 6–16) $7.00

For Professionals (must be ordered on letterhead):
Implementing Token Economies in the Home and in Institutional Settings $125.00

Site License:

For professional use only. Grants copyright permission for unlimited use at one site, including a computer disk (specify either 5¼″ or 3½″ and the IBM word processor that you use) with the instructions and both manuals (IBM format). The instructions and the manuals can be personalized with the institution's name and logo, with attribution. $250.00

Please send prepaid orders to:

Overland Press, Inc.
9853 Rosewood
Shawnee Mission, KS 66207
Phone Inquiries: (913) 383-1270

The Home Point System Manual for Children Aged 6 to 16

INTRODUCTION

At certain times, families may find a need for more structure. This could be due to behavior problems in one or more of the children. It could be due to such extenuating circumstances as the prolonged illness of a family member, or a child who has been diagnosed with Attention Deficit Hyperactivity Disorder. Whatever the case, the Home Point System was developed to help families increase the amount of structure provided for their children. The Home Point System can also be valuable when parents have been too punitive with their children, or when more positive interactions from parents to children just does not come naturally—when the parents need added structure to help them develop a more positive parenting style. There are also some children who have a good deal of difficulty accepting feedback or criticism—children who, when given feedback, are likely to get very aggravated or annoyed with their parents.

The Home Point System has been used with school-age children and adolescents, in families with one to six children, with parents' education ranging from less than high school to postgraduate studies, and with income levels ranging from poverty to upper-income professional. The range of problem behaviors extended from minor, everyday difficulties like getting children to bed at night and getting them to keep their rooms neat, to moderate problems like hitting, tantrums, hyperactivity, and back talk. Our experience is not sufficient to make any recommendations regarding the use of this program with such severe behavior problems as drug addiction. (There is a treatment program that was developed by Dr. Montrose Wolf and his colleagues at the University of Kansas, in Lawrence, Kansas, that has used point systems as one component of a comprehensive treatment program for juvenile delinquents. Dr. Wolf can be contacted at the university for more information on their program.) In the beginning, this program requires dedicated and highly motivated parents who are willing to put forth the effort necessary to teach their children more appropriate ways of behaving.

The program also requires that children be supervised by someone most of the day. We train parents to be teachers. They cannot teach their children if they are not with them. The Home Point System was designed to provide a maximum amount of instruction and feedback to your children through you, the parent. Instruction, feedback, and consequences are the tools you will use to train your child in new, desirable behaviors or to eliminate already present undesirable behaviors. The system's effectiveness in changing behavior will depend on your thoroughness. It will not operate by itself. Its success will depend on the degree to which you actively observe and reward or punish the behaviors you see your child demonstrate.

HOW THE HOME POINT SYSTEM WORKS

The Home Point System is based on two simple, yet thoroughly effective, principles:

- Behavior that is immediately followed by a good, rewarding consequence or event will continue to occur.
- Behavior that is followed by a nonrewarding or punishing consequence will cease to occur or will occur less often.

Like money, points themselves have no value. Points must be given meaning or value in order to become effective. It is only through their power to purchase necessary and enjoyable goods or activities that they gain meaning and become useful. They will always be available for you to give and take. However, points serve as those rewarding or punishing events only when they immediately follow your child's behavior.

Earning Points

Most of us have learned how to make gains in our monetary system and how to avoid or minimize our losses. This learning takes place over a period of time, with many opportunities to gain and lose money. It is through this repetition, the contrast between periods of time when we have a lot and periods of time when we have very little, that we learn how to optimize our income and minimize our losses. While the economy that we live under has a very complex set of rules, a relatively simple set of rules is necessary in order to be able to implement the point system. Within reason, children must be able to earn points at almost any time, day or night. You, as parents, cannot take your child's productive or pleasant behavior for granted. Your children must see the connection between their behavior and their ability to obtain the items and activities that they value. The vehicle that we use to accomplish this is called a point card. Here's an example of what a blank point card looks like.

The point card is similar in function to a checkbook or a savings account book. On it are noted the earnings or deposits and the losses or withdrawals. The net earnings, or the earnings minus the losses, are what the child actually has to spend. As the child progresses throughout the day, he should be earning points at many different times. For example, when your child awakens in the morning, he may be able to earn points

Name_____   Date_____

No. Pts Made	Description	Who Gave Pts	No. Pts Lost	Description	Who Took Pts

= Total Points Earned Today ①   = Total Points Lost Today ②

for getting himself up with his alarm clock (which earns a lot of points), or you may be able to get him up with only one wake-up call (which earns fewer points but is still rewarded). As the morning progresses, the child earns his points by completing his duties or jobs and writing the completed duty or job down on his point card. After writing down the completed duty or job, he must ask you to check his job and sign his point card. It is only after the job and points are written down and signed by the caregiver that the points become his to use or spend at his discretion. The following is an example of a point card filled out in the morning, after a child has completed some of his morning jobs and before he has done anything that's wrong or against your rules.

Thus, Jason got up with mild prompting from you (+10 points), he made his bed (+10 points), he got dressed on his own (+10 points), and he made it to the breakfast table on time (+10 points). When your child earns points, he should be instructed to write the number of points earned in the column marked "Number of Points Made." Under "Description" he should write a brief description of how he earned the points. The column marked "Who Gave Points" is initialed by the adult who awarded the points. For example, if your child is helping you and you say, "Thanks a lot, you've been a big help. Give yourself 20 points," your child would get her card and write 20 under "Number of Points." Then he would write "helping mother" in the "Description" column and bring it to you to initial M (for mother) or D (for dad) in the "Who Gave Points" column, as shown on the completed point card sample. As these jobs were completed, on the left side of the front of the point card, Jason filled out the name of the job, filled in the number of points earned (based on your written list of behaviors to

Name___JASON_____   Date__MONDAY, JUNE 3_____

No. Pts Made	Description	Who Gave Pts	No. Pts Lost	Description	Who Took Pts
10	Up on time	M			
10	Made Bed	M			
10	Dressed	M			
10	Breakfast	M			

= Total Points Earned Today ①   = Total Points Lost Today ②

gain and lose points), and politely asked you to sign his point card. Table B1 shows a list of behaviors and the number of points that each behavior can earn.

These are examples of behaviors that only earn points. These are behaviors you must be aware of and reward consistently, since they are the types of behaviors you would like to see more of every day.

Losing Points

Your child can also lose points for each of the behaviors that are listed on your sheet that details the number of points that can be gained and lost for each behavior. Examples of behaviors that can lose points are shown in Table B2. Behaviors that lose points are those you would like your child to stop doing. For this system to be effective, you must take points away immediately every time one of these behaviors occurs. You should notice that, on the right side of the point card, the child has written down what the behavior was that lost points and how many points were rewarded for handling his emotions well at the time; each point interaction ends on a positive note if possible.

You can see, on the point card, that Jason has earned a number of points for good behaviors; he has lost several points for inappropriate behaviors; and he took most of the point fines well (you can see that the fines were reduced by half).

TABLE B1.   Behaviors That Gain Points

Behavior	Number of points gained
Making bed	+10
Picking up bedroom	+10
Taking bath and cleaning up	+20
Brushing teeth	+10
Doing school work or reading	+30 per ½ hour
Following directions	+10
Volunteering to do something	+10
Telling parents where you are playing	+10
Saying "please" and "thank-you"	+5
Doing errands without complaining	+10
Washing dishes	+30
Drying dishes	+20
Setting table	+20
Cleaning table	+25
Dusting	+20 per room
Sweeping floors (depending on room)	+20 to +40

TABLE B2.   Behaviors That Lose Points

Behavior	Number of points lost
Name calling	−10
Talking back	−10
Fighting	−10
Teasing	−10
Swearing	−10
Interrupting	−10
Wrestling in the house	−10
Leaving clothes lying around	−10
Complaining	−10
Not putting bike away	−10
Leaving property without permission	−10
Arguing	−10
Bringing guest home after school without permission	−20
Improper use of TV, phone	−10
Not getting permission to enter parents' room	−10
Not minding your own business	−10

Name **JASON**   Date **MONDAY, JUNE 3**

No. Pts Made	Description	Who Gave Pts	No. Pts Lost	Description	Who Took Pts
10	UP ON TIME	M	20 10	INTERRUPT	M
10	MADE BED	M	20 10	WHINE	M
10	DRESSED	M			
10	BREAKFAST	M			
10	DISHES TO SINK	M			
10	BRUSH TEETH	M			

___ = Total Points Earned Today ①   ___ = Total Points Lost Today ②

Making Points Powerful

For points to be used as an effective consequence for behavior, earning points (like earning money) must be rewarding for your child; your child must feel like he has indeed gained something. Losing points (like losing money) must be unpleasant or punishing for your child; your child must feel like he has lost something. Points will become meaningful for your child when he is able to use them to buy the "privileges" of having or doing what he desires. Privileges are items or activities usually available in your home or community that your child enjoys and can purchase with his points.

Earning Privileges

As the Point System has developed, we have found a need for two different types of privileges. First, basic privileges are those privileges that most children have access to every day—the types of privileges that most parents would have a difficult time monitoring and restricting access to. This would include answering the telephone, answering the doorbell, watching the same TV shows that the rest of the family is watching, and playing with those toys that are usually left available in the family living area of the home. Extra privileges are those privileges that most children do not have unlimited access to—those privileges that parents should and do restrict access to. I will discuss these two types of privileges separately because they are handled differently in the Point System.

Basic Privileges

Basic privileges ("basics") include using the telephone, using the family room, watching TV, and playing outdoors in the yard (but not off the property). Basics are always purchased as a package. Your child must buy basics before he can buy any extra privileges. Without basics, extra privileges may not be purchased. Basics are always purchased a day ahead of time. For example, if Tuesday's basics cost 80 points, on Monday night your child must have a balance of at least 80 points before he can purchase Tuesday's basic privileges. If your child does not have the necessary points the night before, he must earn double the point value of basics the next day. In our example, basics for Tuesday would now cost 160 points and must be earned before your child has any privileges, including access to any points that may have accumulated in his "bank." Points that are "in the bank" can never be used to purchase basics and may not be spent for anything unless basics have already been earned. The bank will be explained later, along with the use of the cards.

Extra Privileges

Extra privileges can be almost anything your child likes to do. Below is a partial list of possible extra privileges:

Snacks
Riding a bike
Playing with friends
Shopping with Mom
Ride in the car
Playing games
Spending the night with a friend

The privilege to have snacks, for instance, permits your child to have snacks when they are available and when she has paid for them (written them on the point card). Snacks might be available after school or before bed. You should decide what constitutes a snack (for example, one scoop of ice cream, two cookies, or one bottle of pop) and the times they are available. For the points to be of value, your child must be required to spend them for his or her privileges. Privileges must be available as often as possible when your child has the points. Unless the points are worth something— necessary to do fun things—they will not be as effective in changing your child's behavior. Some privileges, after being purchased, are available throughout the day. For example, toys or games need to be purchased only once a day. The only exception would be if your child were to lose his basic privileges. Loss of basic privileges would also result in loss of all other privileges, until the child has his basic privileges back.

USING POINT SYSTEM CARDS

The front of the card is used for the actual record of points gained and lost as these exchanges actually occur. The back is used for extra privileges and for keeping track of the number of points your child has earned or lost. The front of the card is divided into halves, with an "earn" side and a "lost" side. The back has a systematic tracking of points gained, lost, used to purchase privileges, and used to purchase basic privileges for the next day. Also shown is the number of points remaining at the end of the day that can be added to the child's "bank" account.

The following example shows you how to total a card.

Name___JASON_____   Date MONDAY, JUNE 3

No. Pts Made	Description	Who Gave Pts	No. Pts Lost	Description	Who Took Pts
10	Up on time	M	~~20~~ 10	Interrupt	M
10	Made Bed	M	~~20~~ 10	Whine	M
10	Dressed	M			
10	Breakfast	M			
10	DISHES TO SINK	M			
10	Brush Teeth	M			
60	Read	M			
30	Wash Dishes	M			
30	Sweep Kitchen	D			
40	Help with Wash	M			
20	Bath	D			

240 = Total Points Earned Today ①   20 = Total Points Lost Today ②

At the end of the day, your child adds the totals of the "earn" and "lost" columns. In the example, the total points "earned" is 240; the total "lost" is 20. These totals are then written on the back of the card. Any extra privileges your child has bought are written on the back of the card under "Extra Privileges" as they are purchased. At the end of the day they are totaled as shown.

On the right-hand side of the back of the card is the column, "Today's Point Totals." Number (1) in this column is for the total points earned. From the example shown in Table B1, 240 would be entered here. Number (2) is for points lost, which would be 20. When you subtract, you obtain a difference of 220 (3). Now, subtract tomorrow's basic privileges (4) (as an example: 80), leaving a subtotal (5) of 140. Subtract Today's Extra Privileges (6) of 100, which leaves 40 as today's balance (7). This is then added to the previous balance in the bank (8) giving the new balance in the bank (9). The new bank balance on today's card is written on the next day's card in the space reserved for "Previous Balance in Bank." Usually, it is easiest to fill out the next day's card at the same

Basics   Yes   No ④   Today's Point Totals

Extra Privileges   _240_ Earned ①

_20_   _TV_   _20_ Lost (-) ②

_20_   _TV_   _220_ Difference ③

_20_   _SNACK_   _80_ Basics (-) ④

_20_   _BIKE_   _140_ Sub Total ⑤

_20_   _TV_   _100_ Today's Extra Privileges (-) ⑥

____   _____   _40_ Today's Balance ⑦

==================   _200_ Previous Balance in Bank ⑧

_100_ Total for today's extra privileges ⑥   _240_ New Balance in Bank ⑨

time, by writing in the name, date, whether or not basics have been purchased ("Yes" or "No"), and the previous balance in the bank.

The privileges purchased by your children while on the Home Point System will be those you and your children recorded on the list (see Table B3). However, the list may change. You will need to be aware of what your child is doing for fun and add those activities to the list as necessary. Most of the activities children do naturally in their spare time are things they enjoy. Thus, they can be viewed as privileges and added to the list of privileges.

TABLE B3.   Privileges and Their Cost

	Cost in Points
Basic Privileges	
TV, Playing outside in yard, etc.	80 per day
Extra Privileges	
Snacks	10
Tapes and tape player	30
Staying out later to play	1 per minute
Choosing meal	30
Having friends over	
in yard	20
in house	30
Going to a friend's house	30
Riding bike	20
Staying up late	2 per minute
Overnight at a friend's house	200
Toys/games/sports equipment	50 per day
Picking TV program (if OK with parents)	30
Sports activities	100
Parties/dances	150

There will always be jobs that you cannot reasonably expect your child to do on any kind of a regular basis but that you would certainly appreciate having done. These may include, for example:

Cleaning gutters
Washing windows
Washing the car
Raking the yard
Cleaning woodwork

The list of "Extra Jobs" and the "Daily Job Sheet" are necessary so that your child knows what is expected of him or her and what he or she can do for extra points. An extra job may, at times, be assigned if you would like it to be done at a certain time. Your children are not janitors. They should be permitted to have as much spare time as possible. But equally important, they should share some of the responsibilities of the house. This also will give you more time with your children. It is hoped that you can spend your time teaching your children instead of being a maid. The daily jobs will depend on your family needs and do not necessarily need to be the same jobs every day. This will be worked out with you during the first week of the program. The following is an example of a daily job sheet:

	Mon.	Tues.	Wed.	Thurs.	Fri.	Sat.	Sun.
Dust room	Janet	Janet	Joe	Joe	Tom	Tom	Janet
Sweep room	Janet	Janet	Joe	Joe	Tom	Tom	Janet
Clean bathroom	Joe	Joe	Tom	Tom	Janet	Janet	Joe
Dishes	Joe	Joe	Tom	Tom	Janet	Janet	Joe
Trash	Tom	Tom	Janet	Janet	Joe	Joe	Tom

It's best to decide ahead of time what jobs each child will be responsible for each day. The children can pick which jobs they want for the next week at a family meeting (discussed later).

How to Give and Take Away Points

Both giving and taking away points should be pleasant. Here are several things you and your child need to do whenever there is a point exchange.

Rules for Parents

When giving points, remember to:

1. Be near your child and able to touch him (not 20 feet or two rooms away).
2. Look at your child and smile.
3. Use a pleasant voice.
4. Make sure your child is facing you and looking at you.
5. Praise your child by saying something like, "Hey, that's great. You're really doing a nice job. That's really helping me."
6. Reward your child with points and say, "Why don't you write down 20 points for being so good?"

7. Describe the appropriate behavior for your child so that she knows exactly what behavior she is being praised and rewarded for.
8. Pat your child on the back or ruffle his hair occasionally. Kids love it!
9. Have your child acknowledge you by saying something like, "Thanks, Mom," or "OK."

When taking away points, remember the following:

1. Be near your child and able to touch her.
2. Look at your child and smile.
3. Use a pleasant voice. Your child should not be able to tell by the tone of your voice or your facial expression whether you're going to give or take away points.
4. Make sure your child is facing you and looking at you.
5. In a calm manner, explain what was inappropriate. "You interrupted your sister."
6. Be sympathetic. "I know it's hard to lose points, but that's the rule."
7. Give him or her the point fine.
8. Make sure your child takes the fine appropriately (see "Rules for Children" below).
9. Prompting the appropriate responses will sometimes be necessary by saying, for example, "Come on, look at me. That's better."
10. If a point loss is taken very well by your child, it is good to give him back half of the points lost.
11. If your child is too mad or upset to take off the points, don't force the issue. Place your child in time-out (to cool off), and take the points off the card for her. (Time-out is explained later in this manual.)

Rules for Children

When a child is getting points, the following rules apply:

1. The child should be facing his parents, looking at them, and smiling.
2. The child should acknowledge the points by saying, "OK," "Thanks," or something else pleasant.
3. The points should be written by the child on her card within 5 minutes. If they are not, the points aren't counted. If the child is busy, it is acceptable for him to ask his parents nicely to write down the points.
4. The card should be taken to the child's mom or dad, who should be asked within the 5 minutes to sign it; for example, "Mom, would you sign this, please?"
5. After a parent has signed the card, the child should acknowledge it by saying something like, "Thanks, Dad," and returning the card to the place where it is usually kept.

When a child is losing points, the following rules apply:

1. The child should face his parents, look at them, and smile (not frown).
2. The child must acknowledge the point loss by saying, "OK," or "I'll get my card," or something else in a pleasant voice. (Children must keep looking at the parent and be pleasant.)

3. The child must write the point loss on her card. Forgetting to record the point loss doubles the fine after 5 minutes.
4. The child must be pleasant while having the card signed.
5. After a parent has signed the card, the child should acknowledge this by saying, "Thanks, Mom," and returning the card to the place where it is usually kept.

PRACTICE GIVING AND TAKING AWAY POINTS

Once on the Home Point System, families frequently encounter instances where a child has done something to earn points but hasn't done it very well. This is an excellent time to teach your child how to do it correctly by having her practice doing it correctly. Practicing can be done with both social and maintenance (jobs) behaviors.

Practicing with Social Behaviors

If your child becomes unpleasant and talks back when he loses points, the rules in Table B4 will be useful in teaching your child the appropriate response.

Practicing with Maintenance Behaviors

When teaching your child how to do a new job correctly or when giving her feedback on a job poorly done, practicing is essential. For example, if your child is doing the dishes but when you check he is not doing them correctly, the rules in Table B5 will help you teach your child the correct way.

When to Practice

The best time to practice any behavior is during a pleasant time of day. This teaches your child under pleasant circumstances how to respond when things aren't going quite as well. However, prompting and practicing the correct responses are still

TABLE B4. Practicing with Back Talk

1. "You came quickly when I called and I really appreciate that."	Praise a related behavior
2. "But the rule is that you don't talk back after a point loss. I'll have to take off 10 more points for back talk."	Describe fully the inappropriate or inadequate behavior.
3. "Remember, you're suppposed to look at me, be pleasant and say 'OK, Mom.' in a nice tone of voice."	Describe the appropriate behavior.
4. "This way, we'll get along better at home and it will help you take criticism better at school, too."	Give a reason for the appropriate behavior.
5. "Do you understand what you're supposed to do?"	Request acknowledgment.
6. "Say it pleasantly, and give me a big smile like this."	Model: Show child how to do it (parent says "OK" and smiles).
7. "Now you try it."	Practice.
8. "That's right. You're looking at me with a pleasant facial expression."	Praise or feedback during practice.
9. "Great, that's how it's done. You practiced very well. You can have 5 points back of the 10 you lost."	Praise and reward.

TABLE B5.   Practicing with Dishwashing

1. "You're really working steadily, and the table looks really clean. Thanks."	Praise a related behavior.
2. "But, it looks like you haven't gotten all the food off the plates."	Describe fully the inappropriate or inadequate behavior.
3. "It is important that all the dishes are clean with no stuck food left on the plates."	Describe the appropriate behavior.
4. "Because germs can grow on the dishes, and besides, the next time you use the plate you will want it to be clean."	Give a reason for the appropriate behavior.
5. "Do you understand?"	Request acknowledgment.
6. "When food is stuck, a good way to get it off is to use a scraper instead of the cloth, like this."	Model: Show child how to do it.
7. "Now you try it."	Practice.
8. "Great. You're doing a much better job getting them clean now."	Praise or feedback.
9. "When you get done, come get me, and you can get your points plus 10 for practicing. You're really doing great now."	Praise and reward.

important after a rule violation or a poorly done job has occurred. When there has not been a rule violation, you can practice using make-believe violations and make-believe time-out. This is also a good way for your children to earn points. For example:

MOTHER: Jim, let's practice how you're supposed to take a point loss and you can earn 10 points.

JIM: Sure.

MOTHER: Jim, I'm glad you stayed in the house like I asked. Thank you. But, please take 20 points off for throwing the ball in the house. Remember, the rule is that all ball throwing must be done outside.

JIM: Sure, Mom (*with pleasant facial expression and tone of voice*).

MOTHER: That was great! If you can remember to do that the next time you really lose points, I'll give you back half of the points you lost.

JIM: Gee, thanks, Mom.

CHECKING JOBS

Checking jobs, whether daily or extra work, is a vital aspect of this program. It not only helps you teach your children the right way to do things, it provides a good opportunity for you to interact with your child. The rules that apply to practice situations also apply to checking jobs. If the job has been done correctly the first time, you needn't go through all the steps. Instead, make sure you specifically praise the things done well and give points. The following rules will make assigning and monitoring jobs more pleasant for you and less time consuming for your child.

Rules for Children When Doing Jobs

1. Take all necessary equipment (cleanser, broom, and so on) with you before you start the job.

2. Once you have started, don't leave the job. (Each time you do a job without stopping to chat or play, you will earn extra points. But each time you leave a job or are stalling, your mother can take away 10 points.)
3. When you are finished, put all equipment back where it belongs.
4. As soon as your job is done, have it checked. "Dad, will you please check my job?"
5. Be present when your job is checked. By doing this, you can find out exactly what you did properly or discover what else needs to be done.
6. Be pleasant. If you are told that the job has not been done properly, and you act as though you are mad, you will only lose more points.
7. When you receive points for a job, write them down immediately and have your card signed.

Rules for Parents When Checking Jobs

1. Be sure you check periodically (10-minute rule) to see whether your child is working hard or playing. Reward working hard with praise and sometimes points; punish playing with a small point loss whenever necessary.
2. Be sure to reward and praise working at a job until it is finished. Give a fine for leaving the job. Ending stalling will make jobs a lot easier for you and your child.
3. When you're asked to check a job, do it immediately or as soon as possible. Your child must be with you when you check. This is a good time for teaching both maintenance skills (doing the job correctly) and social skills (taking both pleasant and unpleasant criticism well).
4. Always start out by praising a related behavior or part of the job. (Practicing) "I'm really glad you started your job on time, but it looks a little sloppy. You forgot . . ." or, "Hey, the bed looks great. Good job, but you forget to empty the waste basket."
5. Check to see that equipment is put away correctly.
6. Don't reward your child for a job improperly done. This only increases the likelihood that her next job will not be done satisfactorily. If he hasn't done a good job, tell him pleasantly, and specify what remains to be done.
7. When checking jobs, you should use both the components for giving or taking away points and the components for practicing. These are two important aspects of this program. Use them—it will make your job as teacher, parent, and friend a lot easier.

Points for Jobs

The number of points given for a job should be decided beforehand. That way you can reward with extra points a job done especially well and fine a poorly done job. However, all jobs must be done as specified—a poorly done job is not acceptable and must be done again. For this reason, it is good to define how a job is done, then write the description on the job list so that you can look at it whenever a question comes up. The following example describes the job of cleaning the bathroom.

Cleaning Bathroom—60 points

1. Clean all porcelain with cleanser (be sure to rinse it clean).
2. Clean soap out of soap trays.
3. Polish all chrome and mirrors.
4. Wipe off tile walls with damp cloth.
5. Sweep floor with broom.
6. Empty waste basket.

By writing it down, you'll know what to look for when checking a job. Definitions may need to be changed periodically. Just be sure you write the changes on the sheet and inform the children. If all the items above have been done the first time your child asks you to check the bathroom, praise her and give her the full number of points (60 points in the example used above). If the job is not done correctly, go through the practice components and tell him that if he corrects the faulty job components, he can get half of the points possible (30 points). Be sympathetic but firm. Encourage him to do the job right this time so that he can get the 30 points. If, when checked again, the job still has not been done correctly and it's not because the child doesn't know how, place the child in time-out (without loss of privileges) to think about it. After time-out, have her again do the items that weren't done correctly. Be sure to practice each time. If, after time-out, your child cooperates and corrects the job, give him points for correcting the job. If she will not cooperate, place her in time-out again. Most children will do what is required of them rather than sit in time-out. However, once in a while a child will test both you and the rules. Don't give in to such tests; it may only make it harder to convince your child that you and the rules are here to stay. These steps are to be followed when checking jobs:

	If Job Done Right	*If Job Done Wrong*
First check	Full points	Do again
Second check	Half points	Time-out; do again
Third check	Zero points	Time-out; do again (you may, at this time, give points for becoming more pleasant)

Monitoring Your Child: The 10-Minute Rule

It is important that you be aware of what your child is doing. Periodic checks should be made so that you can reward (give points and praise) such appropriate behavior as reading, playing quietly, or working on a job, and punish (take away points) inappropriate behavior like fighting or getting into things. You don't have to check every 10 minutes exactly. However, the checks should be done at intervals somewhere between 5 and 20 minutes each. This rule should not be used to harass your child. When you go to see what he is doing, don't interrogate him. Instead, look at his behavior and either praise and give points, or take away some points and give him feedback. If your child is quietly engaged in a privilege, such as listening to the stereo in her room with the door closed, you don't need to open the door every 10 minutes to see what she is doing.

PUNISHMENT: WHEN POINTS DON'T WORK

On at least two different occasions you will need an effective alternative when the loss of points isn't effective. One alternative that we have found to be very effective is what we call "time-out." "Time-out" means the temporary revoking of all privileges and social interaction. Traditionally, this has been done by having a child stand in a corner or go to his room. We have changed this somewhat. The time-out place should be a dull, but not ugly, place (no closets or dark rooms!). The best places are a living-room chair, a kitchen chair, or a front step (if the child is outside).

Time-Outs When Your Child Has No Points

In this case, time-out is used when your child has lost as many or more points than he has gained. This may occur at any time during the day. In other words, when your child's card balance is zero or below, he must go to time-out. To indicate a time-out on the point card, draw a line across the card. This lets your child start fresh after time-out. First, practice time-outs when your child is not upset so that it will be easier for him when a time-out actually happens. For example, on a pleasant day your child can earn chips for practicing time-out.

Time-Out Procedure

When your child has lost all of her points, a time-out will be necessary when undesirable behavior occurs. Time-out is recommended because, if the child doesn't have any points, there's no way that she can pay a point fine.

1. Explain to the child that he has lost too many points and has a point balance below zero.
2. Take the child to the selected spot.
3. Tell your child that she must stay in this spot for 5 minutes and must be quiet. Do not start the time until your child is quiet, and if at any time there is noise, the time begins when he is quiet again. It is wise to use a timer so that both you and your child know when the time is up.
4. When the initial stay in time-out is completed, your child then has the choice either to work or to stay in the corner. Most children will choose work.
5. Your child must work until she has earned double the point value of basics. If your child's basics cost 80 points, she must work until she has earned 160 points.
6. If your child had been engaging in basic privileges before going to time-out, he may rebuy them for double their point value.
7. Should your child not want to work for basics or misbehave while earning basics back, she must go to time-out.

Rules for the Child in Time-Out

1. While a child is in time-out, no points can be earned or lost. If undesirable behavior occurs while the child is working his or her way out of time-out, he or she goes back to time-out for the designated time.

2. Social interaction is forbidden during time-out. Instruct other family members to observe this, and fine the other children each time they interact with anyone in time-out.
3. Ignore all inappropriate behavior that may follow placement of your child in time-out. Inform your child that the 5-minute time-out starts only when she is quiet. If the child leaves time-out, place her back in the designated time-out spot.

Time-Out for an Angry or Upset Child

There will be times when it is obvious that the points are not working because your child is too mad or upset. If you have to fine your child twice within a short period of time or if your child refuses to take off points, a cooling-off period is necessary. Time-out will provide this cooling off. The following conversation provides an example of when time-out should be used.

FATHER: Janice, you were really good about getting home on time, but you forgot to hang up your coat. Remember, the rule is that we all hang up our coats as soon as we get home. Take off the 10 points and then hang up your coat.

JANICE: I don't want to do it right now.

FATHER: I know it's hard sometimes, but we all have to follow the rules. That's back talk. Remember, you're supposed to say, "OK, Dad," then go do it. Take 10 points off for back talk, and we'll try it again.

JANICE: I'm not going to.

FATHER: Right now you're a little mad, so you will have to go to time-out and cool off. If you do it right away, I'll give you 10 points. That's right—I'll take the 20 points off for you. You're really being quiet; that's great. I'll set the timer now.

10 HELPFUL HINTS FOR PARENTS

1. Nothing good is free. For points to be powerful and useful as consequences for behavior, it is absolutely necessary that all privileges be purchased with points.
2. If it bothers you, it's bad. If your child does something that annoys you, it probably annoys other adults too. Explain this to your child, set a point consequence, fine this behavior, and reward a more appropriate one. Thus, any behavior that bothers you should probably be modified. You should define it, instruct your child, and provide feedback for it.
3. It is absolutely necessary that you have a baby-sitter you can call on short notice. There will undoubtedly be a time when, 5 minutes before a family outing, one of your children will lose his privileges. Because it's not fair to make the rest of the family stay home, you'll need someone to stay with your child or somewhere to take him. If you allow your child to participate in a privilege that he can't purchase, you are only weakening the whole system.
4. Don't be discouraged when a behavior doesn't change overnight. It usually

means that you aren't being consistent enough and are letting things go by too often, or the payoff (privilege) isn't big enough. You have to be consistent with both taking off points and giving points. Don't get discouraged.

5. Prompting is very helpful for teaching your child new skills and for avoiding a show of temper. Prompt the right response before you tell her what she did wrong. Example: "Jack, I'm going to tell you something that might make you a little angry, but if you keep looking at me, stay pleasant, and take it well, you'll earn an extra 30 points." Try it—it works.

6. When point fines are given, remember that you can express sympathy with your child's unfortunate situation while at the same time being firm in applying the point losses. Reassure the child who is receiving a lot of point fines that when you take away points, it doesn't mean you are mad; it only means she is behaving in a manner that is unacceptable.

7. Don't use nagging, unenforceable threats, warnings, emotional pleading, or anger as methods of changing behavior. We know these do not work. Also, parental nagging, tantrums, and anger make life very unpleasant for the whole family. Firm but emotional, even sympathetic, feedback seems to work best.

8. Points and praise go together. Points are not powerful just because they are points. They must be made powerful. *That is the secret to the effectiveness of your point system*. To make points powerful, they must be the only way that the child can get his or her privileges. When you give points, also give praise. And, if it is worth a few words of praise, it couldn't hurt to give a few points.

9. There may be times when your child does something you consider a major misdeed. Any serious rule violation should be handled with point fines. There is no need to nag or repeatedly remind your child of the serious violation. Every new job that is assigned to pay off the fine will remind your child of this rule violation.

10. Do not avoid fines. It is important that children learn to take criticism appropriately. Avoiding fines so that your child does not become upset means you are not dealing with an important learning experience.

FAMILY MEETINGS

Family meetings are used in the Home Point System so that your children can actively participate in the system by having a voice in the way the system works. During or after dinner is usually a convenient time for family meetings, since most families are together at this time and the meeting does not have to compete with other daily activities. At the beginning, family meetings are held once a week with the health-care practitioner present. This helps both the parents and children learn ways to conduct the meeting. Initially, rules and point fines for breaking rules are discussed to make sure everyone understands them, not whether they like or approve of them. Later, family meetings serve as a place where your children can voice their opinions and complaints, if done in the correct manner, without loss of points. If a child brings up a complaint, he should follow the steps listed below.

1. Use a pleasant voice.
2. Have a pleasant facial expression.
3. State the complaint briefly without using derogatory words.
4. Give a possible solution.
5. Encourage others' opinions.

One of the parents takes the responsibility of conducting the family meeting. However, both parents give points for appropriate behavior and take away points for inappropriate behavior. Since this is for the parents as well as for the children, parents may also bring up complaints or discuss rules. Parents, too, must follow the steps above for discussing complaints.

Rules for Conducting a Family Meeting

1. Have all of the children bring their cards to the meeting.
2. Ask if anyone has anything to bring up.
3. Start with one child, then go to the next. This will help avoid confusion.
4. Prompt the child, if necessary, to bring up a subject in the correct manner.
5. Give feedback as to whether she is doing it correctly.
6. Reward bringing up serious matters and appropriate remarks.
7. Fine inappropriate remarks.
8. Keep order in the meeting by fining children for interrupting or displaying other inappropriate behavior.
9. Ask for other opinions and solutions.
10. Call for a vote.
11. Move on to the next child.

It is important that parents remember that a child cannot be fined because of his complaint. He can only be fined if he does not discuss it in the correct manner. Parents may find it necessary to overrule a decision made in a family meeting. This, however, should only be done with the health-care practitioner's knowledge and after the reasons have been explained fully to the children.

Additional Examples of Point Values

Behavior	Points Earned
Brush teeth	+10
Clear own dishes to sink	+10
Clear table	+20
Close drawers	+10
Comb hair before school	+10
Dress self without dawdling	+10
Dust a room	+20
Flush toilet	+10
Fold laundry	+10
Follow direction first time	+10
Get up willingly	+10
Good manners	+10
Homework per ½ hour	+20
Lights/TV off when done	+10
Pick up room	+10
Put belongings away	+10
Put clothes in hamper	+10
Volunteer for job	+10
Wash face once a day	+10

Point Losses (with half back if done nicely!)

Behavior	Points Lost
Arguing	−40
Back talk	−40
Clothes on floor	−20
Complaining	−20
Interrrupting	−40
Not listening	−40
Slamming door	−20
Stalling, dawdling	−40
Yelling in house	−20
Leaving dinner table before finished	−20

MONEY (one each week)

1 point per penny for first $1.00
5 points per penny for second $1.00
10 points per penny for third $1.00
20 points per penny for each additional $1.00
Daily School Note: Lose 100 if not brought home
                        20   Acceptable social behavior
                        20   Work on assignments
                        20   Hand in assignments
                        20   Agree with note
                        10   Grade = C
                        20   Grade = B
                        30   Grade = A

Making photocopies of this manual violates copyright law. If you would like to have more copies of the manual, please order them.

For parents:

Home Chip System (Ages 3–7)	$7.00
Home Point System (Ages 6–16)	$7.00

For Professionals (must be ordered on letterhead):
Implementing Token Economies in the Home and in Institutional Settings $125.00

Site License:

For professional use only. Grants copyright permission for unlimited use at one site, including a computer disk (specify either 5¼″ or 3½″ and the IBM word processor that you use) with the instructions and both manuals (IBM format). The instructions and the manuals can be personalized with the institution's name and logo, with attribution. $250.00

Please send prepaid orders to:

Overland Press, Inc.
9853 Rosewood
Shawnee Mission, KS 66207
Phone Inquiries: (913) 383-1270

Index